A Concise Handbook of
Respiratory Diseases

third edition

A Concise Handbook of
Respiratory Diseases

t h i r d   e d i t i o n

Sattar Farzan, MD
Clinical Professor of Medicine, State University of New York at Buffalo
Attending Physician, Erie County Medical Center
Attending and Consultant, Buffalo VA Medical Center
Consultant and Visiting Teacher, Buffalo General Hospital
Teaching Attending, Sisters of Charity Hospital
Buffalo, New York

with the assistance of
Doris A. Farzan, RN, MS

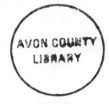

APPLETON & LANGE
Norwalk, Connecticut/San Mateo, California

0-8385-1225-9

Copyright © 1992 by Appleton & Lange
A Publishing Division of Prentice Hall
Copyright 1978 and 1985 by Reston Publishing Company, Inc.
A Prentice Hall Company

92 93 94 95 96 / 10 9 8 7 6 5 4 3 2 1

Prentice Hall International (UK) Limited, *London*
Prentice Hall of Australia Pty. Limited, *Sydney*
Prentice Hall Canada, Inc., *Toronto*
Prentice Hall Hispanoamericana, S.A., *Mexico*
Prentice Hall of India Private Limited, *New Delhi*
Prentice Hall of Japan, Inc., *Tokyo*
Simon & Schuster Asia Pte. Ltd., *Singapore*
Editora Prentice Hall do Brasil Ltda., *Rio de Janeiro*
Prentice Hall, *Englewood Cliffs, New Jersey*

Library of Congress Cataloging-in-Publication Data
Farzan, Sattar, 1932–
    A concise handbook of respiratory diseases / Sattar Farzan, with
the assistance of Doris A. Farzan.—3rd ed.
      p.   cm.
    Includes bibliographical references and index.
    ISBN 0-8385-1225-9
    1. Respiratory organs—Diseases—Handbooks, manuals, etc.
I. Farzan, Doris A.
    [DNLM: 1. Respiratory Tracts Diseases.   WF 140 F247c]
RC731.F37 1992
616.2—dc20
DNLM/DLC
for Library of Congress   91-17209
                                         CIP

Acquisitions Editor: Stephany Scott
Production Editor: Sandra K. Huggard
Designer: Janice Barsevich

PRINTED IN THE UNITED STATES OF AMERICA

THIS BOOK IS DEDICATED TO THE MEMORY OF MY PARENTS

CONTENTS

This revision of *A Concise Handbook of Respiratory Diseases* was undertaken after careful planning and following a thorough and critical examination of the previous edition. The author's aim was to produce a most accurate, up-to-date, and informative book on respiratory diseases while maintaining the text's distinctive features of conciseness and readability. Suggestions by several readers and reviewers of the text were most helpful in this project. To assure both accuracy and up-to-dateness, the revision necessitated a thorough and meticulous search of pertinent medical literature. As with the previous two editions, the educational needs of the readers, especially the students and trainees in respiratory care, were constantly kept in mind throughout the revision process. The length and depth of discussions were held proportional to the practical importance of the subject matters.

All of the chapters have undergone a considerable amount of revision, mainly by addition of the most recent developments in respiratory medicine and advances in related technology. Structurally, the text has been divided into twelve sections, each encompassing related chapters and appendices. Section I contains information on patient data collection through history taking, physical examination, laboratory tests, and monitoring. A brief discussion on exercise test is added to Chapter 2. Section II deals with common infectious diseases involving the respiratory tract. Because of the increasing importance of acquired immunodeficiency syndrome (AIDS) in pulmonary infection, a separate chapter is devoted to AIDS. Section III focuses on obstructive airways diseases, including a chapter on upper airway obstruction. Chapter IV addresses restrictive lung diseases, and Section V contains chapters on environmental lung diseases and tobacco smoking. Section VI is devoted to a study of pulmonary aspiration and atelectasis. Section VII examines neoplastic diseases of the lung. Circulatory disorders that affect the lungs and the effects of lung diseases on circulation are discussed in Section VIII. Section IX focuses on diseases of the pleura and chest wall, as well as trauma and surgery of the chest. Disorders of respiratory control, which include neuromuscular and central nervous system diseases, are the subjects of Section X. Respiratory failure, including respiratory distress syndrome of the newborn, is the focus of Section XI. Mechanical ventilation, included in Chapter 25 (respiratory failure), is discussed in more detail in this section. The latest methods of ventilatory support are succinctly addressed. Useful and practical information on predicted normal values on various pulmonary function tests and other respiratory physiologic data are compiled in eight appendices in Section XII. The bibliographies are thoroughly revised and brought up-to-date with the addition of many recent original studies and review articles. Several useful tables and illustrations are added for further clarification of related subjects. The glossary remains a convenient source of information at the end of the book.

I wish to acknowledge the useful suggestions and encouraging comments by many readers who assisted me in this endeavor. I also would like to thank the editorial staff at Appleton & Lange, especially Stephany Scott and Sandra Huggard for their thoughtful direction and cooperation.

Sattar Farzan, MD

Respiration, in a broad sense, is the combination of various physical and chemical processes by which oxygen is supplied to the living cell for its metabolic needs and carbon dioxide, a product of oxidation, is removed from it. In simple organisms, such as protozoa, the exchange of these gases is by the basic physical process of diffusion that takes place directly between them and their environment. However, in larger and more complex organisms, including man, it is accomplished by more elaborate coordinated functions of (1) the *circulatory system*, which provides a means of carrying these gases in a special medium, the *blood*, and (2) the *respiratory system*, which obtains the necessary oxygen from and eliminates the carbon dioxide to the atmosphere. Although all these functions are essential for cellular respiration and should always be taken into account in dealing with respiratory diseases, in this book we shall be primarily concerned with the *respiratory system*.

The primary function of the respiratory system, the delivery of oxygen to and removal of carbon dioxide from the blood, is accomplished and regulated by an intricate set of structures. These include (1) the lungs, which provide the gas-exchanging surface; (2) the conducting airways, which convey the air in and out of the lungs; (3) the thoracic wall, which supports and protects the lungs and, at the same time, acts as a bellows through the ability to change its volume; (4) the respiratory muscles, which create the energy necessary for the movement of air in and out of the lungs; and (5) the respiratory centers with their sensitive receptors and communicating nerves, which control and regulate ventilation.

The transfer of oxygen and carbon dioxide between the blood in the pulmonary capillaries and the alveoli takes place through an extremely thin but vast membrane by diffusion. The difference in the partial pressures of these gases across the alveolar-capillary membrane determines the direction of movement: oxygen moves from the alveoli to the capillaries, and carbon dioxide moves from the capillaries to the alveoli.

The flow of air in and out of the lungs with each breath, known as ventilation, keeps the alveolar gases at a fairly constant concentration, thus preventing the exhaustion of oxygen and accumulation of carbon dioxide. The air, like any fluid, flows from a region of higher pressure to one of lower pressure. During inspiration, contraction of the inspiratory muscles increases the thoracic volume and hence reduces the intrathoracic pressure. The reduction of the intrathoracic pressure enlarges the alveoli, expands the alveolar gas, and, therefore, lowers its pressure to less than atmospheric. Air flows from the outside (higher pressure) to the alveoli (lower pressure) until pressures equalize. At the end of inspiration, potential energy created by contraction of the inspiratory muscles is stored in the elastic tissues of the lungs and chest wall. During expiration, relaxation of these muscles allows the lungs and thorax to recoil, resulting in reduction of their volumes. Pressure in the alveoli becomes higher than atmospheric, causing the air to flow from the alveoli (higher pressure) to the outside (lower pressure) until the pressures become equal. For further increase in alveolar pressure, such as during cough, the expiratory muscles are also activated.

The flow of air in and out of the lungs encounters only a small amount of resistance. The inspired air is warmed, humidified, and filtered in the upper air passages before reaching the lower airways and alveoli.

The regulation of ventilation is operated by a complex system of sensitive interconnecting structures that sense the need for adjusting ventilation under various physiologic conditions. The activities of respiratory muscles are controlled through their nerve supply by the respiratory centers, which receive and integrate impulses from various receptors and other neurologic centers.

Respiratory dysfunction may result from structural and functional abnormalities in *any* of these components of the respiratory system. Not only the lungs, but also the airways, thoracic wall, respiratory muscles, and related areas of the nervous system should be considered in dealing with respiratory disorders. This monograph adheres to this important principle.

Clinical Manifestations, Diagnostic Studies, Functional Assessment, and Monitoring

CHAPTER *1*

The Patient with Respiratory Disease

Patients with respiratory disease, as with any other medical condition, consult health-care professionals mainly because they, their family members, or friends have noted or suspected a certain deviation from normal health. They may be suffering from uncomfortable symptoms or fear a serious and potentially incapacitating illness. Naturally, they expect a clear and satisfactory explanation of their condition and look for relief and reassurance.

A patient is not just a collection of certain symptoms, signs, damaged organs, and disturbed function. He is human, and has feelings, emotions, hopes, and fears. Health professionals dealing with a patient should use not only their scientific knowledge and technical skill, but also their human understanding, sympathy, and tact. Developing a good rapport with the patient by gaining and maintaining his confidence and demonstrating concern and compassion are essential for successful patient care.

Proper care of the patient with respiratory disease necessitates identifying the specific problems and diagnosing the underlying organic or functional disorder. This can be achieved only after adequate information is obtained from

various sources and by various means. Taking a history, doing a physical examination, obtaining radiographic studies, assessing the various functions, and performing other diagnostic procedures are methods used to provide this information.

TAKING A HISTORY

The history should contain all the pertinent facts about the patient's illness. The characteristics of the main complaint and other associated **symptoms** should be ascertained. The date and the time of the onset of these symptoms, their severity and duration, the circumstances leading to or aggravating them, and the factors alleviating them should be determined. Other essential parts of a thorough history taking include the state of the patient's health prior to the present illness; previous diseases, surgeries, and injuries; occupational and environmental history; allergies; health of family; smoking and other habits; and intake of medication.

Despite remarkable progress in methods of objective evaluation and the availability of sophisticated laboratory tests for patients with respiratory diseases, the importance of history taking has not diminished. This is particularly true in regard to the occupational and environmental history, which is crucial in evaluating the patient with respiratory disorder and, in many instances, is the key to a correct diagnosis.

The common and important symptoms of respiratory diseases are limited in number. These symptoms are cough, expectoration, dyspnea, hemoptysis, chest pain, and wheezing.

COUGH

Cough, one of the important body reflexes, is primarily intended to maintain airway patency by eliminating materials accumulated or deposited on the mucosa of the respiratory tract, such as tracheobronchial secretions, blood, aspirated substances, and other foreign bodies. However, not infrequently, cough is produced by irritation of the airways with nothing to be expectorated. Hyperreactivity of the irritant receptors on the respiratory tract mucosa, resulting from inflammation or other pathologic processes, may enhance the cough reflex to the extent that even a mild irritation can trigger it. The most sensitive areas of the respiratory tract for the cough reflex are the larynx, carina, trachea, and major bronchi. In addition to the airways, irritation of the pleura, tympanic membrane, and occasionally other viscera may produce cough.

The cough reflex is mediated through sensory nerve endings of cranial nerves X (vagus nerve), IX (glossopharyngeal nerve), and occasionally V (trigeminal nerve), and motor nerves of the larynx and respiratory muscles. The reflex center is in the medulla. Cough also may be initiated and partially inhibited voluntarily. The mechanism of cough is as follows (see Fig. 1–1): after a rapid inspiration of a fairly large amount of air, the glottis is tightly closed by the vocal cords for a short period of time while the expiratory muscles, particularly the abdominals, contract vigorously. The intrathoracic pressure is markedly increased, and the trapped air in the lungs is compressed. The sudden opening of the glottis results in an explosive outflow of air with high velocity, carrying the secretions or other materials with it. Transient narrowing of the large intrathoracic airways upon opening of the glottis, which results mainly from inward bulging of their membranous portion, contributes to clearing of these airways. The characteristic noise of cough is due mostly to vibration of vocal cords and sometimes to vibration of secretions. The normal function of the larynx is essential for effective cough and expectoration. In tracheotomized patients, the effectiveness of cough is markedly diminished. The ability to take a deep breath and to create a high expiratory pressure determines the force and the efficacy of cough.

Although a very common symptom, cough has limited diagnostic value; however, it may be the only indication of a serious bronchopulmonary disease. The most common and clinically significant cause of acute cough is viral tracheobronchitis. Other acute inflammatory disorders of the respiratory tract of infectious or noninfectious etiology are most often associated with cough. Alteration of the surface epithelium, by exposing the nerve endings, makes the airways very sensitive to the cough-provoking effect of commonly occurring mild irritants such

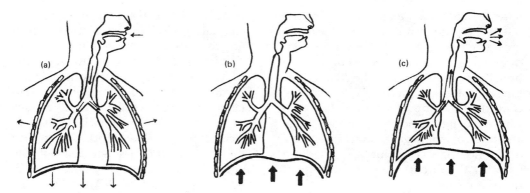

Figure 1–1. Mechanism of cough. (a), Rapid inspiration of fairly large amount of air. (b), The glottis is tightly closed while the expiratory muscles, particularly the abdominals, contract; the intrathoracic pressure is markedly increased and the trapped air in the lungs is compressed. (c), The sudden opening of the glottis results in an expulsive outflow of air with high velocity, carrying the secretions.

as dusts, cold air, rapid or deep breathing, talking, and even laughing. In addition, increased tracheobronchial secretions stimulate coughing. Acute cough may also result from inhalation of irritant gases or aspiration of liquid or solid matters. Heart failure not uncommonly may cause cough.

Chronic cough, defined as a cough lasting for over 3 weeks, usually indicates structural changes of the respiratory tract or persistence of other cough-producing factors. Cough is so prevalent among smokers that they are often oblivious to its presence. Only changes in the characteristics of cough or expectoration may concern them. Such changes are frequently due to an infection, but it may be an indication of the occurrence of a malignant neoplasm, a fairly common disease of smokers. When there is no clinically or radiographically identifiable reason for chronic cough, determination of its cause becomes quite a challenge. Airway **hyperreactivity,** the hallmark of asthma, is a common cause of chronic or recurrent cough in otherwise healthy persons;

therefore, it may be the sole manifestation of asthma. Chronic postnasal drip should also be considered as a possible cause. Recurrent aspiration and chronic left-side heart failure may be the culprit. Foreign-body aspiration should always be kept in mind in differential diagnosis of chronic cough.

After an initial episode of an acute cough spell or choking sensation at the time of aspiration, cough may restart and persist long after the incident. The **angiotensin**-converting enzyme inhibitors such as captopril and enalapril, drugs used for treatment of hypertension and heart failure, may result in a dry annoying cough, which stops after their discontinuation. A **psychogenic** or even intentional cough should be seriously considered when organic causes are properly excluded.

The intensity of cough has no relationship to the severity or seriousness of underlying bronchopulmonary disease. It is not unusual for a patient with serious, even fatal, pulmonary disease to have minimal or no cough. On the other hand, a mild viral infection involving the trachea or the bronchi may cause the most troublesome cough. In certain conditions, the cough may have characteristic features. For example, the characteristics of cough in pertussis (whooping cough) and croup are quite distinctive. Chronic cough productive of very large amounts of sputum is often indicative of bronchiectasis. Voluntary hawking (clearing the throat) is a common sign of postnasal drip.

Although cough is very important in protecting the lungs, clearing the airways, and assuring their patency, it may be an annoying symptom when dry and nonproductive. Moreover, it may occasionally prove to be harmful. Spread of infection, airway injury, hemoptysis, pneumothorax, rib fractures, syncope, and aggravation of heart failure have been attributed to both severe and persistent cough. At times the mechanical irritation of cough itself brings about more coughing.

Respiratory therapists and nurses have the opportunity as well as the responsibility to observe and report the type of cough and expectoration of the patient. From the therapeutic point of view, an effective cough is important in adequate tracheobronchial hygiene. In many patients it is important to encourage cough and expectoration by appropriate instruction, particularly when they are unable to do so spontaneously. This may or may not be combined with measures such as intermittent positive pressure breathing (IPPB), humidity therapy, or postural drainage.

EXPECTORATION

Expectoration is defined as the act of coughing up and spitting out material raised from the respiratory tract. This material is called *sputum.* Normally, sputum consists of secretions formed continuously by the mucous glands and the goblet cells of the tracheobronchial tree. Forming a thin mucous blanket, these secretions move slowly toward the pharynx with the help of **cilia**. Cilia are microscopic hairlike processes, which extend from the free surfaces of the mucosal lining cells and vibrate rhythmically, propelling the overlaying mucous coating. With proper balance between its formation and elimination, a thin protective layer of mucus is maintained for trapping and removing impurities of inspired air, while excessive accumulation of secretions is prevented.

In pathologic conditions increased tracheobronchial secretions may be due to the stimulation of normal secretory cells or to an increase in the number of these cells. In acute situations, increased sputum production is mainly the result of transient stimulation of mucous glands and goblet cells, while their chronic irritation, in addition, causes their hyperplasia. Chronic bronchitis is a good example; prolonged irritation of bronchial glands and cells by cigarette smoke results in an increase in their numbers and activities.

In addition to mucus, expectorated material may contain other fluids transudated or exuded from the various sites of the respiratory tract, including the alveoli. It may contain white blood cells accumulated for the purpose of defense against infection, necrotic material from tissue death, blood, aspirated vomitus, and, rarely, other indigenous or foreign matters.

The quantity of expectoration varies from scant to several hundred milliliters or more per day. Since information regarding the amount of sputum may be valuable in certain clinical situations, it is sometimes necessary to collect the sputum expectorated for 24 hours for measurement of its volume as well as for other studies. It should be remembered that some people, particularly children and sometimes women, have difficulty in expectorating and have a tendency to swallow their sputum.

The gross appearance of sputum may give a clue to the underlying condition. Its color varies from white, yellow, and green to brown or red, and its consistency from watery to thick and even solid. Mucus should be differentiated from mucopurulent or purulent secretions. Yellow sputum generally is indicative of the presence of large numbers of white blood cells, which are the major component of pus. Green discoloration signifies the production of an enzyme from stagnant pus cells. Red or brownish sputum is usually due to the presence of red blood cells. It is not only important to ask the patient to describe the characteristics of his sputum, including color, odor, thickness, and amount; but it should also be carefully observed by the physician, nurse, or therapist. Examination of sputum is discussed further in Chapter 2.

DYSPNEA

Dyspnea is an uncomfortable awareness of breathing generally believed to be due to increased work of ventilation out of proportion to the level of activity. However, the clinical observation that dyspnea develops with respiratory muscle fatigue and weakness suggests that an increase in the efferent neuronal output, rather than actual muscular work of breathing, is the mechanism by which this distressful symptom develops.

The disagreeable awareness of breathing may range in intensity from a mild discomfort to extreme distress. Dyspnea, like pain, is a *subjective* symptom, and thus likely to be influenced by the patient's reaction, sensitivity, and emotional state. The degree of dyspnea, therefore, may be quite different in two individuals with similar conditions.

Although dyspnea is a subjective symptom, the patient may be described as dyspneic when there is enough objective evidence to indicate labored and distressful breathing. Patients having a severe asthma attack or with acute pulmonary edema readily appear dyspneic, as they breathe with difficulty and seem in obvious distress. However, a simple increase in rate or depth of breathing, disturbances of rhythm, or changes in other characteristics of respiration do not necessarily indicate dyspnea. In these situations the terms that exactly characterize the breathing patterns should be used. Various patterns of respiration are discussed on page 160.

Dyspnea as a result of increased work of breathing is seen under numerous clinical conditions. Some of the basic causes are increased airway resistance, such as in upper airway obstruction, asthma, and other chronic obstructive pulmonary diseases; reduced pulmonary compliance as a result of pulmonary fibrosis, congestion, edema, and a variety of other parenchymal lung diseases; mechanical interference with the expansion of the lungs due to massive pleural effusion or pneumothorax; and abnormality of chest wall and respiratory muscles resulting in inefficient and wasteful respiratory efforts.

Dyspnea due to heart disease usually is directly related to changes in the lungs as a result of pulmonary congestion and/or edema characteristic of cardiac failure. Inadequate blood supply to the exercising muscles, including the respiratory muscles, is another factor in producing shortness of breath in heart failure. In patients with severe physical debility, the weakness of respiratory muscles is the main cause of their breathlessness. The same is true in severe anemia, in which there is also increased work of breathing.

Certain patients may complain of shortness of breath with no evidence of organic disease to explain it. These patients often suffer from an anxiety state or panic disorder and have a tendency to hyperventilate. They usually state that they are unable to get enough air and frequently sigh. The psychogenic nature of dyspnea becomes more evident when such patients indicate that they are more aware of this symptom at rest than during physical activity. This is the opposite of the organic causes of dyspnea, in which the severity of shortness of breath is directly related to the amount of exertion.

In evaluating for dyspnea, it is important to identify the circumstances in which patients develop this symptom. Breathlessness may occur with certain body positions. **Orthopnea** refers to dyspnea on lying down, which is a characteristic symptom in heart failure. However, some patients with advanced pulmonary disease may also be more short of breath on lying flat. Bilateral diaphragmatic paralysis is another cause of orthopnea. **Platypnea** is the opposite of orthopnea, in which dyspnea on upright position improves by lying down. It is usually due to certain vascular abnormality of the lung.

Trepopnea indicates that the patient breathes more comfortably when lying on one side or the other. **Paroxysmal nocturnal dyspnea** is the sudden onset of shortness of breath in the middle of the night in a cardiac patient after he has been in bed for a few hours. It probably results from acute and usually transient pulmonary congestion or edema.

The majority of patients with cardiopulmonary disease have *exertional* dyspnea. The amount of exertion resulting in dyspnea helps in determining its severity. A patient who becomes short of breath on walking a short distance on a level surface has a more severe condition than if he were dyspneic on climbing stairs. The change of dyspnea with progression of disease or response to treatment is also judged by the change in the amount of exertion required to induce shortness of breath. It should, however, be remembered that with a slow deterioration of lung function, patients may adjust their physical activities in order not to experience dyspnea. In chronic pulmonary disease, such as emphysema, patients become short of breath with less and less effort, with the progression of the disease, so that, in the advanced stage, they become dyspneic even at rest. A recent increase in dyspnea in the patient with chronic respiratory disease is indicative of an acute event. This may be due to increased airway resistance such as with bronchospasm, secretions, and infection or reduced pulmonary compliance such as with pulmonary congestion or edema. Other causes of sudden dyspnea, which may also occur in otherwise healthy individuals, include spontaneous pneumothorax, pulmonary embolism, and upper airway obstruction.

HEMOPTYSIS

Although **hemoptysis** means spitting blood (*hemo-*, blood; *ptysis*, spitting), it generally refers to the expectoration of blood that originates from the respiratory tract below the pharynx. Blood-tinged or blood-streaked sputum, which may be equally serious, is not usually called hemoptysis. Thus hemoptysis signifies coughing up of an easily quantifiable amount of blood, pure or mixed with sputum. The amount of bleeding indicates the severity of hemoptysis. Massive hemoptysis is the expectoration of 600 milliliters (mL) or more of blood within 24 hours.

Few symptoms force a patient to seek medical advice as readily as hemoptysis. This alarming symptom not only may be life-threatening by its own merit, but it frequently indicates a serious underlying disease, which may be a real challenge to diagnose. The causes of hemoptysis are multitudinous, and almost any pulmonary lesion may result in hemoptysis. A significant number of patients may actually have no demonstrable evidence of cardiopulmonary disease to explain this symptom. The three major basic underlying pathologic conditions are infection, neoplasm, and cardiovascular disorders.

Common infectious causes of hemoptysis are pneumonia, tuberculosis, bronchiectasis, and lung abscess. Fungus infection and parasitic lung diseases may also result in hemoptysis. The latter conditions are some of the most frequent causes of pulmonary hemorrhage in endemic areas of the world.

Among the neoplastic diseases of the lung, bronchogenic carcinoma is the most common cause of hemoptysis. Approximately 50% of patients with lung cancer will have bloody expectoration in the course of their disease. Benign endobronchial tumors may also bleed readily.

Certain cardiovascular diseases manifest with hemoptysis. Pulmonary embolism is frequently associated with bleeding from the respiratory tract. Vascular malformations of the lung should be suspected in patients with hemoptysis without obvious cause. Heart failure may be accompanied by hemoptysis. Among the valvular heart diseases, mitral stenosis is well known for its propensity for hemoptysis.

The immediate danger of hemoptysis is related to airway obstruction. This risk is much greater than that of blood loss. If the rate of bleeding is more than its removal by expectoration or suctioning, the lungs will be flooded. The spread of infection, particularly from a tuberculous lesion, is another potential complication of hemoptysis.

In a patient who gives a history of spitting blood, it should be determined whether the blood is actually coming from the respiratory tract. It is not uncommon for the frightened patient to be confused regarding the source of bleeding. Therefore, it should be ascertained that blood is actually coming from the airways and is not vomited from the gastrointestinal tract. Furthermore, bleeding from the nose, mouth, and throat should be looked for and properly excluded.

Once it is determined that the source of bleeding is the respiratory tract below the pharynx, the rate of bleeding and the amount of blood loss should be estimated from the patient's history, close observation, vital signs, and blood count. The nurse or respiratory therapist will have the opportunity to observe the patient and report the occurrence and the characteristics of bloody expectoration.

In the management of the patient with hemoptysis, the immediate task should be directed toward maintaining a patent airway. The patient's bedside should be equipped with a suction machine, tracheal intubation set, and equipment for respiratory assistance. Bed rest, reassurance, mild sedation, and close observation are measures that should be followed. If the bleeding side is known, the patient is positioned with that side dependent. Hemoptysis will usually stop spontaneously, but occasionally operative procedures will be necessary.

Although a careful history, physical examination, and chest x-ray are most helpful in identifying the cause of hemoptysis, bronchoscopy frequently will be required. In some instances, for a more definitive diagnosis, specialized radiologic examinations such as radioisotopic studies or angiography will be necessary.

CHEST PAIN

Chest pain is one of the symptoms that causes alarm to the patient and concern to the health-care team. It may be due to a variety of conditions, ranging from a transient and insignificant event to a most serious and life-threatening medical catastrophe. As with pain anywhere else, the patient's pain response is unpredictable. The same disease with similar severity may cause minimal discomfort to one patient and excruciating pain to another.

The thorax is made of and contains many structures that may be the site of origin of pain. The thoracic wall is the most common source of chest pain; skin, muscles, nerves, and bones may be its cause in association with various clinical conditions. The lung parenchyma itself is insensitive to painful stimuli, and only the parietal layer of pleura is very pain sensitive. Its direct or indirect involvement by various pathologic processes is a frequent cause of chest pain. Pain in pneumonias and other inflammatory diseases of the lung is usually due to pleural reaction. In lung cancer, the chest pain is frequently indicative of pleural and/or chest-wall invasion. However, certain patients with lung cancer will have a heavy sensation in the chest without such an invasion.

Pulmonary arterial hypertension sometimes causes chest pain, which may be due to increased tension of arterial walls or secondary to myocardial ischemia from right ventricular strain. The sudden and transient chest pain of pulmonary embolism probably occurs through a similar mechanism. However, more persistent "pleuritic" pain following pulmonary embolism is secondary to pleural reaction. In acute inflammation of the trachea and major bronchi (tracheobronchitis), a scratchy feeling behind the sternum is common.

Pleuritic pain refers to chest pain that is produced or aggravated by deep breathing and other chest-wall movement. It is not exclusive to pleural disease, but may also be a manifestation of painful conditions of the chest wall. The lack of chest pain does not exclude the presence of lung disease; many serious pulmonary lesions produce no pain.

Other intrathoracic organs and structures may be the source of chest pain. Pain originating from the heart and its major blood vessels is a common occurrence, particularly the pain of myocardial ischemia (deficient blood supply), which is known as angina pectoris. Myocardial infarction; **pericarditis;** rupture, dissection, or distension of the aorta; disease of the mediastinum; and esophageal disorders are other important causes of chest pain.

Because of the multiplicity of causes of chest pain, it is often a diagnostic challenge. A careful history, thorough physical examination, proper radiographic studies, electrocardiography, and other appropriate tests usually will help to identify the underlying cause of chest pain.

OTHER RESPIRATORY SYMPTOMS

Wheezing, as a symptom, is heard by the patient as a whistling sound in association with asthma. It may also be present in conditions such as acute bronchitis and other causes of bronchial narrowing. Many patients are aware of the presence of wheezing, but others may not notice it. **Auscultation** of the chest will be necessary to detect or confirm the wheezing. This will be discussed in the Physical Examination section below. **Stridor** is a noisy breathing characterized by a harsh inspiratory sound secondary to narrowing of an extrathoracic portion of the upper airway. Abnormal *snoring* is usually a complaint of a roommate or bed companion rather than the snorer. This symptom is important in evaluation for sleep-related respiratory disorders (Chapter 24).

Hoarseness, varying from roughening of the voice to its total loss, is indicative of laryngeal disease, such as inflammation, tumor, vocal cord paralysis and overuse or misuse of vocal cords, or it may be secondary to tracheal intubation.

PHYSICAL EXAMINATION

The physical examination of patients with pulmonary disease should not be limited to the respiratory tract, but should include other organ systems. This will not only enable one to detect concomitant abnormalities, but will also help to identify conditions that may be the cause or result of respiratory disorders. For example, recognition of **signs** of heart disease may explain a patient's breathlessness, or demonstration of peripheral thrombophlebitis will suggest pulmonary embolism in a patient with a compatible clinical picture. Clubbing of fingers and toes (Fig. 1–2) may be a manifestation of lung disease, or cyanosis of fingers and lips may suggest respiratory pathology. The determination of body temperature and other vital signs is indispensable in evaluating patients with respiratory disease.

Remarkable progress in various diagnostic techniques, particularly radiology, and their ready availability have resulted in slackened emphasis on the importance of physical diagnosis. We believe that this is unfortunate. Taking a good history and performing a proper

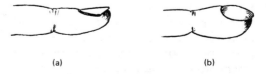
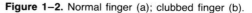

(a)   (b)

Figure 1–2. Normal finger (a); clubbed finger (b).

physical examination will provide valuable information not only necessary for accurate diagnosis, but essential for rational choice and more precise interpretation of diagnostic procedures.

The four fundamental components of the physical examination that are applicable to the examination of patients with respiratory disease are *inspection, palpation, percussion,* and *auscultation.*

Inspection

In performing a physical examination we use our sense organs, the most important being our eyes. Examination by looking is called inspection, which is the most informative phase of a physical examination. This applies to the examination of most areas of the body, as well as the respiratory system. Students of the health sciences should develop the ability and the habit of becoming astute observers, and they should familiarize themselves with simple and easily acquired techniques of inspection. By simple inspection, a great amount of valuable information can be obtained on a patient's general health. His general appearance, developmental and nutritional state, color, complexion, degree of illness and distress, posture, gait, and behavior can be readily assessed.

Inspection in relation to the respiratory system should include observation of the patient's chest and its movement. Shape of the chest and its symmetry, deformities, breathing pattern, rhythm, rate, sighing, use of accessory respiratory muscles, chest excursion, symmetry of expansion, paradoxical movements, retraction between the ribs and above the clavicles, and presence of scars of prior surgery and previous tracheotomy should be carefully noted.

Of particular importance is the observation of paradoxical movement of the chest and the abdomen which is a fairly common, but often overlooked, finding in ventilatory failure in patients with a weak or fatigued diaphragm. Instead of simultaneous expansion of the abdomen and the chest during inspiration, the abdominal wall is sucked inward while the thorax is expanding (see Fig. 1–3).

Observation of the patient while he takes a deep breath will give some idea about the ventilatory ability of the lungs. Bedside performance of a forced expiratory maneuver may give a rough estimate of the degree of airway obstruction. Respiration should be observed for its

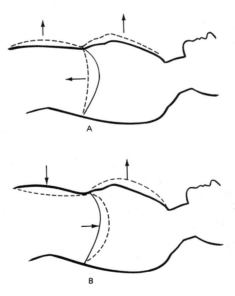

Figure 1–3. Relationship between abdominal and rib cage motions with respiration. Dashed lines and arrows denote directions of movements of the chest wall, diaphragm, and abdomen on inspiration. Normally, the movements of the chest wall and abdomen are in the same direction (A). With a paralyzed or weak diaphragm, there is a paradoxical motion: while the rib cage is expanding, the abdomen is being sucked in (B).

rate and rhythm without the patient's awareness; otherwise the pattern and rate of breathing might change. This can be done by pretending that the examiner is counting the pulse or making some other observation while actually he or she is concentrating on the patient's respiration. Respiratory patterns are discussed on page 16.

Palpation

In palpation, the tactile sense is used to determine the physical characteristics of organs and tissues. Their shape, size, consistency, tenderness, temperature, smoothness or roughness, movement, and movability are thus examined.

Palpation of the chest is mainly used for evaluation of the degree and symmetry of respiratory movements and for determination of *vocal* **fremitus.** For the purpose of elicitation of thoracic expansion and comparison of two sides, the hands are placed symmetrically over the patient's chest at various locations, and the movement of the underlying chest wall is felt while the patient is taking deep breaths (see Fig. 1–4). Vocal fremi-

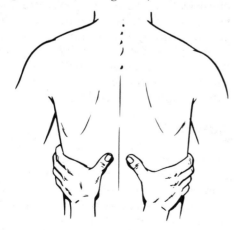

Figure 1–4. Palpation of the chest for an evaluation of its expansion.

tus is the tactile perception of vibration set by the larynx upon phonation and transmitted to the chest wall. It is determined by placing the palms lightly on the patient's chest while he is repeating certain words or numbers in a loud, deep voice. The significance of this examination lies in the comparison of two corresponding sides of the chest.

Reduced ventilation of a lobe or a whole lung due to various pathologic conditions will result in reduced thoracic expansion over that area. The presence of air or fluid between the lung and chest wall, or any obstacle to transmission of voice vibration, including airway obstruction, will cause diminution or absence of vocal fremitus. On the other hand, the consolidation of lung tissue without obstruction to its bronchus, as in pneumonia, will facilitate the transmission of vibration and, thus, will increase vocal fremitus.

Palpation will also allow the examiner to locate the position of the trachea, elicit tenderness, evaluate any masses or swellings, and detect subcutaneous accumulations of air (subcutaneous emphysema).

Percussion

Examination by percussion has been compared to a radar or sonar detection system. Tapping on the chest produces vibration of the chest wall and the underlying lung, which is reflected and picked up by the examiner's auditory and tactile senses. The note and the loudness of sound will depend on the force of percussion and the characteristics of the underlying tissues. Percussion over solid or liquid-containing organs, such as the liver or the heart, results in a low-amplitude, high-frequency short sound without any **resonance;** this is a *dull* percussion note. On the other hand, percussion over an air-containing viscus, such as the lung, produces a *resonant* note, which has a higher amplitude, lower pitch, and longer duration.

The most commonly used method of percussion is as follows: the palmar surface of the middle finger of one hand is firmly applied against the chest wall, while the tip of the middle finger of the other hand strikes upon it with short, quick, and uniform vertical blows, delivered from the wrist (Fig. 1–5). This is repeated by changing the location of percussion to various regions of the chest, always comparing corresponding areas of two sides. The vibrations produced by percussion are not only heard but also felt by the fingers applied over the chest.

Percussion notes vary among normal individuals, and in the same individual over different areas of the chest. This is because of variations in the thickness of the tissues surrounding the lungs in different people and different lung regions and also because of the presence and the position of other intrathoracic structures, as well as unevenness of the thickness of the underlying air-containing lung tissues. However, with few exceptions, the percussion note is equal over the symmetrical areas of the two hemithoraces. That is why percussion notes should be compared over the two corresponding sides. Because of the presence of the liver, the right lung base is dull to percussion. The height of this dullness helps in the estimation of liver size. The position of the heart in the chest, which is close to the anterior wall and somewhat to the left, makes this area relatively dull to percussion.

Increased lung inflation, as during deep inspiration or in patients with emphysema and asthmatic attacks, will cause increased resonance (hyperresonance). Sometimes the presence of a large amount of air in the pleural cavity (**pneumothorax**) will result in a tympanitic note (like the sound of a drum). The replacement of air in the lung by solid tissue or liquid material will reduce the resonance. Over a completely airless lung, or when there is a significant amount of fluid in the pleural cavity, percussion notes will be dull.

Percussion is also useful for delineation of the level of the diaphragm, which roughly corresponds to the line on the chest wall where the normal resonance changes to dullness. Diaphragmatic excursion during a maximum respiratory cycle can be determined by measuring the difference between the levels of the diaphragm at the end of a deep inspiration and after a complete expiration.

Auscultation

Sense of hearing is an important tool for the examination of the respiratory system. The vibration produced by percussion is primarily perceived as sound. Laryngeal disease is usually suspected by a change in voice quality. *Stridor*, a harsh, high-pitched, and loud inspiratory sound, is an important diagnostic

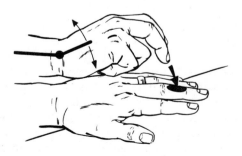

Figure 1–5. Technique of percussion.

sign of upper airway obstruction. Sounds of coughing in certain respiratory diseases, such as whooping cough, are characteristic. In asthmatics during an attack, wheezing may be heard at a distance. Although all these sounds are appreciated by hearing, *auscultation* is commonly referred to as the act of listening for sounds within the body either by the direct application of an ear over the area or, more conveniently, by a *stethoscope*.

The movement of air in and out of the lung normally produces sound vibration as a result of turbulence of flow with sudden changes in the lumen of the airways and their direction. Breath sounds have two basic components, which are discussed below (see Fig. 1–6).

1. **Bronchial** sounds, which are produced in the proximal airways, that is, the larynx, trachea, and large bronchi, have a higher pitch and are harsh and loud. They are heard equally well during both inspiration and expiration, with a distinct short pause in between. Pure bronchial breath sound is closely approximated by the sound heard when the stethoscope is applied directly over the trachea.

2. **Vesicular** sounds are soft and have a lower pitch and hissing quality. These sounds are heard mostly during inspiration, dying away rapidly in the early part of expiration. Vesicular sounds, without interfering bronchial sounds, are best heard in the lower lung fields. The long-held general view that vesicular sounds are produced by the passage of air through the bronchi-

oles and alveolar ducts has recently been questioned. There is increasing evidence that they are large airway sounds that are filtered on their way through the lungs, resulting in reduction and elimination of their certain components.

In the upper lung regions, the breath sounds are a combination of or intermediate between the bronchial and vesicular sounds. They are known as **bronchovesicular** sounds. Under normal conditions, pure bronchial breath sounds should not be heard in any lung areas, and bronchovesicular sounds are considered abnormal in the lower lung fields.

The transmission of breath sounds will depend on the physical characteristics of the tissues through which they traverse. They are usually louder in children and lean individuals, but they are diminished and appear distant in obese people. Presence of air or fluid in the pleural cavity will interfere with the transmission of breath sounds. Reduced ventilation of the lung units will also cause diminution of breath sounds. In certain pathologic conditions where transmission of bronchial sounds is facilitated, bronchial breath sounds will

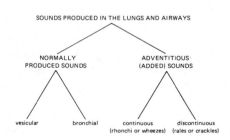

Figure 1–6. Major sounds originating from the lungs in normal and diseased states.

be heard. Consolidation of the lung with pneumonia is a typical example of this phenomenon.

In addition to the breath sounds mentioned above, other sounds may be produced in the lungs under certain abnormal conditions. As they do not occur normally, they are **adventitious,** or added sounds (Fig. 1–6). The adventitious sounds produced by air flow are divided into continuous sounds, or **rhonchi,** and discontinuous sounds, or **rales.** Rhonchi, also known as wheezes, are produced by the passage of air through bronchi that are narrowed by swelling, secretions, bronchospasm, foreign body, or a growth. They have a more or less musical quality with a distinguished pitch and are mostly heard during expiration. Rhonchi due to secretions usually will change or disappear with coughing.

Rales, also known as crackles, are brief and explosive rather than musical, and are heard mostly during inspiration. Although the mechanism of their production is not entirely clear, they are often related to the presence of fluid inside the bronchi and the collapsed distal airways and alveoli. Depending on their site of origin, rales have various qualities. They are divided into fine, medium, and coarse. Fine rales are probably the result of opening of the distal small airways with the flow of air during inspiration. Medium and coarse rales are produced by the passage of air in fluid-containing bronchi. It seems that the courser the rales, the larger are the airways where air and fluid come in contact.

In describing these sounds, other qualities such as their intensity, location, and timing in the respiratory cycle should be noted. As the intrathoracic airways are narrower during expiration, the rhonchi are best heard during this phase of respiration; however, they are not limited to it. During an asthma attack they may be heard during both phases of respiration, but more during expiration. Rhonchus is a Latin word for wheezing and, therefore, they are synonymous. In general usage, however, higher-pitched rhonchi are referred to as wheezes. A phenomenon, in which there is an alteration of transmitted voice sounds is known as **egophony** (bleeting sound of a goat). It is characterized by change of a long *E* sound to a long *A* sound while listening with a stethoscope. It occurs when there is a combination of pulmonary consolidation with pleural effusion.

Another important adventitious sound is the *pleural rub.* This is a grating sound produced by movement and friction of roughened pleural surfaces. It is a diagnostic sign of pleuritis.

RESPIRATORY PATTERNS

Valuable information can be obtained by the careful observation of breathing patterns. In normal individuals at rest, the respiration is more or less regular, at a rate between 12 and 20 per minute (in adults), and the respiratory movements are evident over both the chest and abdomen. Although as a general rule males have predominantly *diaphragmatic* or abdominal breathing and females tend to use **costal** breathing, there are wide individual variations even among a healthy population. Normally, inspiration lasts about half as long as expiration.

Changes in respiratory patterns may be related to the rate, depth, rhythm, ratio of expiration to inspiration, and alternation between abdominal and rib cage breathing.

Rapid breathing, known as **tachypnea** or **polypnea,** is usually indicative of reduced pulmonary or thoracic compliance, and is seen in such conditions as pneumonia, pulmonary congestion and edema, and a variety of other restrictive chest diseases. It may or may not result in increased **alveolar** ventilation, depending on the depth of breathing and the volume of dead space. This can be judged more accurately by the arterial carbon dioxide tension. **Bradypnea,** on the other hand, is abnormal slowness of the respiratory rate. It is seen in patients with respiratory center depression, such as in narcotic drug overdoses. In extreme situations there may be **apnea,** which is the absence of respiration for at least 10 seconds. Apneic episodes are frequently observed during sleep, and are hallmarks of sleep apnea syndrome (see Chapter 24, page 328).

Increased respiratory depth, frequently accompanied by rapid rate, is characteristic of **Kussmaul's breathing,** which is seen in patients with severe metabolic acidosis. Increased depth of breathing is indicative of increased alveolar ventilation unless dead-space ventilation is significantly high. The amount of alveolar ventilation can only be accurately determined by alveolar or arterial carbon dioxide and its rate of elimination. *Hyperventilation* generally refers to excessive *alveolar* ventilation. The causes of hyperventilation are discussed on page 24.

Shallow respiration is usually due to restrictive pulmonary or thoracic conditions. It is almost always compensated by an increased rate of breathing. Conditions resulting in "stiff" lungs,

and impairing thoracic expansion and, therefore, causing shallow respiration, are numerous. Severe pulmonary fibrosis and other parenchymal diseases, marked thoracic deformities, massive pleural effusion, increased intraabdominal pressure, significant chest-wall or pleural pain, and respiratory muscle weakness or fatigue are among conditions that may be associated with shallow, rapid breathing.

In severe obstructive bronchopulmonary disease, the ratio of expiration to inspiration may be significantly increased. This is commonly seen in patients during asthma attacks or with advanced emphysema.

Disturbances of respiratory rhythm are usually due to central nervous system diseases affecting the regulation of respiration. Although other less common respiratory arrhythmias may occur, the most significant and prevalent abnormal respiratory rhythm is the periodic breathing of Cheyne-Stokes.

Cheyne-Stokes respiration is characterized by alternate waxing and waning of the depth and the rate of breathing. Typically, periods of apnea of various durations are interposed between the cycles. The apneic period is terminated by respirations of gradually increasing depth and frequency until a peak is reached, which is followed by gradually diminishing respiratory effort until the next apneic phase. Cheyne-Stokes respiration may occasionally be observed during sleep in normal persons, particularly newborns and the elderly. It commonly occurs in high altitudes or following forced hyperventilation.

The clinical importance of Cheyne-Stokes ventilation, however, is related to its association with certain central nervous system disorders and cardiac failure. Both abnormal response of the respiratory centers and prolonged circulation time have been implicated in its production. Frequently, it seems that the combination of these two mechanisms is operative. It is the disturbance of *coordination* of factors, which normally control the rhythmic respiration, that results in periodic breathing. It appears that hyperexcitability of the respiratory centers alternates with their depression. Toward the end of apnea a rise in arterial PCO_2 and, more importantly, a fall in arterial PO_2 stimulate the central and peripheral **chemoreceptors** to a point of overshooting hyperventilation. The latter results in the restoration of oxygenation and the reduction of arterial PCO_2, which in turn suppresses ventilatory drive to the point of its complete cessation (apnea), and the cycle repeats itself. This instability in ventilatory control systems may be the result of prolonged circulation time, which causes a delay in sensing the chemical changes in the blood returning from the lungs. Frequently, however, there is impairment of the sensitivity of the ventilatory control centers.

SYSTEMIC MANIFESTATIONS OF RESPIRATORY DISORDERS

Significant alteration of respiratory function may result in systemic manifestations, primarily through the impairment of oxygenation and/or carbon dioxide elimination. Since the regulation of arterial oxygenation and carbon dioxide removal is the main function of the lungs, its derangement is the most important indication of abnormal respiratory function. Because of its signifi-

cant functional reserve, however, the respiratory system is capable of regulating and maintaining the arterial blood gases despite the presence of pathologic conditions. Therefore, the lack of an abnormality in the blood gases does not exclude respiratory disease.

Hypoxemia and Hypoxia
Hypoxemia means low blood oxygen, and commonly refers to decreased arterial blood oxygen tension (PO_2) or saturation below normal levels. **Hypoxia** is a more general term, and signifies low oxygen in tissues or cells resulting from inadequate oxygen delivery to meet their oxidative requirements. **Anoxia,** which means absence of oxygen, is the extreme degree of hypoxia.

The adequate oxygenation of tissue depends on its blood supply containing a sufficient *amount* of oxygen. The amount of oxygen carried in the blood is a function of its oxygen tension, or saturation, and hemoglobin available for its transport. Low hemoglobin levels in anemia and reduced available hemoglobin for binding oxygen in carbon monoxide poisoning are conditions in which the arterial blood oxygen content is decreased, while its partial pressure remains normal. Therefore, tissue hypoxia may result not only from arterial hypoxemia, but also from the reduction of tissue blood supply and from diminished oxygen-carrying capacity of the blood. Moreover, delivery of oxygen to tissues is also influenced by the affinity of hemoglobin to oxygen. This particular and important characteristic of hemoglobin determines its ability to bind and release oxygen under various circumstances, and is the basis for construction of the oxygen-hemoglobin dissociation curve. The subject of oxygen transport is discussed further on page 44.

The basic respiratory *causes of hypoxemia* are reduced inspired oxygen tension, alveolar hypoventilation, impairment of diffusion, ventilation-perfusion mismatching, and venous-to-arterial shunting.

Reduced inspired oxygen tension is usually due to the low atmospheric pressure of high altitudes. As the oxygen concentration does not change with altitude, its partial pressure is directly proportional to the atmospheric pressure. Low inspired oxygen results in reduced alveolar and, hence, arterial oxygen tensions.

Hypoxemia of alveolar hypoventilation is also due to reduced alveolar oxygen concentrations. Decreased alveolar ventilation results in the accumulation of carbon dioxide and the proportional reduction of oxygen. (See the alveolar air equation in Appendix D.)

Impairment of diffusion across the alveolar capillary membrane may be due to increased thickness of this membrane or its reduced surface area. The resulting hypoxemia is further enhanced by exercise, because the increased blood flow through the pulmonary capillary diminishes the time available for oxygen uptake by the blood. In most **interstitial** lung diseases, there is a diffusion defect. Concomitant ventilation-perfusion abnormality, however, probably plays a more significant role in causing hypoxemia.

The most common cause of hypoxemia in pulmonary diseases is *ventilation-perfusion mismatching.* As a result of variations in the mechanical properties of different lung units, their ventilation will differ significantly. If their blood flow does not adjust to match ventilation, hypoxemia will result (Fig. 1–7). The poorly ventilated units will have low alveolar oxygen; therefore, blood coming from these units will not be adequately oxygenated. The mixture of this blood with the well-oxygenated blood coming from well-ventilated units

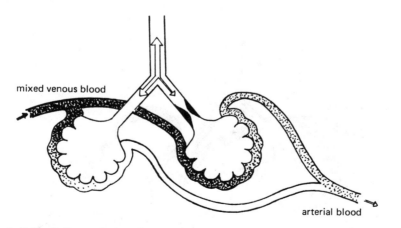

mixed venous blood

arterial blood

Figure 1–7. Ventilation-perfusion mismatching resulting in hypoxemia. Blood returning from the alveoli on the left is well oxygenated as a result of their adequate ventilation. Because of decreased ventilation of the alveoli on the right, their blood is poorly oxygenated. Mixture of well-oxygenated with poorly oxygenated blood results in arterial hypoxemia.

will result in hypoxic blood. Excessive ventilation of these units cannot, therefore, correct hypoxemia resulting from reduced ventilation of other lung units.

In *venoarterial shunting*, the unsaturated venous blood mixes with well-oxygenated arterial blood, lowering its oxygen content. The shunting may be between the heart chambers or large blood vessels in certain congenital cardiovascular diseases; but in respiratory disorders it takes place inside the lungs. Intrapulmonary shunting may reasonably be considered as a form of ventilation-perfusion abnormality in which ventilation in certain lung units is absent; thus blood flowing through them is not exposed to any oxygen and remains as venous blood. The mixture of such blood with well-oxygenated blood will reduce its oxygen content (Figs. 1–8 and 1–9). Hypoxemia due to shunting is not fully corrected by inhalation of high oxygen concentrations, whereas hypoxemia from other causes will be. The administration of 100% oxygen is used for the calculation of

shunt fractions in many clinical situations (see Appendix H).

Marked reduction in venous blood oxygen content in patients with low cardiac output or increased metabolism aggravates arterial hypoxemia resulting from pulmonary causes, particularly shunting (Fig. 1–10).

The most reliable indicator of hypoxemia is the arterial blood PO_2 determination. Most symptoms and signs of hypoxemia will not be present unless it is severe.

Cyanosis is commonly considered as an important sign of hypoxemia. This time-honored clinical sign, however, is fraught with pitfalls and misinterpretations. Cyanosis by definition is the bluish discoloration of skin and mucous membranes due to the presence of an adequate amount of deoxygenated or *reduced* hemoglobin or certain other hemoglobin compounds in the *capillary blood*. Discoloration due to deposition of certain pigments can be readily differentiated from true cyanosis by pressing over the discol-

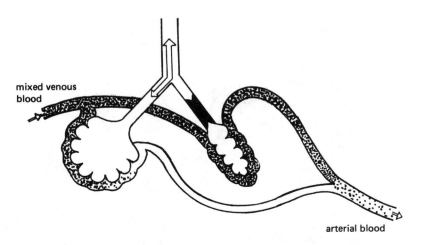

mixed venous
blood

arterial blood

Figure 1–8. Hypoxemia resulting from intrapulmonary shunting.

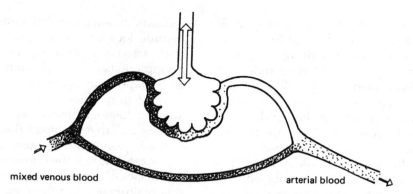

Figure 1–9. Hypoxemia resulting from venoarterial shunting.

ored area; cyanotic skin blanches; a pigmented one does not.

It has been estimated that the presence of at least 5 grams (g) of reduced hemoglobin, 1.5 g of methemoglobin (a hemoglobin compound with ferric instead of ferrous iron), or 0.5 g of sulfhemoglobin (derived from the combination of ferric iron of methemoglobin with hydrogen sulfide) in 100 mL of *capillary* blood is required for the occurrence of cyanosis. The latter two hemoglobin compounds may be occasional causes of cyanosis, whereas cyanosis

due to unoxygenated blood in the capillaries is a common occurrence.

Several factors result in increased amounts of reduced hemoglobin in capillary blood. Arterial hypoxemia causes cyanosis when the oxygen content is low enough to result in a significant amount of reduced hemoglobin. The capillary blood flow and the extraction of oxygen by tissues will, however, determine how much more hemoglobin will be deoxygenated while in the capillaries. This is one of the reasons that some patients appear more cyanotic

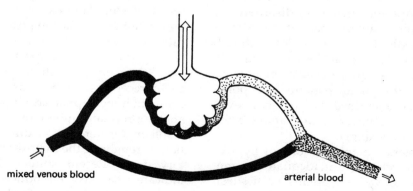

Figure 1–10. Effect of very low venous blood oxygen on arterial hypoxemia with venoarterial shunting. With the same degree of shunt, the severity of arterial hypoxemia depends on venous blood oxygen content.

than others with the same degree of arterial hypoxemia. Arterial hypoxemia need not even be present for the development of cyanosis. Marked reduction in capillary blood flow will allow for enough oxygen extraction by the tissues for cyanosis to appear. Bluish discoloration of the nose and fingertips in very cold weather is a common observation.

In clinical conditions in which peripheral blood flow is diminished as a result of systemic shock or local factors, cyanosis may be observed. This type of cyanosis, in which the arterial blood oxygen content is normal, is called *peripheral* cyanosis, in contradistinction to *central* cyanosis in which arterial blood oxygen is low. Although this differentiation can be unequivocally made only by measurement of arterial blood PO_2, it may also be made in some instances on clinical grounds. Cold extremities with diminished pulse in cyanotic areas, but normal color in warm regions, suggest peripheral cyanosis; warm extremities and more uniform distribution of cyanosis suggest a central type. It should, however, be emphasized that in many clinical situations cyanosis is the result of both arterial hypoxemia and circulatory disorders.

Severely anemic patients may have a markedly low arterial PO_2 without apparent cyanosis, as these patients will not have enough reduced hemoglobin. On the other hand, patients with polycythemia (increased hemoglobin level above normal) may seem cyanotic even without hypoxemia.

Systemic manifestations of hypoxemia are related to inadequate oxygen delivery to various organs or tissues. Hypoxemia, however, may not be associated with tissue hypoxia, particularly when it is of long duration. There are individuals, such as inhabitants in high-altitude locations, who despite significant arterial hypoxemia are entirely asymptomatic. Several compensatory and adaptive mechanisms, such as an increase in red blood cells and an alteration in hemoglobin-oxygen affinity as well as a change in blood flow, will assure adequate tissue oxygenation.

As the brain is the organ most sensitive to lack of oxygen, symptoms of cerebral malfunction are the most common manifestations of hypoxemia. Acute cerebral hypoxia usually results in impaired judgment, clumsiness, and a feeling of drunkenness. If severe, mental confusion, coma, and death will occur. Chronic longstanding hypoxia manifests with fatigue, apathy, reduced attention, drowsiness, and muscle twitching.

Hypoxia has a significant effect on the cardiovascular system. It increases the cardiac output and heart rate. Cardiac arrhythmias are common in severe hypoxemia. It dilates peripheral and cerebral blood vessels, and is a potent constrictor of the pulmonary arteries. Chronic pulmonary hypertension and cor pulmonale are important complications of longstanding hypoxemia. As a result of stimulation of red blood cell production, chronic hypoxemia may cause secondary polycythemia.

Hypoxemia is an important respiratory stimulant through the peripheral chemoreceptors. In patients with concomitant hypercapnia, administration of an inappropriate amount of oxygen may result in further carbon dioxide retention by removing the hypoxemic ventilatory drive. Recent studies, however, indicate that oxygen-induced hypercapnia is primarily due to further impairment of gas exchange when the ratio of dead space to total ventilation increases.

Severe hypoxemia resulting in inadequate tissue oxygenation may cause anaerobic metabolism (metabolism in the absence of oxygen). The waste product of such metabolism includes lactic acid, accumulation of which results in metabolic acidosis.

Hypercapnia

The metabolic production of carbon dioxide and its elimination by the lungs determine its partial pressure (PCO_2) in arterial blood. Normally the lungs are capable of regulating their ventilation, through a very sensitive control system, according to the amount of carbon dioxide production. As a result, arterial carbon dioxide tension is maintained within a narrow normal range. **Hypercapnia** or **hypercarbia** is an increase in arterial blood PCO_2 above 45 torr, the upper limit of normal.

Effective alveolar ventilation is that portion of ventilation which participates in gas exchange; it is inversely related to arterial blood PCO_2. Doubling alveolar ventilation will result in halving the arterial blood PCO_2, and vice versa. Effectiveness of alveolar ventilation, therefore, is judged by arterial blood carbon dioxide tension. Hypercapnia then indicates inadequate alveolar ventilation in relation to metabolic production of carbon dioxide.

There are numerous causes of carbon dioxide retention. These are discussed in Chapter 25.

Variable degrees of hypoxemia are always present in patients with hypercapnia, unless a high concentration of oxygen is administered. In clinical situations, therefore, the manifestations of hypercapnia are often combined with manifestations of hypoxemia. A clinical picture of pure hypercapnia may be experimentally demonstrated in individuals breathing CO_2 mixtures. Increased pulse rate and blood pressure, dizziness, headaches, mental clouding, visual difficulty, muscle twitching and tremor, and mental depression are frequently observed. Severe hypercapnia may result in loss of consciousness, which is commonly known as *CO$_2$ narcosis*. Carbon dioxide dilates cerebral blood vessels, resulting in increased blood flow to the brain. It has a constricting effect on pulmonary vessels.

An acute accumulation of carbon dioxide results in an increased hydrogen ion concentration (**acidosis**), which is at least partly responsible for most of the harmful effects of CO_2 retention. Slow and gradual increases in the PCO_2, as seen in patients with chronic ventilatory failure, will allow for metabolic compensation by the elevation of serum bicarbonate and, therefore, will prevent or at least slow down the changes in pH. This is further discussed in Chapter 2.

In patients with acute respiratory failure, when there is a combination of hypercapnia and hypoxemia, a clinical picture characterized by headaches, somnolence, mental confusion, weakness, fatigue, irritability, and involuntary muscle movements is commonly observed. In more severe cases, loss of consciousness, paralysis, coma, and death may supervene.

Hypocapnia

Hypocapnia is the reverse of hypercapnia and signifies low arterial blood carbon dioxide tensions. It indicates an increased ventilation out of proportion to the metabolic production of carbon dioxide. This excessive alveolar ventilation is commonly known as *hyperventi-*

lation. Although hyperventilation may be suspected clinically, it can only be confirmed by demonstration of a low arterial blood PCO_2.

Acute reduction of arterial blood PCO_2 results in respiratory alkalosis, which at least partly is responsible for clinical manifestations of the *hyperventilation syndrome.* They include light-headedness, fatigue, irritability, inability to concentrate, sense of unreality, tingling, muscle twitching, and impaired consciousness. The most common cause of hyperventilation is anxiety reaction, including panic attack, but it may also be due to central nervous system disease, severe anemia, shock, high fever, septicemia, alcoholic intoxication, severe liver disease, aspirin poisoning, and several other conditions.

Increased ventilatory response to metabolic acidosis is an important compensatory mechanism for controlling excessive accumulation of hydrogen ions. Lack of respiratory compensation of metabolic acidosis is indicative of significant ventilatory impairment.

In chronic hyperventilation, metabolic compensation by reduction of serum bicarbonate will result in the correction of pH.

In many patients with respiratory disease, particularly in patients with hypoxemic respiratory failure, hyperventilation may be part of the clinical picture. It may be due to hypoxemic stimulation of the chemoreceptors, but it is often due to increased responsiveness of certain reflexes originating in the lungs. Hyperventilation as a result of mechanical ventilation is a common occurrence, which may be inadvertent or intentional.

BIBLIOGRAPHY

Anthonisen NR. Hypoxemia and O_2 therapy. *Am Rev Respir Dis.* 1982; 126:729–733.

Branch WT, McNeil BJ. Analysis of the differential diagnosis and assessment of pleuritic chest pain in young adults. *Am J Med.* 1983; 75:671–679.

Burki NK. Dyspnea. *Clin Chest Med.* 1980; 1 (1):47–55.

Cockcroft A, Adams L, Guz A. Assessment of breathlessness. *Q J Med.* 1989; 72:669–676.

Cohen CA, Zagelbaum G, Gross D, et al. Clinical manifestations of inspiratory muscle fatigue. *Am J Med.* 1982; 73:308–316.

Farzan S. Cough and sputum production. In: Walker HK, et al eds. *Clinical Methods.* 3rd ed. Boston, Mass: Butterworth; 1990; 207–210.

Forgacs P. The functional basis of pulmonary sounds. *Chest.* 1978; 73:399–405.

Glauser FL, ed. *Signs and Symptoms in Pulmonary Medicine.* Philadelphia, Pa: Lippincott; 1983.

Goldman, JM. Hemoptysis. *Emerg Med Clin North Am.* 1989; 7:325–338.

Irwin RS, Curley FJ, French CL. Chronic cough: the spectrum and frequency of causes, key components of the diagnostic evaluation, and outcome of specific therapy. *Am Rev Respir Dis.* 1990; 141:640–647.

Loudon RG. The lung exam. *Clin Chest Med.* 1987; 8:265–272.

Loudon RG, Murphy RLH Jr. Lung sounds. *Am Rev Respir Dis.* 1984; 130:663–673.

Pratter MR, Curley FJ, Dubois J, Irwin RS. Cause and evaluation of chronic dyspnea in a pulmonary disease clinic. *Arch Intern Med.* 1989; 149:2277–2282.

Schneider RR, Seckler SG. Evaluation of acute chest pain. *Med Clin North Am.* 1981; 65 (1):53–66.

Sebastian JL, McKinney WP, Kaufman J, Young MJ. Angiotensin-converting enzyme inhibitors and cough. *Chest.* 1991; 99:36–39.

Tobin MJ, Chadha TS, Jenouri G, et al.

Breathing patterns. *Chest.* 1983; 84:202–205, 286–294.

Wasserman K, Casaburi R. Dyspnea: physiologic and pathophysiologic mechanisms. *Annu Rev Med.* 1988; 39:503–515.

Wedzicha JA, Pearson MC. Management of massive hemoptysis. *Respir Med.* 1990; 84:9–12.

Weinbergerger SE, Schwartzstein RM, Weiss JW. Hypercapnia. *N Engl J Med.* 1989; 321:1223–1231.

Wolkove N, Dajczman E, Colacone A, Keisman H. The relationship between pulmonary function and dyspnea in obstructive lung disease. *Chest.* 1989; 96:1247–1251.

CHAPTER 2

Diagnostic Methods, Functional Assessment, and Monitoring

The diagnosis of respiratory diseases and the evaluation of their functional effect can be frequently made by appropriate history taking and physical examination. However, in most instances, applicable laboratory, radiographic, and/ or bedside procedures are necessary for a definitive diagnosis, accurate functional assessment, and close monitoring. This chapter deals with these ancillary studies. It should be emphasized that information obtained by history and physical examination is essential for their proper selection and effective utilization. The results of these studies should always be interpreted in light of clinical information and by considering their accuracy, sensitivity, and specificity.

SPUTUM EXAMINATION

Expectoration is a significant manifestation of many respiratory disorders, and information obtained from sputum examination may be necessary for their diagnosis and management. Sputum examination is particularly helpful in the evaluation of respiratory-tract infections

for bacteriologic identification and selection of the proper antibiotic. It is important in assessment of therapy in patients with tuberculosis, chronic bronchitis, asthma, lung abcess, and many other pulmonary diseases. The diagnosis of lung carcinoma and several other conditions is frequently made by or suspected from sputum examination.

Obtaining a proper sputum sample is most important for a successful sputum examination. It is most commonly done by collecting the *expectorated* sputum in a sterile bottle. Unfortunately, this simple task is often fraught with misinformation and mishandling. The respiratory therapist or nurse should be well informed about the proper technique for sputum collection. The sputum sample must represent secretions from the lower respiratory tract; nasal secretions and saliva are not acceptable. The patient should be observed and helped during the sputum collection. First, the mouth should be cleared of food particles and rinsed with water. The patient is then asked to take a few deep breaths, and, at the end of the last inspiration, he is instructed to perform a series of gentle, short coughs. Often, following several deep breaths, the secretions will be mobilized more proximally, and the ensuing cough will be more effective in expelling them. The patient should be cautioned not to swallow the sputum, but rather to expectorate it into the specimen bottle. This procedure is repeated until an adequate sample is obtained. It is often easier to collect sputum in the morning upon the patient's arising.

Sometimes it is not possible to obtain a sputum sample by cough and expectoration because of dry cough or the thick and tenacious nature of the secretion. The use of aerosolized solutions, such as saline, propylene glycol, acetylcysteine, and others, may help in inducing sputum production and expectoration. Systemic hydration is important in dehydrated patients for sputum production. Sputum induction in patients with acquired immunodeficiency syndrome (AIDS), when *Pneumocystis carinii* pneumonia is suspected, is a simple and effective way of making a specific diagnosis (see Chapter 6).

Tracheobronchial suctioning, through the nose or the mouth, is an important way of obtaining a sample of secretions, particularly in obtunded or debilitated patients. Occasionally, secretions are obtained by transtracheal aspiration. With local anesthesia and sterile technique, a small catheter is passed via a large-bore needle inserted into the lumen of the trachea, entering percutaneously through the cricothyroid membrane. The secretions aspirated with this technique, which bypasses the mouth and the pharnyx, are most suitable for anaerobic bacterial culture. With the use of fiberoptic bronchoscopy, usually an adequate amount of

secretion can be obtained. It also allows for the study of samples selectively collected from desired lobar or segmental bronchi. Aspiration of the stomach by a nasogastric tube, before arising in the morning, may yield tracheobronchial secretions swallowed during the preceding night. This method is used to obtain a sample for identification of tubercle bacilli in patients suspected of having pulmonary tuberculosis, but unable to expectorate, or as a supplement to sputum examination. Gastric aspiration is particularly useful in children who have difficulty in producing sputum.

Once an adequate sample is collected, its gross characteristics should be observed; this may provide important information as discussed earlier on page 7. The specimen should be taken to the appropriate laboratory for its desired examination. This should be done promptly when bacteriologic studies are intended. Sputum is usually examined for its cell content, particularly the amount and the type of white blood cells. The presence of alveolar macrophages in sputum is an important indication that its origin is the lung. **Squamous** epithelial cells indicate the presence of secretions from areas above the larnyx, and thus are unsuitable for bacteriologic examination. Significant numbers of polymorphonuclear neutrophils suggest bacterial infection, whereas eosinophils often are indicative of an allergic process such as asthma. Bacteriologic studies will include smear and special staining, as well as culturing on special media, depending on the organisms that are suspected. Sputum is also examined for malignant cells in patients suspected of having neoplastic lesions of the respiratory tract.

RADIOGRAPHIC EXAMINATION OF THE CHEST

Radiographic examination plays a most important role in studying patients with respiratory disorders and in diagnosing unsuspected lung diseases. Without a chest x-ray, examination of such patients is considered incomplete. A number of pulmonary conditions will be either undiagnosed or misdiagnosed without radiographic study. Many cases of pulmonary malignancy, early tuberculosis, and a variety of other lesions may be completely unrecognized until discovered by a chest x-ray. Radiographic examination is commonly used for screening asymptomatic individuals to detect tuberculosis and, sometimes, other lung diseases.

In patients with respiratory disease, x-ray examination enables better identification of a lesion, more correct assessment of its extent, and its more precise localization. It also helps in following the patient's progress and response to therapeutic measures. In addition, x-ray film is an important medical document, particularly useful as a comparison for future studies.

Principles of Radiographic Study of the Chest

Because of differences in the density of its various structures, the chest is very suitable for radiographic examination. There is enough contrast between most of these structures to allow for their delineation on the x-ray film. The air-containing lungs, having the least density, do not significantly interfere with the passage of roentgen rays, causing dark prints on the film; the bones, because of their high density, impede the traverse of x-rays, and therefore prevent its impression on the film, which remains white. The heart, blood vessels, mediastinum, and diaphragm, which have a density greater than air but less than bone, cause differing shades of white and gray on the x-ray film. In addition to their density, the thickness of various structures is an important factor in affecting the x-ray penetration.

The ribs and other bones can be easily identified from the surrounding soft tissue and the lungs. The silhouette of the heart and its major blood vessels, which are flanked by the lungs, is clearly outlined. The diaphragm, with its underlying abdominal organs, contrasts with the air-containing lungs above it. The trachea, because of its air content, is visualized in the middle of the upper mediastinum. The pulmonary blood vessels are traceable from the hili, branching and tapering toward the lung periphery.

Because of the superimposition of certain structures and for better localization of the lesions, usually at least two radiographic views are obtained: (1) Posteroanterior (PA) or occasionally anteroposterior (AP). (2) Lateral (right or left). Sometimes other projections such as obliques may be necessary.

The standard posteroanterior projection, which is the cornerstone of radiographic examination of the chest, is obtained by placing the patient in front of the radiographic cassette so that the front of the chest touches it. The x-ray tube is located behind the patient at a distance of about 2 meters. The beam of radiation from the x-ray tube passes through the patient's back in a direction perpendicular to the surface of the film. This is intended to minimize distortion and magnification effects. The x-ray is usually taken at the end of inspiration while the patient is temporarily holding his breath. The exposure time, voltage, and current are individualized according to the patient's age, thickness of the chest wall, and particular purpose of the study.

Reading a Chest X-Ray. In reading a radiographic picture of the chest, the following observations are made (Figs. 2–1 and 2–2):

1. Soft tissues surrounding the bony thorax, including breast shadows.
2. Bony structures; counting and identifying the individual ribs, looking for fractures, deformity and other lesions; spinal curvature.
3. Diaphragm, its position, comparing the two sides (usually the right hemidiaphragm is slightly higher than the left), its contour, sharpness of its angles with the chest wall (**costophrenic** or CP angles). A small amount of pleural effusion would obliterate these angles.
4. The mediastinum, including the heart, its position, width, and contour; heart size, configuration, and the ratio of its width to the inner thoracic diameter (cardiothoracic ratio is normally less than ½). In a PA projection of the chest, the outline of the mediastinum on the right side is made by (from above downward) the innominate vein, superior vena cava, right atrium, and, sometimes, the inferior vena cava. On the left, it is made by (from above downward) the subclavian vessels, aorta, pulmonary artery trunk, and the left ventricle (Fig. 2–3).
5. The lungs, their volume, background density, shadows of various lesions; pulmonary blood vessels, their size and direction; hili, their position, size, and sharpness. The background lung density is normally due to the presence of blood in the pulmonary capillaries, while the larger vessels create the visible lung markings. Normally, the bronchi, beyond a short distance from the tracheal bifurcation, are not visible. The hilum in a chest film refers to the area of the lung where the pulmonary blood vessels converge; it also contains some lymph nodes, which are not normally discernible, but they may become quite large and readily identifiable in certain pathologic conditions. The right hilar position is normally slightly lower than the left.
6. Pleura, its thickness, presence of fluid or air in the pleural cavity; interlobar fissures. Normally, the pleura does not cast any identifiable shadow, but the fissures may be seen as linear densities. The major fissures are usually seen on a lateral chest x-ray film; the minor or horizontal fissures may be seen on both PA and lateral views. Presence of a small amount of fluid causes blunting of the normally sharp angle between the diaphragm and the chest wall (CP angle). A lateral decubitus film (taken across the table while the patient is lying on his side) may be necessary to confirm the presence of fluid.

The characteristics of any abnormality observed on a chest x-ray film should

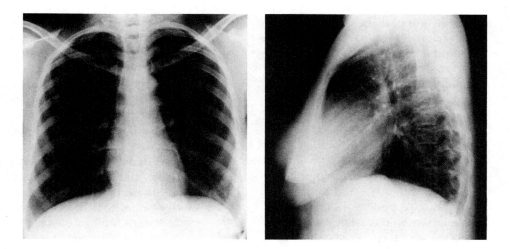

Figures 2–1 and 2–2. Normal posteroanterior and lateral chest roentgenograms.

be described (for example, its location, density, size, configuration, and effect on the lung and other adjacent structures). Adequate knowledge of bronchopulmonary segments is necessary for proper localization of lesions seen on a chest radiograph.

There are numerous descriptive radiologic terms. Some of the important ones used in interpretation of a chest x-ray are as follows.

- **Radiolucency** is the property of being radiolucent, that is, allow-

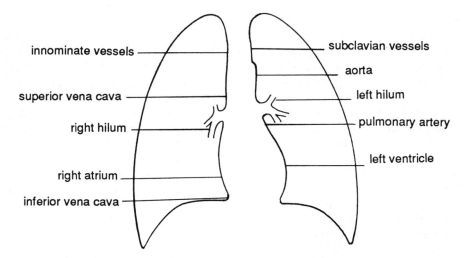

Figure 2–3. Components of the mediastinal borders in a normal chest.

ing for the passage of x-rays. This is a relative term used in defining darker areas on a chest x-ray, such as radiolucency of an emphysematous lung or radiolucency of the inside of a cavity.

- **Radiodensity** is the opposite of radiolucency. It is used to describe dense shadows that look whiter on x-ray film.
- **Consolidation** is a pathologic term that indicates a solid-appearing lung due to pneumonia. It is also used in radiology to describe a radiodensity characteristic of pneumonia.
- **Infiltration** is a loose radiologic term that usually indicates any ill-defined radiodensity, often due to an inflammatory process.
- **Interstitial density** describes density due to thickening of the interstitial tissue of the lung, which often appears as diffuse ground glass, reticular (netlike), or nodular shadow. Coarse reticular density is usually called **honeycombing. Miliary** density refers to the diffuse punctate shadows such as seen in miliary tuberculosis.
- **Alveolar** or **air-space density** is due to the presence of denser substances replacing the air in the alveoli. Alveolar edema gives rise to this type of radiographic change. Pulmonary consolidation is a confluent air-space density.
- **Homogeneous density** is characteristic of uniformly dense lesions, such as a solid tumor, fluid-containing cyst, or collection of fluid in the pleural space.
- **Pulmonary mass** is a large, 6 cm or more in diameter, demarcated ra-

diodensity. It often indicates a neoplastic lesion. **Mediastinal mass** is a similar shadow in the mediastinum.
- **Pulmonary nodule** is a smaller, less than 6 cm, circumscribed density, which may be single, and then is called a solitary pulmonary nodule or "coin" lesion.
- **Pleural density** is a radiodensity due to pleural inflammation, fluid, tumor, or scarring.
- **Cavity** refers to a radiolucent lesion surrounded by denser tissue. It is due to a localized necrotic lung lesion that has sloughed off. It is the hallmark of a lung abscess. A fluid level may be seen inside a cavity.
- **Air cyst** is a thin-walled radiolucent area surrounded by more or less normal lung. It is also called a **bulla. Bleb** refers to a superficial lung bulla abutting the pleura.
- **Calcification** indicates the presence of calcium salt deposited in certain lesions. It has a density similar to bone.
- **Volume loss** signifies reduction of volume of a whole lung or part of it as seen on a chest x-ray film. Depending on its location, it is usually manifested by displacement of the mediastinum, trachea, diaphragm, hilum, and interlobar fissures toward the involved area and approximation of the ribs.
- An air **bronchogram** outlines the air-containing bronchial tree beyond its normally visible portion. It results from an infiltration or consolidation that surrounds the bronchi, making their contrasting air columns visible.

Computerized Tomographic Scanning

An important innovation in diagnostic radiology in recent years is the development of an imaging technique in which radiologic and computer technologies are combined to enable the reconstruction of pictures showing transverse cross sections of the body as thin slices. As in standard radiographic study, computerized **tomographic** scanning (CT scan) is based on contrasting various structures in the slice that have different specific gravities. This contrast may be enhanced by the intravenous injection of a radiopaque material, which increases the density of tissues proportional to their vascularity.

Thoracic CT scan is supplementary to the standard radiographic studies. It is most useful for additional delineation of mediastinal structures, intrapulmonary nodules, and pleural disease; and for staging intrathoracic malignancies. CT scan helps to quantify the density of intrathoracic lesions, to differentiate between vascular and neoplastic shadows, and to detail abnormalities not demonstrated by standard radiographs. The introduction of high-resolution techniques has improved these capabilities and has made a more detailed study of diffuse lung disease possible.

The more recently introduced technique of magnetic resonance imaging (MRI) has been occasionally used for studying pathologic conditions of intrathoracic organs. Although it has certain advantages over CT scan, it has shown no significant additional diagnostic benefit. Absence of ionizing radiation, lack of need for injection of contrast material, and its ability to produce sagital and coronal views in addition to transverse sections are its major advantages over CT scan. Presently, MRI of the chest is limited to situations in which the patient is allergic to iodinated contrast material and for definition of lesions not adequately identified on CT scan.

Bronchography

Bronchography is radiography of the lung after instillation of a radiopaque medium into the tracheobronchial tree. The contrast material, by outlining the lumen of the airways, will allow the study of certain tracheobronchial abnormalities, such as obstructing lesions and bronchiectasis. The latter condition is the main indication for bronchography which, in addition to confirmation of diagnosis, permits evaluation of its severity and extent and helps to select patients for surgical intervention. Recognition of involved lobes and segments will allow for more effective use of postural drainage in bronchiectasis. Since the advent of the fiberoptic bronchoscope and the introduction of newer imaging techniques, the need for bronchography for diagnosis of lung cancer and other endobronchial lesions has significantly diminished.

Pulmonary Angiography

Pulmonary **angiography** is the radiographic study of pulmonary vessels, which are opacified by injection of a contrast material into a peripheral vein, vena cava, right chambers of the heart, or the pulmonary artery. The main purpose of this study in pulmonary medicine is to investigate for obstructive lesions. It is particularly useful in pulmonary embolism whenever the diagnosis is in doubt and confirmation is essential for a major therapeutic decision. Occasionally, pulmonary angiography is done for investigation of hemoptysis of unknown cause, for evaluation of vascular malformation, and for study of patients with lung cancer for its resectability.

Radionuclide Lung Scanning

The radioisotope scanning in respiratory disease is an important diagnostic tool, particularly in thromboembolic disorders. **Perfusion** lung scanning, which is the most commonly used radioisotope study, examines the distribution of blood flow to different lung regions. It is usually done by intravenous injection of a substance tagged with radioactive material. Human albumin, which is processed to form into particles or microspheres large enough to be blocked in the pulmonary capillaries, is the most commonly used vehicle. It is labeled with radioactive technetium (99^mTc) or other radionuclides. After injection, radioactivity of the lung fields is studied by a counter or, more conveniently, by a special camera over the anterior, posterior, and both lateral surfaces of the chest.

A defect in a lung scan is indicative of perfusion impairment, which may be primary and due to obstruction of a branch of the pulmonary artery, such as in pulmonary embolism, or secondary and due to reduction or cessation of perfusion as a result of a diseased lung. It is always necessary, therefore, to have a concomitant chest x-ray film for proper interpretation of a lung scan.

A *ventilation* lung scan with a radioactive gas, such as xenon, or aerosolized radioactive material, such as radiolabeled albumin or sulfur colloid, is used for determining the distribution of ventilation in various lung regions and also for ascertaining whether or not

reduced perfusion is the result of diminished ventilation of a corresponding lung region.

ENDOSCOPY–BRONCHOSCOPY

One of the important methods of examination of the respiratory tract is **endoscopy,** which is direct inspection inside the suspected areas. Viewing the upper airways, with instruments such as a rhinoscope to look inside the nasal passages, laryngoscopic mirror to inspect the nasopharynx, hypopharynx, epiglottis, and vocal cords, and direct laryngoscope for visualization of the larynx and passage of an endotracheal tube, is a form of endoscopy. However, the most important endoscopic examination of the respiratory tract is by a bronchoscope, which, in addition to its main purpose of looking inside the bronchi, will allow for examination of the upper air passages.

The development of the *fiberoptic bronchoscope* has revolutionized the field of endoscopic examination by its ease of insertion, acceptability by the patients, and versatility in visualizing all segmental and subsegmental bronchi.

In the fiberoptic bronchoscope, as in any fiberscope, tightly packed fiberoptic bundles (specially processed fiberglass) transmit the light from an external high intensity light source, and other similarly made bundles, with the help of an objective lens, return the visual image to the eyepiece of the instrument. Its tip is remotely controlled and can be directed to any desired position. The flexible optic fibers, straight or bent, will allow the transmission of light and optical image from one end to the other in any position and direction. A small channel inside the scope permits instillation of anesthetics, suctioning, and passing of a brush or biopsy forceps. The diameter of a fiberoptic bronchoscope, despite all these functioning parts, is very small (5–6 mm). Its advantages over the older rigid bronchoscope are, therefore, quite evident.

The *rigid bronchoscope* is made of a straight metallic tube with a light at its end. It is still used in some instances, such as for removal of certain foreign bodies, suctioning large amounts of thick and inspissated secretions, and studying the source of severe or massive hemoptysis. Otherwise, the flexible fiberscope has replaced the rigid bronchoscope.

Fiberoptic bronchoscopy is usually done under local anesthesia with mild or no sedation. The bronchoscope may be passed through the mouth, nose, or a tracheal tube. The upper air passages, vocal cords, trachea, **carina,** and bronchi down to the subsegmental bronchi are methodically studied. Observation is made on the characteristics of **mucosa,** secretions, orientation of airways, external compression, and internal obstructing and nonobstructing lesions. Material for bacteriologic, pathologic, and cytologic studies is often obtained during bronchoscopy.

Indications for bronchoscopy are:

1. Clinically or radiographically suspected bronchial obstruction. Bronchoscopy not only identifies the cause of obstruction but it may also be therapeutic when it is due to retained secretions.
2. Evaluation of suspicious lesions, particularly when carcinoma or other endobronchial lesions are suspected. Bronchoscopic biopsy and other techniques for obtaining pathologic samples are done when such lesions are found.
3. Investigation of patient for hemoptysis.
4. Preoperative evaluation for lung resection.
5. Suspected foreign-body aspiration and its removal.
6. Bronchial suctioning when secretions cannot be cleared by simpler means.
7. To obtain bacteriologic and pathologic specimens in a variety of localized or diffuse lung diseases, in which a specific diagnosis is not possible by less invasive methods.

Specimens are usually procured bronchoscopically by suctioning, bronchial washing, endobronchial or transbronchial biopsy, needle aspiration, and bronchoalveolar lavage (BAL). By allowing to sample intraalveolar contents, BAL is most useful for the diagnosis of *Pneumocystis carinii* pneumonia in AIDS patients (see Chapter 6).

Thoracentesis and pleural biopsy are discussed in Chapter 21. Description of other methods of obtaining pathologic samples, such as mediastinoscopy, **transthoracic** needle aspiration, and thoracoscopic or open lung biopsy is beyond the scope of this book.

PULMONARY FUNCTION STUDIES

As the main functions of the lungs are oxygenation of blood and removal of carbon dioxide from it, determination of arterial blood gases seems to be the most important functional evaluation of the respiratory system. In view of the significant reserve capacity of lung function, however, alteration of blood gases need not be present with reduction of functioning lung units. For instance, surgical removal of a significant portion of the lung may have no effect on the arterial blood oxygen and carbon dioxide if the remaining lung continues to maintain adequate alveolar ventilation and blood perfusion for gas exchange, while other studies, such as measurement of lung volumes, diffusion, compliance and maximum voluntary ventilation, will be abnormal. Therefore, although abnormal blood gases are generally indicative of impaired respiratory function, normal values do not necessarily signify normal lungs.

Numerous tests may identify functional impairment of the respiratory system at a more or less early stage of respiratory disease. Commonly performed pulmonary function studies are measurements of lung volumes, forced expiratory flow rates, diffusing capacity, maximum inspiratory and expiratory pressures, and arterial blood gases. In some instances, the assessment of regional ventilation and perfusion, the determination of closing volume, exercise test, and the measurement of compliance are also done.

No single test of lung function would be adequate for proper and accurate measurement of functional capability of the respiratory system; it is usually necessary to perform several of these studies concurrently in patients with, or suspected to have, respiratory disorders. These tests are especially useful for identifying various *patterns* of functional impairment, assessing the severity of functional defects, evaluat-

ing disability, determining suitability for certain jobs or activities, and following the progress of disease and its response to therapeutic measures. Pulmonary function studies, however, have limited usefulness for diagnosing a specific disease entity.

In this section, certain principles and clinical uses of pulmonary function tests are discussed without a description of their technical aspects. Predicted normal values, nomograms, and formulas are presented in Appendix B.

Lung Volumes

Total lung capacity is the volume of air in the lungs at the end of a maximum inspiration; it is made up of four volumes (Fig. 2–4):

1. **Residual volume** (RV) is the volume of air that remains in the lungs after a maximum expiration.
2. **Expiratory reserve volume** (ERV) is the maximum volume of air that can be exhaled after expiration of tidal volume.
3. **Tidal volume** (TV) is the volume of air inspired and expired with each normal breath.
4. **Inspiratory reserve volume** (IRV) is the maximum volume of air that one can breathe in after inspiration of tidal volume.

Combining two or more of these volumes makes the following four capacities (Fig. 2–4):

1. **Functional residual capacity** (FRC) is the total of residual volume and expiratory reserve volume; therefore, it is the volume of air remaining in the lungs at the end of expiration of tidal vol-

ume. This is the *resting end-expiratory position*.

2. **Inspiratory capacity** (IC) is the sum of tidal volume and inspiratory reserve volume; therefore, it is the maximum volume of air that can be inspired from the resting end-expiratory position.

3. **Vital capacity** (VC) is the total of expiratory reserve volume, tidal volume, and inspiratory reserve volume, or the sum of expiratory reserve volume and inspiratory capacity. It is the maximum volume of air that can be exhaled by forceful effort following a maximum inspiration.

4. **Total lung capacity** (TLC) is the sum of RV, ERV, TV, and IRV, or total of IC and FRC, or sum of VC and RV.

Lung volumes and capacities that do not include the residual volume can be easily measured from a spirometric

tracing (Fig. 2–4) obtained by a simple spirometer or by one of the currently available electronic, computerized systems. The Wright respirometer is used as a bedside method for measurement of vital capacity and tidal volume. This small gadget is particularly useful when frequent measurements of vital capacity and tidal volume are necessary in the management of patients with respiratory failure.

Special equipment will be required for measuring residual volume and, therefore, FRC and TLC. One of the following three methods can be used for these measurements.

Closed circuit helium equilibration is the most commonly used method. A closed circuit made of the patient's lungs and airways, connecting tubings, and a special spirometric container with a known concentration of helium is the basis for this method. As helium is not absorbed to any significant degree, its concentration at the end of equilibration

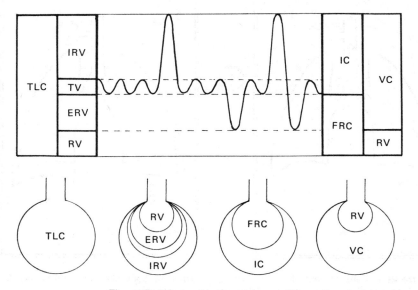

Figure 2–4. Lung volumes and capacities.

allows the calculation of the lung volume (usually FRC from which the equilibration is accomplished). As this method measures the volume of gases in direct communication with the bronchi, it does not include the volume without such communication.

With the help of a **plethysmograph** (body box), total intrathoracic gas volume can be measured. The principle of this method is based on Boyle's law on the relationship between changes of pressure and the volume of a gas. The subject sits inside the airtight box, equipped with a sensitive manometer, breathing air about him with a mouthpiece connected to another manometer. At a desired position of the respiratory cycle (usually FRC), the mouthpiece is occluded by a remotely controlled shutter while the patient continues to breathe

against an obstruction (Fig. 2–5). This will result in a reduction of intrathoracic pressure measured by the manometer between the patient's mouth and the shutter, while the pressure inside the body box, read from its manometer, increases as a result of thoracic expansion. From these pressure changes the original thoracic gas volume is calculated, using Boyle's equation.

With the *nitrogen washout method*, the amount of nitrogen in the lungs at FRC is measured after it is washed out by breathing 100% oxygen. The FRC is then calculated from the volume of nitrogen, which is about 80% of the total gas in the lungs at the beginning of the test.

Ventilation

The volume of air inspired, or expired, every minute at a resting state is called

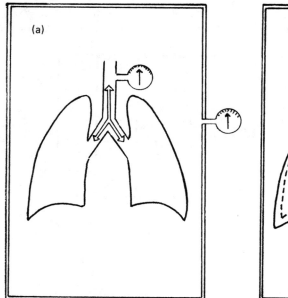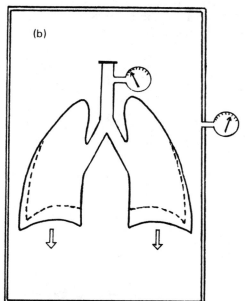

Figure 2–5. Measurement of intrathoracic gas volume by body plethysmography. (a), Quiet breathing with airway open; (b), inspiration against closed airway.

resting minute ventilation. It is the product of tidal volume and rate of breathing (provided that tidal volumes are equal and the rate is regular). For the bedside need, the Wright respirometer is quite adequate and easy to use. The problem with measurement of minute ventilation is due to the fact that, once the patient is aware of his breathing, it is no longer a purely unconscious process; therefore, both the rate and the depth of breathing may change.

Minute ventilation is composed of *deadspace ventilation* and *alveolar ventilation.* The space occupied by the air that does not exchange with capillary blood is called *dead space;* and the remainder of the air volume that is in the alveoli, and which therefore participates in gas exchange, is called *alveolar space.* Ventilation of these two spaces is called, respectively, dead-space ventilation and alveolar ventilation.

Anatomic and Physiologic Dead Spaces.

The anatomic dead space is the internal volume of the conducting airways from the nose and mouth down to the respiratory bronchioles. It is usually estimated from the body height or weight. The physiologic dead space is more closely related to the efficiency of ventilation, as it includes not only the volume in the conducting airways, but also the volume of gas ventilating the alveoli that do not contribute to gas exchange with blood. It is measured by Bohr's equation described in Appendix F. Dead-space ventilation is determined by multiplying physiologic dead space by the respiratory rate.

Alveolar Ventilation.

Effective alveolar ventilation is part of the minute ventilation that participates in gas exchange; therefore, it is the difference between minute ventilation and dead space ventilation. Alveolar ventilation can also be calculated from an equation derived from carbon dioxide elimination and arterial PCO_2 (see Appendix E).

Distribution of Ventilation: Closing Volume.

Normally, alveolar ventilation in various lung regions is not uniform but shows a gradual vertical decrement from the base of the lungs to their apexes when the subject is in a standing or sitting position. In pathologic states there is a marked derangement of distribution of ventilation. Maldistribution of ventilation is often suspected by physical examination or radiographic studies. For its more precise determination, however, certain laboratory tests are necessary. The ventilation lung scan (page 34) is one such method. Regional differences of distribution of ventilation can also be determined by single-breath nitrogen test, which is the basis for measurement of closing volume.

Pleural pressure at the lung bases is positive at the end of maximal expiration (residual volume), thus exceeding the airway pressure and leading to closure of distal airways. In normal young individuals, the small airways at the lung bases do not start to close until the volume of the lungs is reduced to less than functional residual capacity (FRC). The volume of the lungs at which the small airways begin to close is known as *closing volume.* This volume normally is between FRC and residual volume.

The small airway closure occurs at higher volumes with aging and various pathologic conditions. The closing volume is, therefore, increased in these situations, reaching and even surpassing the FRC. Determination of closing volume is a particularly sensitive test for identification of obstructive lung disease at its early stage, when the usual flow studies are not conclusive.

The principle of measurement of closing volume is based on variation of the concentration of a tracer gas continuously determined throughout a slow vital-capacity expiration. Nitrogen existing in the lungs after a vital-capacity inspiration of pure oxygen may be conveniently used for this purpose. This method is referred to as a *single-breath nitrogen test*. Throughout the slow expiration to the residual volume position, the concentration of nitrogen and volume of expired air are measured and recorded. The curve thus obtained will demonstrate changes in nitrogen concentrations at various lung volumes, showing four different phases (Fig. 2–6). Phase I represents gas from dead space only, which is filled with oxygen without nitrogen; phase II shows a rapid rise in nitrogen concentration, and represents a mixture of dead space and alveolar gas; phase III is the alveolar plateau with slight fluctuations and a small positive slope; and phase IV dem-

onstrates a sudden increase in the nitrogen concentration due to closure of airways in the dependent lung regions and contribution of alveoli relatively rich in nitrogen (upper lung zones). The beginning of phase IV, therefore, represents the closing volume.

An increase in closing volume, especially when it is larger than the FRC, indicates premature closure of intrapulmonary airways as a result of narrowing of small airways or reduced elastic recoil. Closing volume is considered to be a sensitive indicator of small airway disease, which is thought to represent the early stage of pathologic changes in smokers. The slope of phase III provides information on distribution of ventilation; the more uneven the distribution, the steeper the slope.

Forced Expiratory Flow Rates

The volume of a forceful expiration in relation to time, measured from a maximal inspiratory position, allows for the evaluation of air flow in the respiratory tract. It is the most commonly performed pulmonary function study essential for the assessment of airway resis-

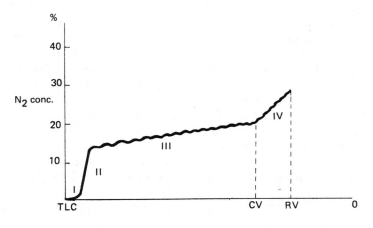

Figure 2–6. Measurement of closing volume (CV) by single-breath nitrogen test.

tance. This test is usually done by a recording spirometer.

The subject initially takes a maximally deep breath, holds it for a short while, and then expires as rapidly and forcibly as possible into the spirometer, which records volume versus time (Fig. 2–7). The tracing thus obtained is called a *forced spirogram* and the total volume expired is known as *forced expiratory vital capacity*. The analysis of the forced spirogram is one of the most useful pulmonary function studies. Measurements of specifically selected portions of the curve will allow the determination of flow rates at different times of forced expiration. FEV_1, one of the most important measurements, is the forced expiratory volume in the first second. The volumes expired in the first 0.5, 0.75, 2.0, or 3.0 seconds can also be calculated. The values obtained are either expressed in an absolute term or a percentage of vital capacity.

Maximum expiratory flow rate (MEFR), also known as $FEF_{200-1200}$, refers to the flow rate for the liter of forced expired air after the first 200 mL. *Maximum midexpiratory flow* (MMF), commonly known as $FEF_{25-75\%}$, is the flow rate for the middle two quarters of the forced vital capacity.

Peak expiratory flow rate, which is the highest flow at any time during a forced expiration, is usually measured by a peak flow meter. It can also be determined from a maximum expiratory flow–volume curve (see below).

The measurement of flow rates is particularly helpful in evaluating patients for airway obstruction. Reduced flow rates are indicative of *obstructive ventilatory impairment*.

Maximal Expiratory Flow–Volume Curve. By studying a forced spirogram, it is evident that the flow rates are higher shortly after the beginning of expiratory effort, when lung volume is large, and decrease progressively toward the end as lung volume diminishes. Plotting expiratory flow rates, measured instantaneously, against lung volume (a forced vital capacity maneuver) will result in a curve known as the *maximal expiratory flow-volume curve* (Fig. 2–8). The summit of the curve indicates the peak expiratory flow, which takes place earlier at a volume close to total lung capacity (TLC), followed by progressive reduction of flow until it ceases at the residual volume. As in the forced spirogram, the maximal expiratory flow-

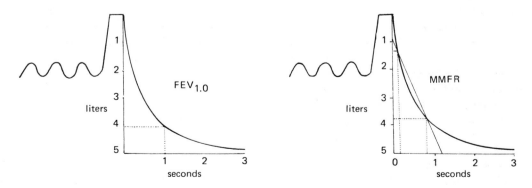

Figure 2–7. Forced expiratory spirogram in a normal individual.

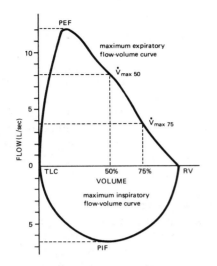

Figure 2–8. Maximum flow-volume loop made of maximum expiratory and inspiratory flow-volume curves.

volume curve measures the forced vital capacity and gives information on airway function. It offers, however, an added feature for better understanding of airway dynamics.

The airflow in the early portion (about the first one-third) of the curve, which includes the peak flow, is markedly influenced by the intrathoracic pressure and, therefore, is effort dependent. In the remaining portion (last two-thirds of the curve) the maximum flows are reached rapidly with an effort of less than one-third of the maximum expiratory muscle force, and therefore cannot be increased by further effort. This can be explained by narrowing of the airways with increasing intrathoracic pressure, which offsets the beneficial effect of higher driving pressure, and thus limits the airflow. The mechanical characteristics of the airway influence the position and the configuration of this portion of the maximal expiratory flow-

volume curve and allows determination of airway abnormalities. For a numerical recording, flow rates at 50% and 75% of the expired vital capacity, respectively known as $\dot{V}_{max50}$ and $\dot{V}_{max75}$, are more commonly measured.

Flow-Volume Loop. Maximal inspiratory flow can also be measured by taking a forceful inspiration from the position of residual volume. Its recording, plotted against lung volume, produces the inspiratory flow-volume curve. When combined with the expiratory flow-volume curve, it makes a loop known as the flow-volume loop (Fig. 2–8). The inspiratory limb is fairly symmetrical with the peak flow occurring at midpoint. Peak inspiratory flow is normally less than peak expiratory flow. The maximal-effort flow-volume loop is especially helpful for diagnosis as well as characterization of obstruction of central or upper airways, as will be discussed in Chapter 7.

Diffusing Capacity

Diffusion is the random molecular motion by which matter is transported from a region of higher to one of lower concentration. In the lungs, the net movement of gases by diffusion between the alveolar air and the capillary blood takes place as a result of their pressure gradient: oxygen moves from the alveoli into the pulmonary capillaries, and carbon dioxide moves in the opposite direction.

Diffusing capacity is defined as the movement of a gas (in milliliters, or mL) that crosses the alveolar-capillary membrane every minute for each millimeter (mm) of mercury (mm Hg) pressure difference of that gas in the alveoli and capillaries. Its unit, therefore, is mL/

min/mm Hg. Although it is the diffusing capacity of oxygen that is clinically important, because of the closeness of diffusion behavior of carbon monoxide (CO) to oxygen, the former is more widely used for measurement of diffusing capacity.

Both single-breath and steady-state methods, commonly used for determination of CO diffusing capacity (DL_{co}), are based on the same principle. For its calculation, two measurements are necessary: the amount of CO passing from the alveoli to the blood each minute, and the difference between its partial pressure (PCO) in the alveoli and pulmonary capillaries. The amount of CO transferred is measured by determination of the difference of CO concentrations in inspired and expired air. As the amount of CO used for the test is small and it is taken up by the hemoglobin as soon as it enters the blood, PCO in the capillary blood will be negligible. Therefore, the mean alveolar PCO is the only other measurement needed in the equation:

$$D_L CO = \frac{mL\ CO\ transferred/min}{mm\ Hg\ mean\ alveolar\ PCO}$$

The mean alveolar PCO is determined by sampling the alveolar gas.

Diffusing capacity is affected by several physiologic as well as pathologic factors. The concentration of hemoglobin in blood, the volume blood in pulmonary capillaries, the rate of blood flow, the surface area where the capillary blood and alveolar air are in close proximity, and the characteristics of the alveolar-capillary membrane, particularly its thickness, are all important in this regard. Therefore, alteration of diffusing capacity does not indicate a specific anatomic or physiologic abnormality. It may be reduced in a variety of

pathologic conditions of the lung. In a patient with known pulmonary disease, however, measurement of diffusing capacity is one of the more useful methods for assessment of its severity, follow-up of disease progress, and determination of response to therapy. It may also be helpful as a sensitive test in demonstration of an abnormality when the result of other studies is equivocal, as in sarcoidosis or in the early course of *Pneumocystis carinii* pneumonia in AIDS.

Maximum Inspiratory and Expiratory Forces

Assessment of the strength of inspiratory and expiratory muscles in respiratory disorders is of paramount importance, particularly in conditions known to affect these muscles. In recent years, the realization that inspiratory muscle weakness and fatigue play a significant role in perpetuating respiratory failure from various causes has resulted in a renewed interest in this area. In evaluating the need for mechanical ventilatory support, in following patients on ventilators, and in serving as a guideline for proper weaning time and method, the measurement of respiratory muscle strength has become a common practice.

The simplest method for determining respiratory muscle strength is the use of a special manometer capable of measuring both negative and positive pressures (Fig. 2–9). The inspiratory and expiratory forces are measured during static effort when no air is flowing. For determining the maximum inspiratory pressure (PI_{max}), the subject, after breathing out fully, holds the wide mouthpiece of the manometer tightly against the lips and makes a greatest possible inspiratory effort. The maxi-

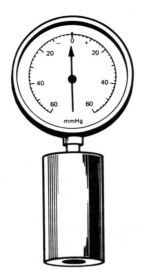

Figure 2–9. Manometer for measuring maximum inspiratory and expiratory pressures.

mum expiratory pressure (PE_{max}) is obtained by exhaling forcibly, after a full inspiration. The values, usually in cm H_2O, are read directly. For more accurate results, the best of three consecutive PI_{max} and/or PE_{max} efforts is chosen and recorded.

ARTERIAL BLOOD STUDIES

As was briefly mentioned earlier, the main function of the respiratory system is to maintain arterial blood oxygen and carbon dioxide within a physiologic range. It is also essential for regulation of acid-base balance. Measurement of the arterial blood oxygen, carbon dioxide, and pH, therefore, seems to be a most logical approach to evaluation of respiratory function. However, because of the large pulmonary reserve and effective adjustment of ventilation and perfusion within the lungs, normal

blood gases and pH do not exclude the presence of pulmonary disease. Their abnormality, on the other hand, unless due to extrapulmonary conditions such as right-to-left cardiac shunt or metabolic derangement, is a definite indication of impaired respiratory function. Arterial blood studies performed routinely consist of the measurement of **partial pressure** of oxygen (PO_2), partial pressure of carbon dioxide (PCO_2), and pH. The bicarbonate level and the oxygen content are usually calculated. Because of the importance of these studies in respiratory disorders, the basic concepts on the transport of oxygen and carbon dioxide in blood as well as acid-base balance will be briefly discussed.

Oxygen Transport

When a liquid is in equilibrium with a gas, the partial pressure of that gas will be the same in the liquid as in the gas form, regardless of its solubility or other factors. Water exposed to air, for example, will have the same *partial pressure* of oxygen and nitrogen as in the air, which is the product of barometric pressure and the fractional concentration of the respective gas. At sea level, the partial pressure of oxygen and nitrogen will be 760×0.2093 and 760×0.79, respectively. However, the *concentration* or the *amount* of gas in a liquid will be determined not only by its partial pressure, but also by its *solubility* in that liquid.

Concentration of a gas in simple solution has a linear relationship with its partial pressure at any particular temperature; that is, if partial pressure is doubled or tripled, the concentration will also double or triple (Fig. 2–10). In a liquid containing a gas in some other form in addition to simple solution, the relationship between the partial pres-

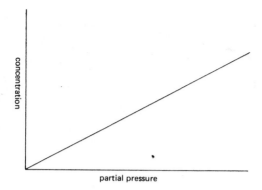

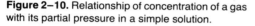

Figure 2–10. Relationship of concentration of a gas with its partial pressure in a simple solution.

sure of the gas and its concentration will not be linear. The presence of hemoglobin in blood makes it behave quite differently from other liquids in regard to the amount of certain gases that it can hold under various partial pressures. This is particularly applicable to oxygen, which is carried in the blood by both of the following mechanisms:

1. In simple solution, in which the amount of oxygen carried has a linear relationship with its partial pressure. Each 100 mL of blood carries about 0.003 mL of oxygen per mmHg (**torp**) at body temperature in simple solution. At a partial pressure of 100 torr, the amount of oxygen in solution in 100 mL of blood at body temperature will be 0.3 mL.

2. Hemoglobin has the particular ability to carry oxygen as a chemical compound, oxyhemoglobin (HbO_2). Although the amount of oxygen carried this way is also dependent on its partial pressure, the relationship is not linear. This is due to the following two factors: (a) As in any chemical reaction, the amount of oxygen that can have chemical reaction with a finite amount of hemoglobin will be limited. (b) The affinity of hemoglobin for oxygen increases once it is partly combined with oxygen.

The particular characteristics of the chemical combination of oxygen with hemoglobin result in a special relationship between PO_2 and oxygen saturation of hemoglobin. This relationship is demonstrated by a curve referred to as the *oxygen–hemoglobin dissociation curve* (Fig. 2–11). It is evident from this curve that increasing the partial pressure of oxygen will have a different rate of increase in oxygen saturation depending on the area of the curve. The slope of the curve is small at the very beginning of the curve, then increases rapidly at the middle, and then progressively diminishes to an almost horizontal position toward the end.

The oxygen *content* of arterial blood is a function of the saturation of hemoglobin and the amount of hemoglobin. Each gram of hemoglobin, once fully saturated, contains 1.39 mL oxygen; therefore, 100 mL of blood with a hemoglobin content of 15 g will be able to combine and carry about 20 mL of oxygen when saturated. With an arterial partial pressure of 90 to 100 torr, the hemoglobin will be 96.5 to 97.5% saturated. The amount of oxygen carried in solution will be very small (0.3 mL) at this partial pressure.

The oxygen-hemoglobin dissociation curve has great importance in understanding various phenomena associated with oxygen transport and delivery. As can be seen from the upper part of the curve, reduction of partial

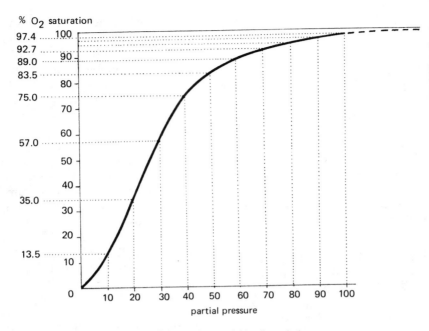

Figure 2–11. Oxygen–hemoglobin dissociation curve.

pressure of arterial oxygen, as seen in many clinical situations, does not result in a proportional reduction of its oxygen content as happens with gases in simple solution. For example, the reduction of arterial PO_2 from 100 torr to 60 torr will diminish its saturation from 97.5 to only 89%, and therefore, a significant amount of oxygen will still be available to the tissues. On the other hand, the steep portion of the curve will allow a larger amount of oxygen utilization without resulting in a dangerously low capillary blood PO_2. Such a low PO_2 occurs in the capillary blood of the tissues with high oxygen extraction.

Under various physiologic and pathologic conditions, the oxygen–hemoglobin dissociation curve changes, shifting its position to the right or left. A right shift indicates a reduced hemoglobin affinity for oxygen; that is, the

oxygen content of blood will be reduced with the same partial pressure. A left shift will result in an increased affinity and, therefore, a higher oxygen content with the same PO_2 (Fig. 2–12). A right shift facilitates release of oxygen at the tissue site, and left shift will have the opposite effect.

Factors known to cause changes in the oxygen–hemoglobin dissociation curve include pH and temperature. Both high hydrogen ion concentration (low pH) and elevated temperature result in right shift of the curve; alkalosis and low temperature shift it to the left. A special phosphorus compound present in red blood cells affects the oxygen affinity of hemoglobin. The substance is 2,3 diphosphoglycerate (2,3 DPG), which in high concentrations shifts the dissociation curve to the right and, therefore, facilitates oxygen delivery to tissues.

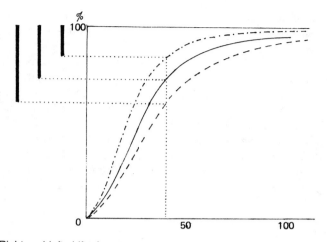

Figure 2–12. Right and left shift of oxygen-hemoglobin dissociation curve. Solid bars demonstrate the amounts of oxygen extracted from fully saturated arterial blood at the tissue sites: right shift facilitates release of oxygen (longest bar); left shift will have the opposite effect (shortest bar).

Among the conditions known to increase red cell 2,3 DPG, prolonged hypoxemia as a result of residence at high altitudes or cardipulmonary disease and chronic anemia are well known. Storage of blood in a blood bank is a good example in which the red cell 2,3 DPG is reduced.

P_{50} refers to the partial pressure of oxygen at which the hemoglobin is 50% saturated (Fig. 2–13). Normally, P_{50} is about 27 torr. It is evident that with the shift of the dissociation curve to the right, P_{50} will be increased, whereas it will be reduced with a shift of the curve to the left. Factors that result in the reduced affinity of hemoglobin for oxygen, such as acidosis, high temperature, or increased 2,3 DPG, cause a right shift of the oxygen–hemoglobin dissociation curve, and therefore the P_{50} will increase; on the other hand, factors resulting in increased oxygen affinity, such as alkalosis, low temperature, or reduced 2,3 DPG cause a left shift of the curve,

and thus reduce the P_{50}. At the tissue sites, in addition to acidosis, which causes a right shift of the oxygen–hemoglobin dissociation curve, a high concentration of CO_2 also facilitates the unloading of oxygen (**Bohr effect**).

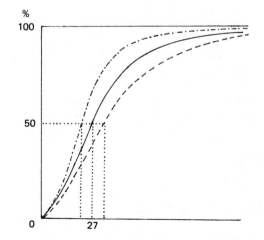

Figure 2–13. P_{50}. Right shift of oxygen–hemoglobin dissociation curve will increase the P_{50}; left shift will reduce the P_{50}.

Carbon Dioxide Transport

Carbon dioxide, although a very soluble gas, is carried in blood mostly in chemical combination; only small amounts remain in simple solution. Once CO_2 diffuses to the capillary blood from its site of production, most of it moves inside the red blood cells, facilitated by O_2 unloading (**Haldane effect**). In plasma, very small amounts of carbon dioxide react with water to form carbonic acid, which then dissociates into bicarbonate and hydrogen ions: $CO_2 + H_2O \rightleftharpoons H_2CO_3 \rightleftharpoons HCO_3^- + H^+$. Some of the dissolved CO_2 in plasma reacts with amino groups of plasma proteins, forming **carbamino compounds.** Hydrogen ions produced by these reactions are buffered by plasma buffering systems (see below). Part of the carbon dioxide remains in simple solution in plasma.

In the red cells, a small amount of CO_2 remains in physical solution; and some forms carbamino compounds with hemoglobin; but most of the CO_2 reacts chemically with water inside the red cells, forming carbonic acid, which immediately dissociates to HCO_3^- and H^+. The presence of an enzyme, **carbonic anhydrase,** is essential for this reaction. Hydrogen ion is buffered by hemoglobin; this buffering effect is enhanced by loss of oxygen from hemoglobin. Bicarbonate ions, accumulated within red cells, create a concentration gradient between the red cells and plasma, which results in its diffusion into plasma.

The transfer of HCO_3^- (an anion) from the red cell to plasma is not accompanied by the transport of cation (positively charged ion); as a result, another anion, Cl^-, passes from plasma to red cells in order to maintain electrical neutrality. This process is known as the *chloride shift.*

At the pulmonary capillary, the reverse of the above reactions takes place, and CO_2 is thus eliminated. As mentioned earlier carbon dioxide loading and oxygen unloading in tissue capillaries are mutually helpful; low O_2 improves CO_2 uptake, and high CO_2 facilitates unloading of oxygen; the reverse is true in pulmonary sites.

The transport of a significant amount of CO_2 from its site of production to the lung is accomplished with only minor change in blood pH, because of this particular CO_2 transport mechanism.

Acid-Base Balance

Elimination of CO_2 by the lungs is of utmost importance in regulation of acid-base status of the body. The amount of hydrogen ion eliminated by the lungs far exceeds the amount excreted by the kidneys. Therefore, the respiratory system has a crucial role in acid-base balance.

An acid is defined as a molecular or ionic compound that is capable of donating a hydrogen ion (proton); a base is a substance capable of receiving a proton. H_2CO_3 is a weak acid and HCl is a strong acid; HCO_3^- is a strong base, and Cl^- is a weak base, since the former readily takes up H^+ but the latter does not.

When a weak acid is in solution in the presence of its salt, which is almost completely ionized, that solution will resist a change in pH when a strong acid or alkali is added. Such a mixture constitutes a **buffer** *pair* or *system*. From the law of mass action, the following equation of buffers is derived:

$$H^+ = K \text{ (dissociation constant)}$$
$$\times \frac{\text{acid}}{\text{salt (or base)}}$$

This equation was suggested by Henderson over half a century ago.

Hydrogen ion in blood and some other body fluids has a very low concentration; in arterial blood it is about 40×10^{-9} Eq per liter. In dealing with extremely large or small numbers, use of a logarithm becomes very convenient. The negative logarithm of hydrogen ion concentration, termed as pH by Sorensen, is more commonly used to express this concentration. The normal arterial blood pH of 7.4 is the negative logarithm of 40×10^{-9}.

Hasselbalch converted the Henderson equation into the logarithmic terms, expressing H^+ in terms of pH as proposed by Sorensen. The equation was thus changed to

$$pH = pK + \log \left(\frac{\text{base}}{\text{acid}} \right)$$

which is known as the Henderson-Hasselbalch equation.

The CO_2–bicarbonate buffer pair, among other buffer systems in the blood, is most convenient for studying the acid-base balance of the blood. With this buffer system, which has a pK of 6.1, the Henderson-Hasselbalch equation is written as follows:

$$pH = 6.1 + \log \frac{HCO_3^-}{(CO_2)}$$

In this equation, (CO_2) represents the total of physically dissolved CO_2 (99%) and hydrated CO_2 (1%). It is, therefore, directly dependent on the partial pressure of carbon dioxide (PCO_2). The equation may be rewritten as

$$pH = 6.1 + \log \frac{HCO_3^-}{\alpha(PCO_2)}$$

α is the solubility of carbon dioxide, which is 0.0301. From this equation, any of its three components can be calculated if the other two are known.

The equation demonstrates that it is the *ratio* of HCO_3^- to PCO_2 that determines the pH, rather than the absolute amount of each. The numerator is an indication of metabolic changes; the denominator is an indicator of ventilatory function. Normally, with a bicarbonate value of about 24 mEq per liter and (CO_2) of about 1.2, the ratio in arterial blood will be 20/1, or a pH of 7.4. Despite the continuous production of carbon dioxide and other metabolic end products, the respiratory system and the kidneys are normally able to keep the arterial PCO_2, bicarbonate, and pH within normal physiologic range. The protection of pH and its maintenance in a narrow range takes priority over the normalization of bicarbonate ion and PCO_2. Other protective mechanisms operative for this purpose include tissue and blood buffering activities and the exchange of ions between the plasma and the red cells. As long as the $HCO_3^-/\alpha(PCO_2)$ ratio remains at 20/1, regardless of absolute values of bicarbonate and PCO_2, pH will stay normal. Only when this ratio is altered will the pH change; with a lower ratio, the pH will be reduced (**acidemia**); and with a higher ratio, it will be increased (**alkalemia**).

The arterial blood pH is considered normal when it is between 7.35 and

7.45. Thus, *acidemia* means an arterial blood pH of less than 7.35 and *alkalemia* signifies a pH higher than 7.45. **Acidosis** and **alkalosis,** by current convention, indicate the primary process that initiated an alteration in arterial blood pH. The term "respiratory" is used when the initial event is a change in carbon dioxide; and nonrespiratory or "metabolic" term is applied when an acid-base disorder is initiated by an alteration in plasma bicarbonate. Each of these primary processes brings about *secondary* or *compensatory* changes in an attempt to minimize alterations in blood pH.

Primary metabolic operations result in a secondary ventilatory response that affects PCO_2. Primary respiratory disturbances induce metabolic responses in two steps: an immediate effect through the buffering mechanism and the exchange of ions between the intracellular and extracellular fluid compartments; and a slow response (several hours to a few days) through the change in the renal excretion of H^+ and HCO_3^-. There-

fore, there are six simple acid-base disorders (see Fig. 2–14).

Secondary or compensatory responses in simple acid-base disturbances are to a certain limit predictable and are proportional to the magnitude of the primary changes. These relationships, which are the basis for designing various acid-base maps and nomograms, are shown in Appendix C.

Simple Acid-Base Disturbances

Metabolic Acid-Base Disorders. When the primary disturbance is in the concentration of bicarbonate, respiratory alteration reflected by a change in PCO_2 is the expected secondary response. In *metabolic acidosis* resulting from the increased production or the reduced excretion of H^+, the plasma HCO_3^- is lowered by its buffering function ($H^+ + HCO_3^- \rightarrow H_2O + CO_2$). Low plasma bicarbonate may also result from its excessive loss from the gastrointestinal tract or through the kidneys, or it may be due to its inadequate production by the kidneys.

SIMPLE ACID-BASE DISTURBANCE	pH	PRIMARY ABNORMALITY	SECONDARY CHANGE
Metabolic acidosis	↓	↓ HCO_3^-	↓↓ PCO_2
Metabolic alkalosis	↑	↑ HCO_3^-	↑ PCO_2
Respiratory acidosis, acute	↓	↑ PCO_2	↑ HCO_3^-
Respiratory acidosis, chronic	↓	↑ PCO_2	↑↑ HCO_3^-
Respiratory alkalosis, acute	↑	↓ PCO_2	↓ HCO_3^-
Respiratory alkalosis, chronic	↑	↓ PCO_2	↓↓ HCO_3^-

Figure 2–14. Six simple acid-base disorders. Primary abnormalities, changes in pH, and secondary responses are shown. Note that secondary changes are more marked (double arrows) with metabolic acidosis, chronic respiratory acidosis, and chronic respiratory alkalosis.

The respiratory response to simple metabolic acidosis is increased alveolar ventilation, which results in reduced arterial blood PCO_2. To a certain limit, patients with a normal respiratory system will be able to increase the alveolar ventilation to such a degree that for every mEq reduction in bicarbonate, PCO_2 will be lowered by 1.2 torr. Significant deviation from this relationship indicates an additional primary acid-base disorder (see below).

Metabolic alkalosis usually results from the excessive loss of hydrogen ions through the gastrointestinal tract or the kidneys (increased production or reduced loss of bicarbonate by the kidneys). Sometimes it may be the result of the administration of alkali or the overcorrection of chronic respiratory acidosis by mechanical ventilation. The respiratory response to simple metabolic alkalosis is a reduction of alveolar ventilation (high PCO_2). The normal response is about 0.6 torr increase in PCO_2 for every mEq increase in plasma bicarbonate, up to a certain limit.

Respiratory Acid-Base Disorders.

Simple *respiratory acidosis* results from increased arterial PCO_2, which in turn is due to inadequate alveolar ventilation. The causes of respiratory acidosis are discussed in Chapter 25. An acute increase in PCO_2 causes a more marked reduction in pH than if it develops chronically, as metabolic compensation for the former is meager. For each torr increment in PCO_2 acutely, the plasma bicarbonate level increases by 0.1 mEq per liter. For example, an acute increase of PCO_2 to 70 torr from a normal level of 40 torr will result in 3 mEq increase in bicarbonate from the normal level of 24 to 27 mEq per liter. The pH will reduce to about 7.2. In chronic respiratory acidosis, renal compensation will be added, and the pH will be less acid. For every torr increase in PCO_2 in the chronic state, the plasma bicarbonate level will increase by 0.35 mEq per liter. With the above example of a PCO_2 of 70 torr in chronic respiratory acidosis, bicarbonate will increase to 34.5 mEq per liter with a pH of 7.31.

Respiratory alkalosis is due to increased alveolar ventilation. In the acute state, secondary (compensatory) change is small and averages about 0.2 mEq reduction in bicarbonate for every torr decrease in PCO_2. For example, acute hyperventilation resulting in an arterial PCO_2 of 20 will cause the plasma bicarbonate to reduce to 20 mEq, and the pH will be 7.62. In chronic respiratory alkalosis, there is additional renal compensation, which lowers the plasma bicarbonate further, with a reduction of 0.5 mEq bicarbonate for each torr of decrease in PCO_2. With a chronic hyperventilation to a PCO_2 level of 20 torr, the plasma bicarbonate will reach about 14 mEq with a pH of 7.46.

Mixed Acid-Base Disturbances

In practical settings, it is not unusual to encounter combinations of two, or occasionally more, simple acid-base disorders above and beyond compensatory changes. They are referred to as mixed acid-base disorders in which the arterial blood studies show changes of PCO_2 or HCO_3^- that are outside the range expected for the primary disturbance. Many times the mixed disturbance is strongly suspected from the clinical findings. Acid-base maps should be used in the context of clinical information for the interpretation of these disorders. Commonly encountered mixed acid-base disturbances are: chronic respiratory acidosis with metabolic alkalosis; acute respiratory acidosis with chronic respiratory acidosis; acute respiratory acidosis with metabolic acidosis; and metabolic acidosis with chronic respiratory acidosis.

Measurement of Blood Gases and pH

Arterial blood is most frequently used for blood gas and pH analysis. A blood sample is obtained by puncture of an accessible artery in the following order of preference: radial artery, brachial artery, and femoral artery. The blood is collected anaerobically (without air exposure) in a syringe, which has been prepared by rinsing its inside with a solution of heparin. Once the blood sample is obtained, it should be immediately cooled inside an ice-filled container and taken to the blood gas laboratory. Sometimes an indwelling cannula (arterial line) is used when frequent arterial blood sampling is necessary.

Occasionally, venous blood is studied for its gases and pH. A mixed venous blood sample obtained from a catheter in the pulmonary artery is used for determination of arteriovenous PO_2 difference, calculation of venoarterial shunt, and measurement of cardiac output.

Measurement of Blood Oxygen. Before the development of the oxygen electrode, oxygen content of blood was measured by cumbersome, time-con-

suming, and less accurate methods. At the present, partial pressure of oxygen is measured by the *Clark membrane electrode.* The introduction of such an electrode has markedly facilitated measurement of PO_2, and most hospitals are equipped with it.

The Clark electrode (Fig. 2–15) consists of a very thin platinum wire sealed in glass except for its tip, which is covered with a membrane permeable to oxygen. Between the glass-platinum unit and membrane, there is a film of a weak electrolyte solution. A chloridated silver reference electrode (anode) is in contact with the solution. A potential of -0.7 volts (V) applied to the platinum results in the passage of a current that is directly proportional to the availability of O_2 *molecules* at the platinum surface. The availability of O_2 molecules is directly related to the PO_2 of solution (blood) to be tested, which is directly read from a calibrated galvanometer.

From the measured PO_2, oxygen saturation and, if hemoglobin level is known, oxygen content can be calculated.

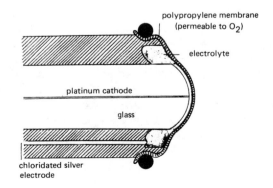

Figure 2–15. Clark electrode for measurement of blood oxygen tension.

Measurement of pH. The measurement of pH is done by a *glass electrode.* The principle of this method is based on the fact that hydrogen ions can pass through the silicate lattice of glass. If a bulb made of a thin glass containing hydrochloric acid is immersed in a solution containing H^+, a voltage develops between the hydrochloric acid in the bulb and the solution outside the bulb. This voltage is directly proportional to the logarithm of the ratio of the two hydrogen ion concentrations. The solution pH is thus read from a voltameter.

Measurement of Carbon Dioxide. Among the methods available for determination of carbon dioxide, the direct measurement of PCO_2 by a special electrode is the most commonly used method, and is also the easiest and most accurate.

Known as the Severinghaus CO_2 electrode (Fig. 2–16), it consists of a glass pH electrode covered with a Teflon membrane. A thin layer of a solution of salt and sodium bicarbonate is held between the glass and teflon membrane by a "spacer" (cellophane or nylon stocking mesh). The Teflon membrane

is permeable to CO_2, but not to H^+. A reference electrode in contact with the solution film permits measurement of the resulting pH, which is directly related to the PCO_2 of the sample to be studied. With proper calibration, PCO_2 is read directly.

Plasma bicarbonate is readily calculated from the Henderson-Hasselbalch equation, or read from a nomogram, once pH and PCO_2 are known.

Other Methods of Monitoring Blood Gases

In addition to intermittent measurements of PO_2 and PCO_2 of arterial blood samples, recent technological development has enabled clinicians to monitor arterial blood gases continuously without subjecting patients to the discomfort and risk of arterial punctures. The knowledge that PO_2 and PCO_2 immediately over a well-perfused and properly heated skin surface approach those of arterial blood has allowed the use of special **transcutaneous** electrodes that measure the oxygen and carbon dioxide tensions of "arterialized" capillary blood. Because of their closer approximation with arterial gas tensions in

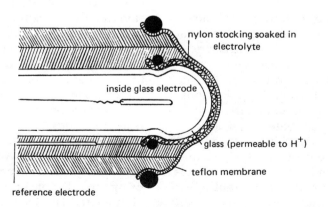

Figure 2–16. Severinghaus CO_2 electrode.

newborn infants, transcutaneous technique has gained popularity in neonatal intensive care units. As the accuracy of correlation of transcutaneous gas tensions with those of arterial blood depends on cardiac output and cutaneous blood flow, low readings in hemodynamically unstable patients should be interpreted with caution and should be confirmed by other methods. Because with increasing age the difference between transcutaneous and arterial blood gas tensions widens, this technique has not been very useful for noninvasive monitoring of adult patients.

Carbon dioxide tension at the end of each expired tidal volume, known as *end-tidal* PCO_2, can be measured by spectrometry or infrared analyzer as an estimate of arterial PCO_2, provided that there is no significant ventilation-perfusion mismatching. This method has the advantage of monitoring the ventilatory status of patients on respirator on a continuous basis. Although end-tidal PCO_2 measurement underestimates the arterial PCO_2 when dead-space ventilation is increased, it may still be relied on for following the trend of changes in ventilation if the physiologic dead space remains constant.

Among the noninvasive innovations for monitoring changes of arterial blood oxygen, *transmission oximetry* is having a significant impact on the practice of pulmonary medicine in increasing numbers of clinical applications. Using the spectrophotometric principle, which differentiates light absorption by oxyhemoglobin and reduced hemoglobin, percentage of O_2 saturation of capillary blood is transcutaneously determined. The nonpulse oximeter, introduced earlier, has been almost completely replaced by much more practical and smaller pulse oximeters. These devices measure the pulsatile change in light transmission in tissues with an adequate blood flow, such as a finger tip or an ear lobe. As the absorption of light by other tissue factors and venous blood is automatically cancelled out, a pulse oximeter senses only the arterial blood flowing to the tissues with each pulse. Individual variability in skin color therefore has little effect on measurements. Because pulse oximetry is becoming almost a routine monitoring method and its wide clinical applications are involving many health professionals in its use, they should become familiar with its indications and limitations. Most pulse oximeters in clinical use show a reasonable accuracy with O_2 saturations between 70% and 100%. When O_2 saturation is below 70%, its accuracy diminishes. Moreover, in patients receiving supplemental oxygen, as during general anesthesia, when PaO_2 levels are high, pulse oximetry cannot be relied on to show significant alteration in oxygen tension if changes in saturation are small. This is related to the shape of the oxygen-hemoglobin dissociation curve; changes in arterial tensions at the horizontal portion of the curve cause only minimal changes in O_2 saturation (see page 46). Monitoring O_2 saturation by oximetry, even in these situations, is useful for warning the clinicians when the impairment of oxygenation becomes severe enough to result in O_2 desaturation.

Intravascular monitoring of oxygen saturation is feasible with the help of fiberoptic filaments and an oximeter using the principle of reflection spectrophotometry. This technology has helped in developing a special form of balloon-floatation catheter, which can be used for the continuous monitoring of mixed-venous blood saturation in the pulmonary artery.

HEMODYNAMIC MEASUREMENTS AND MONITORING

Although the study of pulmonary hemodynamics is part of a thorough evaluation of respiratory function, in practice it is limited to situations in which important therapeutic measures are based on the information derived from such a study. As the hemodynamic measurements necessitate cardiovascular catheterization, they are done in critical care units or in catheterization laboratories. Three basic variables studied are pressure, flow, and resistance. Pressures inside the central veins, right heart chambers, and pulmonary artery are determined by passing a special catheter connected to pressure-sensing and measuring device.

Central systemic venous pressure (CVP) is the most common parameter measured in clinical situations. It not only gives information on the adequacy or deficit of circulating volume, but it also reflects the function of the right side of the heart. CVP is the filling pressure or preload of the right ventricle. It is always elevated in right ventricular heart failure. For measurements of pressures inside the right heart chambers and beyond, a specially designed catheter with a small balloon at its end (Swan-Ganz) is commonly used. This type of catheterization is usually done at the bedside with or without fluoroscopic guidance. The catheter, inserted through a peripheral or central vein

while connected to a pressure monitoring device, is advanced into the right atrium, right ventricle, and pulmonary artery, directed by the blood flow carrying the inflated balloon at the end of the catheter (Fig. 2–17). Pressure waveforms displayed on the oscilloscope indicate the position of the catheter tip, and the pressures are directly displayed or recorded. Once in the pulmonary artery, further advancement of the catheter results in "wedging" of the balloon tip when the pressure waveform similar to one of the right atrium is formed (Fig. 2–18). The pressure recorded at this point is the pulmonary artery occlusion or wedge pressure, also known as pulmonary-capillary pressure, which is a reflection of left atrial pressure (left ventricular filling pressure). With deflation of the balloon, pulmonary artery

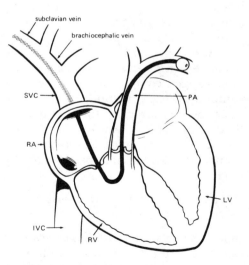

Figure 2–17. Balloon-tipped pulmonary artery catheter that has passed through the right subclavian vein, right brachiocephalic vein, superior vena cava (SVC), right atrium (RA), right ventricle (RV), pulmonary artery trunk (PA), and left pulmonary artery. It is wedged, with the balloon inflated, in a branch of the left pulmonary artery.

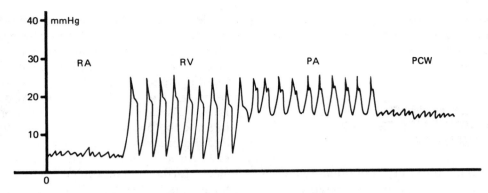

Figure 2–18. Pressure recordings from a balloon-tipped pulmonary artery catheter as it passes through the right atrium (RA), right ventricle (RV), and pulmonary artery (PA) to pulmonary capillary wedge (PCW) position.

pulsations reappear. For continuous monitoring, the catheter is left in this position with the balloon deflated. Blood sampled from the catheter in the pulmonary artery is the mixed venous blood that is used for measuring arteriovenous oxygen content difference and cardiac output.

Although cardiac output can be calculated from arterial and mixed venous oxygen contents and oxygen consumption (**Fick's method**), it can more easily be measured by the thermodilution variant of the Swan-Ganz catheter. As vascular resistance is the pressure change across a vascular bed divided by the flow:

(Resistance = driving pressure/
blood flow),

pulmonary vascular resistance can be calculated from the pressure difference between two areas of the pulmonary vascular bed (driving pressure) and cardiac output. Total pulmonary vascular resistance equals the difference between the mean pulmonary artery and

wedge pressures divided by cardiac output.

SLEEP STUDY

In recent years with better recognition and definition of sleep-related alteration of respiration, especially sleep apnea, evaluation of ventilatory events during sleep has become a common practice. Such a study not only identifies the presence of sleep apnea and other breathing disorders, but it also determines their mechanism, magnitude, and pathophysiologic effects. Proper therapeutic decisions are based on the analysis of the information thus obtained.

As the sleep study comprises several simultaneously recorded events on a polygraphic paper, it is also referred to as **polysomnography**. It usually includes continuous recordings of the following during a night's sleep:

1. Brain waves (electroencephalogram) and eye movements (elec-

trooculogram) for the purpose of determining the stages of sleep.

2. Airflow for detection of apneic episodes, which may be monitored by a **thermister,** CO_2 analyzer, **pneumotachograph,** or tracheal sound recorder.

3. Motion of the abdomen and the rib cage for determination of their mechanical activities and their paradoxical movements.

4. Ear oximetry for displaying the changes in O_2 saturation and its correlation with ventilatory alterations.

5. Electrocardiogram for monitoring the heart rate and rhythm.

Proper analysis and interpretation of these recordings, above all, will allow the diagnosis (or exclusion) of sleep apnea, frequency and duration of apneic episodes, and determination of their cause as well as their effect on the arterial blood oxygenation. Sleep apnea syndrome is discussed in Chapter 24.

BRONCHIAL PROVOCATION TEST

This test measures the bronchial responsiveness to certain agents. It is based on the knowledge that individuals with asthma demonstrate a distinct feature of bronchial reactivity characterized by an exaggerated sensitivity of the airways to the bronchoconstrictive effect of a variety of physical, chemical, and biological agents. Most of these stimuli are nonspecific and affect all asthmatics, while specific response to known **allergens** can be demonstrated only in asthmatics allergic to them. For demonstration of

nonspecific bronchial hyperreactivity, inhalational challenge tests can be performed by a number of techniques, including cold air, hyperventilation, osmotic challenge, and inhalation of a **cholinergic** agent. The most commonly used method is inhalation challenge with the cholinergic agent *methacholine*. After determining the baseline FEV_1 and establishing the control value by inhalation of the dilutent, gradually increasing concentrations of methacholine are administered by inhalation. Trial with each concentration consists of inhalation of five breaths from FRC position followed by measurement of FEV_1 within 1 to 2 minutes. Once a 20% reduction of FEV_1 is achieved, the test is terminated; otherwise it is continued until the inhalation of the last concentration. An inhaled bronchodilator should be given whenever there is an excessive bronchoconstrictive response. The lowest concentration of methacholine that results in a FEV_1 reduction of 20% is known as PC_{20} (provocative concentration to reduce flow rates by 20%). The lower the PC_{20}, the higher is the airway responsiveness to the agent. The bronchial provocation test is most useful in situations in which the history, physical findings, and simpler pulmonary function tests for bronchial asthma are atypical and equivocal, or when the diagnosis of a chronic cough is in question.

EXERCISE TEST

Although the information obtained by history, physical examination, and routine pulmonary function and other laboratory tests is often adequate for detecting the presence of cardiorespiratory impairment and for estimating the degree of disability from it, in some clinical situations a more objective and quantitative functional assessment will be necessary. This is usually accomplished with the help of exercise testing, by which cardiovascular and respiratory responses to varying external workloads are assessed. Dependent on the clinical and physiologic information inquired, exercise testing varies from simple and noninvasive to complex and invasive types. Either a treadmill or a cycle **ergometer** is usually the basis for any exercise testing. A simple test consists of observing the subject perform increasing levels of standardized exercise loads, while measuring pulse rate, respiratory rate, and blood pressure; assessing the subject's appearance; looking for signs of distress; and noting subjective complaints of dyspnea and muscle fatigue. This simple study usually provides an adequate guide to the maximum level of exercise that the subject is able to perform and maintain. Additional useful information can be obtained by pulse oximetry, electrocardiography, and measurement of minute ventilation. Oxygen uptake ($\dot{V}O_2$), including $\dot{V}O_{2max}$, is usually estimated from the mechanical power output and subject's weight. In more complex testing, other data such as arterial and venous blood gases, diffusing capacity, actual O_2 consumption and CO_2 elimination, blood lactate level, cardiac output, and intracardiac and pulmonary artery pressures are also measured.

The major practical indication of exercise testing in pulmonary medicine is for demonstration and quantitation of hypoxemia during exercise in two common clinical situations: (1) in patients with restrictive lung disease with a normal or near normal arterial PO_2 and alveolar-arterial oxygen gradient, and (2) in patients with chronic obstructive lung disease who appear to have disabling symptoms with only a mild to moderate resting hypoxemia. The result of exercise testing would help to determine a need for oxygen therapy with exertion.

BIBLIOGRAPHY

Acres JC, Kryger MH. Clinical significance of pulmonary function tests: Upper airway obstruction. *Chest.* 1981; 80:207–211.

American Thoracic Society. Clinical role of bronchoalveolar lavage in adults with pulmonary disease. *Am Rev Respir Dis.* 1990; 142:481–486.

American Thoracic Society. Indications and standards for cardiopulmonary sleep studies. *Am Rev Respir Dis.* 1989; 139:559–568.

Braman SS, Corrao WM. Bronchoprovocation testing. *Clin Chest Med.* 1989; 10:165–176.

Briscoe WA. Lung volumes. In: Fenn WO, Rahn H, eds. *Handbook of Physiology, II.* Washington, D.C., American Physiological Society; 1965; 1345–1379.

Buist AS. Tests of small airways function. *Respir Care.* 1989; 34:446–452.

Celli BR. Clinical and physologic evaluation of respiratory muscle function. *Clin Chest Med.* 1989; 10:199–214.

Clausen JL. Clinical interpretation of pulmonary function tests. *Respir Care.* 1989; 34:638–645.

Crapo RO, Foster RE II. Carbon monoxide diffusing capacity. *Clin Chest Med.* 1989; 10:187–198.

Dellinger RR. Fiberoptic bronchoscopy in adult airway management. *Crit Care Med.* 1990; 18:882–887.

Felson B. *Chest Roentgenology.* Philadelphia, Pa: Saunders; 1973.

Fulkerson WJ. Fiberoptic bronchoscopy. *N Engl J Med*. 1984; 311:511–515.

Funsten AW, Suratt PM. Evaluation of respiratory disorders during sleep. *Clin Chest Med*. 1989; 10:265–276.

Gardner RM, Crapo RO, Nelson SB. Spirometry and flow-volume curves. *Clin Chest Med*. 1989; 10:145–164.

Goldberg M, Green SB, Moss ML, et al. Computer-based instruction and diagnosis of acid-base disorders. *JAMA*. 1973; 223:269–275.

Hansen JE. Arterial blood gases. *Clin Chest Med*. 1989; 10:227–237.

Kacmarek RM, Cycyk-Chapman MC, Young-Palazzo PJ, Romagnoli DM. Determination of maximal inspiratory pressure. *Respir Care*. 1989; 34:868–878.

Kramer EL, Divgi CR. Pulmonary applications of nuclear medicine. *Clin Chest Med*. 1991; 12:55–75.

Leitman BS, Naiclich DP. Computerized tomography of the chest: indications and basic interpretation. *Hosp Med*. 1990 (August); 114–128; (September); 75–88.

Marini JJ. Lung mechanics determinations at the bedside: instrumentation and clinical application. *Respir Care*. 1990; 35:669–693.

McKelvie RS, Jones NL. Cardiopulmonary exercise testing. *Clin Chest Med*. 1989; 10:277–291.

Narins RG, Emmett M. Simple and mixed acid-base disorders: a practical approach. *Medicine*. 1980; 59:161–187.

O'Quin R, Marini JJ. Pulmonary artery occlusion pressure: clinical physiology, measurement, and interpretation. *Am Rev Respir Dis*. 1983; 128:319–326.

Osgood CF, Watson MH, Slaughter MS, McIntyre NR. Hemodynamic monitoring in respiratory care. *Respir Care*. 1984; 29:25–34.

Ries AL. Measurement of lung volumes. *Clin Chest Med*. 1989; 10:177–186.

Schnapp LM, Cohen NH. Pulse oximetry: uses and abuses. *Chest*. 1990; 98:1244–1250.

Thomas HM, Lefrak SS, Irwin RS, et al. The oxyhemoglobin dissociation curve in health and disease. *Am J Med*. 1974; 57:331–348.

Tobin MJ. Respiratory monitoring. *JAMA*. 1990; 264:244–251.

Weinreb JC, Naidich DP. Thoracic magnetic resonance imaging. *Clin Chest Med*. 1991; 12:33–54.

Wiedemann HP, McCarthy K. Noninvasive monitoring of oxygen and carbon dioxide. *Clin Chest Med*. 1989; 10:239–254.

Zavala DC, Schoell JE. Ultrathin needle aspiration of the lung in infectious and malignant disease. *Am Rev Respir Dis*. 1981; 123:125–131.

Zerhouni E. Computed tomography of the pulmonary parenchyma: an overview. *Chest*. 1989; 95:901–907.

Infectious Diseases
of the Lung

CHAPTER 3

Acute Lower Respiratory Tract Infections

The lower respiratory tract begins at the main carina and comprises the bronchi, bronchioles, alveolar ducts, alveolar sacs, and alveoli. With rare exceptions, bacteria, mycoplasmas, and viruses are the causes of acute infections of the lower respiratory tract in immunocompetent persons. In immunocompromised hosts, however, opportunistic organisms may also be involved. Mycobacteria and fungi usually result in chronic infection. In most instances, the infective agents enter the lower respiratory tract through the airways by inhalation or aspiration. Occasionally, the infection occurs via the bloodstream. Although the inhalation of airborne organisms and the aspiration of contaminated upper airway secretions occur even in healthy individuals, the airways distal to the larynx are normally sterile. Several defense mechanisms prevent the contamination of the lower respiratory tract in the normal host. The filtration action of upper airways, reflexes resulting in the timely closure of laryngeal entry by the epiglottis and the glottis by the vocal cords, coughing, and the mucociliary escalator constitute the primary line of defense. After that, the offending organisms encounter various antibodies present in the mucus and available from the blood, the scavenging alveolar macrophages, and the white blood cells. When the defense mechanisms of the respiratory tract are weakened or inoperative, or when, because of the number and the aggressiveness of the organisms the normal defenses are overwhelmed, infection will result.

Depending on the region of the lower respiratory tract predominantly involved with inflammation, the terms bronchitis, bronchiolitis, and pneumonia are applied.

ACUTE BRONCHITIS

Acute infectious bronchitis is an acute inflammation of the bronchial mucous membrane resulting from infectious agents. Because of frequent involvement of the trachea, the term acute tracheobronchitis may be more appropriate. Bronchitis due to noninfectious causes, such as physical or chemical irritants or allergy, is discussed elsewhere in this book.

Etiology. The most common infectious causes of acute bronchitis are viruses. These viruses are also causative agents of the upper respiratory infections that usually precede acute bronchitis. They include influenza viruses, parainfluenza viruses, adenoviruses, rhinoviruses, and a variety of other viruses. *Mycoplasma pneumoniae* is also a common cause of acute bronchitis. The role of bacterial infection in acute bronchitis, however, is more difficult to define. Primary acute bacterial bronchitis is very uncommon. Whether secondary bacterial infection plays a significant part in previously healthy individuals with viral bronchitis is not clear. Frequent isolation of organisms such as pneumococci, streptococci, and *Hemophilus influenzae* from the sputum does not necessarily indicate that they are acting as pathogenic agents in acute bronchitis. These bacteria are usually cleared without specific therapy. However, in patients with underlying chronic obstructive pulmonary disease, such as emphysema, chronic bronchitis, and bronchiectasis, the role of bacterial infection of the bronchi is more important. Similarly, in elderly and debilitated individuals and patients with cardiac failure or certain other chronic disorders, bacterial superinfection may have more significance.

Acute bronchitis is seen in all age groups. Its incidence is higher during cold seasons.

Clinical Manifestations. Acute tracheobronchitis is usually preceded by signs of upper respiratory tract infection, such as stuffy and runny nose and sore throat. Cough is always present and varies in severity. It is initially dry and very annoying. Cough is more troublesome at night. Exposure to cold, deep breathing, talking, and even laughing may precipitate coughing bouts. The patient may complain of a retrosternal, uncomfortable, scratchy feeling. In a few days, when bronchial secretions are established, cough becomes productive of mucus or mucopurulent sputum. Dyspnea is usually not present, except when there is underlying chronic cardiopulmonary disease. Inflammation of bronchial mucosa is known to result in hyperreactivity of the airways and thus may result in bronchospasm. It is a common precipitating cause of bronchospasm in patients with bronchial asthma.

The physical examination may show evidence of inflammation of the upper respiratory tract. The examination of the chest may be entirely normal. Sometimes scattered wheezing may be heard. A few rales may also be present at the time of increased bronchial secretions. Fever, if present, is usually mild, except in young children, who may have high temperatures.

A chest x-ray, which is normal in uncomplicated acute bronchitis, will be necessary to rule out pneumonia in questionable cases.

Management. The treatment of acute bronchitis is generally symptomatic. Bed rest may be advisable in more severe cases to avoid cold and dry air. The patient's room should be well humidified. Sometimes steam inhalation is beneficial. The role of cough syrups and expectorants is not clearly established in the treatment of acute bronchitis. In cases where the cough is very distressing and interferes with rest and sleep, certain preparations containing codeine or dextromethorphan may be prescribed. Antibiotics are not usually indicated in management of uncomplicated acute bronchitis. They do, however, have an important role in treating acute bronchitis superimposed on chronic obstructive lung disease.

Prognosis. Acute bronchitis without accompanying chronic illness is a self-limited disease and has a good prognosis. In a few patients it may progress to pneumonia or bronchopneumonia. The role of recurrent acute bronchitis in the **pathogenesis** of chronic obstructive pulmonary disease (COPD) has not been unequivocally established. However, it is known to play a significant part in **exacerbation** and progression of COPD.

ACUTE INFECTIOUS BRONCHIOLITIS

Acute infectious bronchiolitis (inflammation of bronchioles) is a serious respiratory infection that is almost exclusively seen in young children, particularly in the first two years of life. Inflammation involves the bronchioles, resulting in their obstruction. Although occasionally bacteria may be the cause, it is most commonly a viral infection. Respiratory syncytial virus is the most important offending organism in causing bronchiolitis in children.

As in acute bronchitis, upper respiratory tract infections frequently precede the onset of bronchiolitis. The onset of disease is heralded by cough and varying degrees of dyspnea. At its early stage, respiratory symptoms are suggestive of an asthma attack. Systemic manifestations of progressive fever and prostration indicate an infectious process.

On *physical examination,* the child appears apprehensive and irritable; respiration is rapid and shallow, often accompanied by expiratory grunt. The child uses his accessory respiratory muscles. In more severe cases, there is marked cyanosis, as well as some pallor. The chest is hyperresonant to percussion; scattered rhonchi and wheezes are heard in both lung fields. When the airway obstruction is more severe, breath sounds are barely audible. Untreated, the child may succumb to respiratory or cardiac failure.

The chest x-ray shows marked hyperradiolucency with or without **parenchymal** infiltration. Arterial blood shows significant hypoxemia. Acute bronchiolitis is sometimes very difficult to differentiate from bronchial asthma.

Management. The treatment of acute bronchiolitis is mainly supportive. The child should be placed in an atmosphere high in humidity and oxygen (children's tent). Adequate fluid by parenteral route should be administered. Bronchodilators may be beneficial; they should be given whenever there is significant bronchospasm or if asthma cannot be excluded. The antiviral drug ribavirin in aerosolized form is effective in the treatment of respiratory syncytial viral disease. It is given for 12–18 hours daily and delivered to an infant oxygen hood by a special small-particle aerosol generator (SPAG). Duration of treatment is between 3 and 7 days. Severely ill patients, not responding to the above regimen, may require mechanical ventilatory support. Antibiotics are frequently administered, despite the fact that bronchiolitis is most often a viral infection and, therefore, not responsive to these therapeutic agents.

PNEUMONIA

Pneumonia is defined as an acute inflammation of the gas-exchanging units of the lungs, which include respiratory bronchioles, alveolar ducts, alveolar sacs, and alveoli. Although it may also result from noninfectious causes, the term *pneumonia* usually applies to acute infection unless otherwise specified.

Etiology. The direct causes of infectious pneumonia are various microorganisms; however, the host factors are most important in its pathogenesis. Pneumonia occasionally occurs in apparently healthy people, but in the majority of cases it is associated with conditions in which there is significant impairment of the lung defense mechanisms mentioned earlier. The contamination of distal airways and alveoli by potentially pathogenic organisms is a prerequisite for the development of pneumonia. A break in the defense mechanisms that normally prevent such a contamination is the major cause. Altered protective reflexes of the epiglottis and the **glottis,** a suppressed or ineffective cough mechanism, impaired mucociliary transport, and obstructed airways are important contributory factors. Impairment of blood supply, abnormal number or function of phagocytic cells and other cells involved in cellular immunity, lack of proper antibodies, and alteration of other elements of the immunologic system deprive the lungs of their second line of defense. In conditions known to predispose to pneumonia, one or often several of these physical and biological

defenses are defective. These conditions include chronic lung disease, alcoholism, seizure disorder and other causes of altered consciousness, malnutrition, neuromuscular diseases, chronic debilitating illnesses, immunologic disorders, malignant conditions and their treatment, major surgical operations, and old age.

Pathogenesis and Pathology. Pathogenic organisms reaching the distal airways and alveoli incite an intense tissue reaction resulting in the outpouring of inflammatory exudates and cells. Interstitial tissue and alveolar spaces are variably involved in the inflammatory process and infiltrated or filled with exudative fluid and migrating cells. White blood cells, particularly neutrophilic granulocytes, and indigenous cells actively phagocytize the organisms and release their enzymes and immunologic mediators, which in turn cause further inflammation and recruitment of more inflammatory cells. Depending on the number and the virulence of the organisms and the body's ability to ward off their onslaught, further progression of the infection may be halted, or it may continue to involve adjacent lung tissue through the airways and/or interalveolar openings. Once a significant portion of the lung is filled with inflammatory cells and **exudate,** it becomes consolidated. Bacteria capable of causing significant destruction or loss of lung tissue result in **necrotizing** pneumonia. Adjacent pleura may also be involved with inflammation resulting in pleural **effusion** which may be invaded by the organisms. *Bronchopneumonia* is a term used to indicate simultaneous involvement of the airways and the lung parenchyma with infection. Inflammation due to viruses and mycoplasmas is predominantly in the interstitial tissue.

Once the infection is brought under control, either spontaneously or by antimicrobial therapy, the resolution of inflammation and healing take place. In situations in which there is no significant tissue necrosis, the resolution without sequelae is expected to be complete and the normal lung function will be restored; whereas when there are significant destructive changes, healing proceeds slowly by deposition of fibrous scar tissue, and there will be measurable loss of lung function.

Pathophysiologic changes with pneumonia are the result of reduced functioning lung volume and alteration of ventilation and blood flow. Mismatching of ventilation with perfusion and intrapulmonary shunting are the causes of arterial hypoxemia commonly seen in pneumonia.

Clinical Manifestations. The onset of pneumonia, which may be abrupt or gradual, is usually heralded by systemic manifestations of infection, such as general malaise, chills, and fever, as well as local symptoms of cough, chest pain, and dyspnea. Upper respiratory symptoms often precede the onset of pneumonia. Expectoration varies depending on the causative organisms, stage of disease, and other factors. It may be scant or totally absent at the beginning but increases with the progression of the disease; at which time it is usually purulent but may also be bloody or rusty in color. Extrapulmonary features, such as mental confusion or disorientation, sometimes overshadow the respiratory symptoms, particularly in the elderly and the alcoholic. In patients with involvement of multiple lobes, either at the presenta-

tion or with the progression of disease, dyspnea and cyanosis predominate.

On physical examination, the patient with pneumonia usually appears quite ill. The common findings are fever, tachycardia, rapid breathing, and abnormalities on the examination of the chest. The latter are variable and may include poor respiratory excursion, dullness to percussion, reduced breath sounds, and inspiratory crackles. Bronchial breath sounds and tactile fremitus, if present, are indicative of a significant area of consolidation. In some patients, particularly with viral or mycoplasmal pneumonia, the physical examination of the chest may be normal despite significant radiographic abnormalities.

Common abnormal laboratory findings are low arterial blood PO_2 and PCO_2 and frequent elevation of the white blood cell count.

Radiographic Findings. The radiographic examination of the chest is usually the clue for the diagnosis of pneumonia. A normal chest x-ray study with at least two properly taken posteroanterior (PA) and lateral projections usually excludes the diagnosis of pneumonia. Radiographic patterns reflect the pathologic changes of the lungs. A homogeneous density involving a large area and showing an air bronchogram is indicative of consolidation (Fig. 3–1). Patches of density along the airways with segmental distribution signify bronchopneumonia. A diffuse reticular density indicates thickening of the interstitial tissue, which is seen in interstitial pneumonia resulting from viral or mycoplasmal infection. In necrotizing pneumonia, radiolucent areas inside the airspace densities are usually seen (Fig. 3–2).

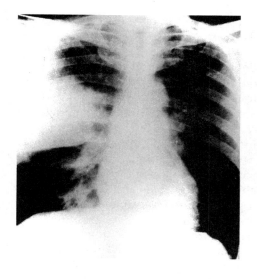

Figure 3–1. Consolidation of the right upper lobe due to pneumococcal pneumonia.

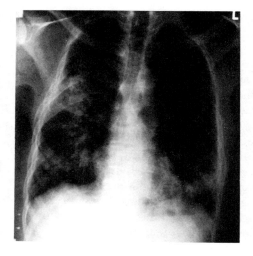

Figure 3–2. Chest radiograph of a patient with bilateral necrotizing pneumonia.

DIAGNOSIS AND CLASSIFICATION OF PNEUMONIAS

A diagnosis of pneumonia is often established with consistent radiographic findings in a proper clinical setting of history and physical examination. The difficulty in clinical practice is the accurate identification of the bacteriologic cause of a pneumonia. Although sputum examination seems to be the most important study for this purpose, it is often fraught with problems arising from improper sampling and interpretation of its results. Moreover, the identification of organisms essential for early therapeutic decision making may be delayed. The circumstances in which pneumonias develop usually determine the most likely organisms involved. This concept is the basis for classifying pneumonias for practical purposes into three broad categories of community-acquired pneumonias, hospital-acquired pneumonias, and pneumonias in an immunocompromised host.

Community-Acquired Pneumonias

Community-acquired pneumonias are, by definition, contracted outside the hospital environment. In bacterial pneumonia, the organism most commonly involved is *Streptococcus pneumoniae* (pneumococcus), which characteristically results in *lobar pneumonia*. The onset of pneumococcal pneumonia is acute and often ushered in by a severe shaking chill followed by a high fever. Signs of consolidation on the physical examination and the chest x-ray film are more commonly observed in pneumococcal pneumonia. The sputum is often purulent and may be rusty in color. On a smear with gram stain, characteristic gram-positive diplococci are often seen inside or along with numerous polymorphonuclear leukocytes. Sputum culture may be positive for *S pneumoniae*, but a negative culture does not exclude the diagnosis. As these organisms may enter the bloodstream, blood cultures are positive in about a quarter of the cases.

Less common bacterial causes of community-acquired pneumonia are *Hemophilus influenzae, Klebsiella pneumoniae, Legionella pneumophila,* and rarely other gram-negative bacteria. In pneumonias developing as a result of aspiration of vomitus following alcoholic intoxication, seizure disorders, or other unconscious states, anaerobic organisms with or without **aerobic** bacteria are the most common causative agents. Although staphylococcus rarely causes pneumonia in otherwise healthy adults, it is not an uncommon cause of pulmonary infection in infants and in adults during influenza epidemics or in intravenous drug abusers. In the latter cases, the organism may reach the lung via the bloodstream. The onset of pneumonias caused by gram-negative bacteria, anaerobic organisms, and staphylococci are less abrupt and the clinical picture is less distinct because of frequent association with other debilitating medical conditions. *H influenzae* pneumonia in chronic obstructive lung disease and Klebsiella pneumonia in alcoholics are examples of this association. Radiographic findings suggesting a necrotizing process and the presence of a significant amount of pleural reaction are strongly suggestive of pneumonia from these organisms. Sputum examination, as in hospital-acquired pneumonias, is important for diagnosis. Unfortunately, a specific diagnosis based solely on sputum examination cannot be made because of the likelihood of its contamination by oral or pharyngeal flora, especially with anaerobic bacteria. How-

ever, the demonstration of large numbers of morphologically distinct bacteria on a properly obtained sputum sample or their predominant growth on culture are highly suggestive of their role in pulmonary infection. Bacteriologic studies from other sources and by various methods discussed earlier (page 28) may be needed. If pleural effusion is present, its removal by thoracentesis is indicated.

The major manifestation of *Legionnaires' disease* is pneumonia, which may be community- or hospital-acquired, and may occur with or without immunodeficiency. It results from the lower respiratory tract infection by inhalation of aerosolized droplets containing the causative organisms, *Legionella pneumophila* and other legionella species. They are small gram-negative bacilli. These organisms are ubiquitous with an affinity for warm water. They are transmitted by aerosolization of contaminated water, as occurs in air-conditioning or cooling towers. The outbreaks of this disease occur mostly during late summer and early fall. Legionnaires' disease starts as an acute pneumonia with high fever and a nonproductive cough, which may rapidly progress, causing hypoxemia and respiratory failure. Extrapulmonary manifestations may suggest the diagnosis. Headache, muscle ache, general malaise, mental confusion, prostration, diarrhea and other gastrointestinal symptoms, and abnormal liver function are commonly present. Radiographic changes have no characteristic features, but they are known to progress rapidly. Once this disease is suspected, the examination of materials such as sputum, bronchial washings or brushings, and pleural fluid will help the diagnosis. Direct immunofluorescent antibody (DFA) staining of these materials is more rapid and considered to be specific, whereas culturing in special media, as well as serologic tests, require more time and are useful for retrospective confirmation.

The most common cause of community-acquired pneumonia in young adults, especially in military recruits, is *Mycoplasma pneumoniae.* This organism is smaller than bacteria, but larger than viruses, and is only identifiable by its cultural characteristics. *M pneumoniae* is commonly associated with mild respiratory infection in children. The infection occurs in several family members and, as small epidemics, among military recruits. Mycoplasma pneumonia is usually preceded by an upper respiratory infection; and its manifestations are cough (often nonproductive), headache, and fever. The examination of the chest usually is normal, or findings are few and less striking than expected from radiographic changes. In an occasional patient, a characteristic bullous lesion on the eardrum may be seen. X-ray findings vary widely in their character and distribution. An interstitial, ill-defined pattern suggestive of viral pneumonia is most common. At times the findings may mimic bacterial pneumonia. The diagnosis is often suspected on clinical grounds and further supported by excluding bacterial infection. The presence of a serum antibody that agglutinates the red cells at a low temperature is the basis for cold **agglutination** test, which may become positive in many patients; however, it is not specific for this disease. More specific tests of complement fixation or culture of the organisms from the sputum will confirm the diagnosis in retrospect.

Viral pneumonias are uncommon in the civilian population with normal immunologic states. A variety of viruses can sporadically cause pneumonia among the general population; however, influenza, chickenpox, and adenovirus infection are better known for their association with pneumonia.

Influenza, generally a self-limited disease, usually affects the cell lining of the respiratory tract, causing local and systemic symptoms of flu. Occasionally a minimal and transient infiltration may be noted in the chest roentgenogram coinciding with flu symptoms. A more severe form of pneumonia that typically presents several days after the onset of influenza is characterized by increasing dyspnea, anxiety, and cyanosis. These symptoms usually begin when flu symptoms seem to be improving. Cough that is often nonproductive may be associated with hemoptysis. Severe influenza virus pneumonia is more commonly seen in patients with heart disease, chronic lung disease, old age, and general debility. It may be complicated by bacterial superinfection.

Chickenpox (varicella), although generally a mild disease in children, may be complicated by primary viral pneumonia in adults. It may be quite severe and life threatening. The diagnosis is often established by a chest roentgenogram associated with the characteristic skin rash of chickenpox, which is always present.

Adenovirus is probably the most common cause of viral pneumonia outside of influenza epidemics. It may be seen sporadically, but often in small epidemic form especially among military recruits. This virus is the most common etiologic agent of acute respiratory disease (ARD), a syndrome characterized by fever, sore throat, cough, hoarseness, and conjunctivitis. Adenovirus pneumonia is usually mild and is always associated with upper respiratory symptoms. Rarely it may be very severe, resulting in hypoxic respiratory failure.

Viral pneumonias like mycoplasma pneumonia have the clinical features of scant physical findings on the examination of the chest despite obvious abnormality on radiographic study. The latter usually shows patchy interstitial density, which in severe form is diffuse and may involve the entire lung fields. In advanced cases with respiratory failure, diffuse airspace densities resembling pulmonary edema may be present. Viral pneumonia is one of the causes of the adult respiratory distress syndrome (ARDS) discussed in Chapter 25.

Community-acquired bacterial pneumonia resulting from aspiration is most commonly due to anaerobic organisms that are a major part of the mouth flora. Necrotizing pneumonia and lung abscess are the usual consequences of aspiration-induced lower respiratory tract infections (see page 75).

Hospital-Acquired Pneumonias

Hospital-acquired or nosocomial pneumonia by definition is contracted during hospitalization. It is a major cause of morbidity and mortality in hospitalized patients. Unlike community-acquired respiratory tract infections, nosocomial pneumonias are frequently due to gram-negative bacteria and staphylococci. Advancement in medical technology; progress in the care of critically ill patients; prolongation of survival of seriously ill and "terminal cases"; extended hospitalization; subjection to a variety of diagnostic and therapeutic instrumenta-

tions; and increasing use of antimicrobials, cytotoxic drugs, and immunosuppressants are some of the causes of predisposition to pneumonia from these organisms. In contradistinction to the healthy population who rarely harbor aerobic gram-negative bacteria in their upper airways, hospitalized patients, particularly when chronically and seriously ill and/or confined to critical care units, are readily colonized with these organisms. A combination of presence of these pathogenic bacteria and defective pulmonary or systemic defense mechanisms—so common in these patients—markedly increases the risk of developing hospital-acquired pneumonia (Fig. 3–3). Poor state of consciousness, aspiration of upper airway secretions, presence of an artificial airway, and laxity in the use of sterile technique for airway suctioning are important precipitating events. Practitioners of respiratory care should be aware of the importance of the respiratory therapy equipment as a potential source of outbreaks of **nosocomial** pneumonia.

Although any pathogenic organism may cause pneumonia in hospitalized patients, the most common agents are

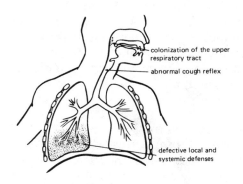

Figure 3–3. Pathogenesis of gram-negative pneumonia.

Klebsiella, Escherichia coli, Enterobacter, Proteus, and *Serratia* among the gram-negative organisms; and *Staphylococcus aureus* and *Streptococcus pneumoniae* among the gram-positive bacteria. Pneumonia developing as a result of aspiration in a hospitalized patient is more often from one or several of these organisms than from anaerobic bacteria.

Clinical manifestations of pneumonia developing while the patient is in the hospital are often less clear and overshadowed by the underlying illness. Nevertheless, it is usually suspected with the occurrence of or increase in fever and the onset of or a change in respiratory symptoms, and confirmed by chest roentgenography. Its bacteriologic diagnosis, however, remains a difficult clinical challenge. Proper collection of sputum and its study by Gram's stain and culture remain very useful, although the interpretation of findings is not always easy. As colonization with the pathogenic organisms without disease is common in hospitalized patients, bacteriologic studies of expectorated sputum may lack specificity, and their results should be assessed in the light of clinical situations. Blood culture and, if present, pleural fluid culture should be obtained. Sometimes, more invasive diagnostic studies such as transtracheal aspiration, bronchoscopy, bronchoalveolar lavage (BAL), percutaneous lung aspiration biopsy, and, rarely, open-lung biopsy may be necessary.

Pneumonia in Immunocompromised Host

As the body's immune system is essential in defending it against ever-present infecting agents, it should not be surprising that infection by a variety of organisms is so prevalent in individuals with immunologic deficiency. Either or both limbs of immunity, known as humoral and cellular, may be deficient (see Chapter 14). Lymphocytes mediate both humoral and cellular immunities through their B-cell and T-cell lines, respectively. The activities of T and B lymphocytes in host defense against infection also involve other cells important in fighting infection. Antibodies produced by the **B lymphocytes** enhance the **phagocytic** activities of polymorphonuclear leukocytes, and the products of **T lymphocytes** activate **macrophages,** which in turn are important in trapping and processing the **antigens.** Although both types of immunodeficiency predispose to infection, certain characteristics differentiate the two. Patients with a defect in humoral immunity lack antibodies and are more susceptible to infection with certain bacteria that are usually extracellular and encapsulated, such as pneumococci, *H influenzae,* and *Klebsiella;* while the individuals with cellular immunodeficiency have recurrent infection with low-virulence or opportunistic organisms, such as fungi, mycobacteria, certain viruses, and *Pneumocystis carinii.*

Immune deficiency may be primary or secondary to a variety of causes. Primary immunodeficiency states are usually congenital, and their manifestations occur early in childhood. There are increasing numbers of patients with secondary immune deficiency as a result of advances in the fields of cancer chemotherapy and organ transplantation. Many malignant diseases such as multiple myeloma and chronic lymphocytic leukemia result in impaired antibody production, whereas others such as Hodgkin's disease cause cellular immune deficiency. Treatment with **cyto-**

toxic drugs or immunosuppressants may depress both humoral and cellular immunity. The production of granulocytic white blood cells is also known to be suppressed by cancer chemotherapy. Chronic debilitating diseases, especially renal failure, and long-term treatment with corticosteroids impair cell-mediated responses. Because of the importance and unique features of the recently recognized entity of *acquired immunodeficiency syndrome* (AIDS), its pulmonary complications, including pneumonia, are discussed separately in this text (see Chapter 6).

Pulmonary infection in the immunocompromised host may result not only from common pathogens but also from unusual and so-called opportunistic organisms. This is the major difference between pneumonia in these patients and that of persons with a normal immunologic state. The unusual microorganisms involved in infection among these patients include, but are not limited to, nocardia, aspergillus, cryptococcus, atypical mycobacteria, legionella, pneumocystis, and cytomegalovirus. Pneumonias from these organisms and common bacteria in immunocompromised patients have no distinguishing clinical or radiographic features; and, therefore, specific diagnosis will depend on demonstration or isolation of the causative agent. As these patients, by nature of their underlying immune deficiency, are unable to ward off their infection, it may be rapidly progressive and fatal. Therefore, an accurate diagnosis in a most expeditious way is essential for instituting early effective treatment. Most patients with common bacterial pneumonia have productive sputum, which should help in bacteriologic diagnosis.

However, many patients, particularly when unusual organisms are involved, have no significant expectoration, or their sputum examination is inconclusive. In this situation, invasive methods will be necessary to obtain material for bacteriologic studies. Blood culture and bacteriologic examination of pleural fluid, if present, should always be done. Transtracheal aspiration, bronchoscopy with brushing and transbronchial biopsy, bronchoalveolar lavage, transthoracic needle aspiration of the lung, and open lung biopsy are the procedures that may have to be resorted to for specific diagnosis. Because of its high yield, some prefer open lung biopsy as the procedure of choice. However, the information obtained from simpler methods may suffice in most instances, especially when the organisms can be readily demonstrated with a special staining method as in infection with *pneumocystis*.

MANAGEMENT OF PATIENTS WITH PNEUMONIA

In view of the many causes of pneumonia, significant variations in its presentation, and widely different respiratory consequences, only a brief discussion of the principles and the objectives of management applicable to pneumonias in general is presented here. Although treatment of the patient with pneumonia should be individualized, the basic therapeutic principles of eradication of infection and supportive, as well as symptomatic, measures are appropriate in every case.

Patients with mild or moderate disease who are not immunocompromised and do not have serious underlying medical conditions are treated as outpatients with proper follow-up. Other patients with pneumonia are managed in the hospital. Adequate hydration, proper nutrition, supplemental oxygen, analgesics, and encouragement of effective coughing are the measures that help in alleviating symptoms and enhancing recovery. There is no therapeutic benefit of intermittent positive pressure (IPPB) treatment, and the indication for postural drainage is limited to situations in which there is a significant collection of secretions difficult to be expectorated by cough alone. In poorly responsive patients, tracheal suctioning may be necessary. In patients who have severe respiratory difficulty and intractable hypoxemia, tracheal intubation and mechanical ventilation will be required.

The choice of antibiotics in the treatment of pneumonia will be more appropriately determined by the information from bacteriologic studies. Viral pneumonias, unless complicated by bacterial superinfection, will not respond to antibiotics. However, some of the antiviral agents may be effective in the treatment of certain specific viral pneumonias. Acyclovir for varicella pneumonia and aerosolized ribavirin for respiratory syncytial virus pneumonia are examples with proven efficacy. Mycoplasmal pneumonia and Legionnaires' disease respond best to erythromycin. Pneumococcal pneumonia and community-acquired aspiration pneumonia are treated with penicillin. Erythromycin is a good alternative to penicillin in the treatment of pneumococcal infection. Clindamycin is the preferred antibiotic for the treatment of anaerobic pneumonia in penicillin-allergic patients. Staphylococcal pneumonia is best treated with a penicillinase-resistant penicillin, such as oxacillin or nafcillin. The alternatives are vancomycin or a cephalosporin. *H influenzae* pneumonia is treated with ampicillin, chloramphenicol, or one of the appropriate cephalosporins. Other gram-negative pneumonias are mostly responsive to aminoglycosides (gentamicin or tobramycin) and many of the third-generation cephalosporins. With pseudomonas infection, antibiotic-sensitivity studies may be necessary for best antimicrobial selection; combination of antibiotics is sometimes necessary. For pneumocystis pneumonia, combination of sulfamethoxazole and trimethoprim (Septra or Bactrim) or pentamidine is the treatment of choice. Management of mycobacterial and fungal infections are addressed in the next two chapters.

It should be emphasized that in practical situations precise bacteriologic diagnosis is not always possible and is often delayed. In these situations antibiotic choice is often empirical and usually the coverage is broad. However, the circumstances in which pneumonia develops, as discussed earlier, are important in deciding the choice of antibiotics. In view of the many organisms that can cause pneumonia in immunocompromised hosts and the seriousness of respiratory infection in these patients, every effort should be made for a specific diagnosis.

Preventive Measures. Despite the availability of very effective antimicrobials for the treatment of respiratory tract infections, pneumonia remains one of the most common causes of hospitalization and death. Therefore, every attempt should be made to prevent its occurrence. Unfortunately, the factors that play major roles in the etiology of pneumonia are host factors that are difficult to alter. An increasing population of the aged, chronically ill, and immunocompromised people is an example that demonstrates the complexity of the problem. However, good public and personal health habits, including proper nutrition and the avoidance or cessation of smoking and excessive alcohol consumption would reduce the incidence of pneumonia, as well as many chronic illnesses that predispose to it. In dealing with hospitalized patients, particularly in critical care units, the role of hospital infection control cannot be overstressed. A vaccine made of pneumococcal capsular antigen is intended to enhance antibody production against 23 capsular serotypes of pneumococci known to cause significant illness in humans. Pneumococcal vaccination is recommended to be given *once* for individuals with sickle cell anemia; persons whose spleen has been removed; the elderly; and patients with chronic lung, heart, or kidney disease. Although patients with altered humoral responses are at a higher risk in developing serious pneumococcal infection, they are unable to mount an antibody response to the vaccine and thus do not benefit from it.

LUNG ABSCESS

Pulmonary abscess is a localized area of **suppurative** lesion associated with **necrosis** of lung tissue. Although small areas of necrosis and microscopic evidence of abscess formation may be present in many pulmonary infections, only those in which abscess is the predominant pathologic process are considered here. Because of its ready communication with an airway, lung abscess will usually present as an air-containing cavitary lesion.

Etiology and Pathogenesis. Almost any pyogenic organism may cause lung abscess; however, the most common causes of community-acquired lung abscess are anaerobic bacteria. They commonly include peptostreptococci, peptococci, fusobacteria, and bacteroides. Staphylococci, streptococci, and most aerobic gram-negative organisms are also fairly common etiologic agents. Aspiration is a frequent preceding event, and most patients present with a history of impaired consciousness or swallowing problems. Bronchial obstruction due to **bronchogenic** carcinoma, foreign body, or other causes is an important local predisposing factor. Increasingly larger numbers of patients, especially among cigarette smokers over 50 years of age, are being recognized in whom the underlying predisposing factor for lung abscess is bronchogenic carcinoma. Occasionally, abscess formation in the lung may be the result of septic embolism from a remote infected site. Other rare causes include penetrating chest wound and suppurative lesion below the diaphragm with extension into the lung.

An area of **pneumonitis** always precedes the formation of an abscess. The time interval between known aspiration and abscess formation averages about 2 weeks. In production of a lung abscess, usually more than one type of organism is involved that often includes anaerobic bacteria.

Clinical Manifestations. The onset may be acute or insidious. The common presenting symptoms of lung abscess include cough, expectoration, fever, chest pain, hemoptysis, and weight loss. The mode of presentation and duration of symptoms prior to hospitalization will determine acuteness or chronicity of illness.

An initially dry or minimally productive cough is soon followed by sudden increase in the amount of expectoration of purulent and often foul-smelling sputum. This coincides with communication of the abscess with the bronchial tree. Fever, which may decrease at this time, continues at a variable level. Hemoptysis, although uncommon, may be sometimes massive and life threatening. Weight loss is common in patients with chronic lung abscess.

In acute lung abscess, there is high temperature, tachycardia, and tachypnea; dullness and impaired breath sounds may be detected over the diseased area; a few rales may also be heard. Patients with protracted lung abscess appear chronically ill; fever is variable and may even be absent; digital clubbing is common.

Radiographic Findings. Prior to cavity formation, the chest x-ray shows a localized area of consolidation. Only after communication with a bronchus and evacuation of part of its purulent contents will the lung abscess manifest its characteristic radiographic picture, which is an area of radiolucency surrounded by variable parenchymal density and containing an air-fluid level (Fig. 3–4). The most common sites for lung abscess are the superior segments of lower lobes and the posterior segments of upper lobes. Abscess in basilar segments is less common; other segments are rarely involved. This predilection is due to the effect of gravity and the direction of the bronchi at the time of aspiration, which commonly takes place in the supine position. The right

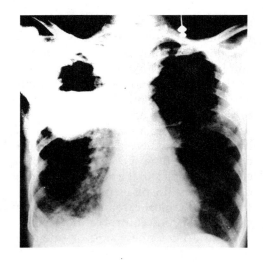

Figure 3–4. Radiographic demonstration of a large lung abscess involving the right upper lobe.

lung is involved more often than the left.

Laboratory Findings. **Leukocytosis** and mild to moderate anemia are frequently present. Sputum examination shows numerous pus cells and necrotic materials. Both gram-positive and gram-negative organisms are seen, which may or may not be representative of bacterial population of the abscess. Because of the significance of anaerobic bacteria in lung abscess and contamination of sputum by the normal anaerobic oral flora, material for bacteriologic study should be obtained by methods bypassing the **oropharynx.** Transtracheal aspiration is one such method. If pleural fluid is present, it should be tapped for bacteriologic study and for the exclusion of **empyema.**

Management. Ever since the advent of antibiotics and their proper use, treatment of lung abscess has been primarily medical. Surgical intervention has been very infrequently necessary. Penicillin, which has been very effective in most cases, is the antibiotic of choice, unless organisms responsible for the lung abscess are resistant to this antibiotic. Then antibiotic choice will depend on the result of culture and sensitivity studies. Some experts recommend clindamycin as the first choice. Antimicrobials should be continued until clinical improvement and roentgenographic clearing or stabilization are achieved. This may take from 3 weeks to a few months.

Adjunctive therapy should include adequate nutrition, treatment of underlying conditions, and *effective drainage* of the abscess. The latter is essential in successful management of pulmonary abscess, and is usually accomplished by proper *postural drainage* with or without other maneuvers. When abscess is large, this procedure should be performed with great caution as the patient may be unable to expectorate the volume of pus that may drain. Postural drainage should be done several times a day, at least initially. As proper positioning is crucial for effective drainage, exact location of the abscess in relation to the bronchopulmonary segments should be ascertained by radiographic studies.

Bronchoscopy is sometimes indicated for diagnostic and therapeutic purposes, mostly in middle-aged or older smokers in whom lung cancer may be the underlying cause of the abscess. Surgical procedures for drainage or resection are resorted to when the patient does not respond to appropriate medical therapy. In very ill and weak patients, tracheostomy may be needed for adequate tracheobronchial toilet or for mechanical ventilatory support. Complicating pleural empyema should be drained.

Course and Prognosis. With proper management, lung abscess will show clinical and radiographic improvement in a majority of cases. In acute abscess, the size of the cavity diminishes rapidly and closes in a short period of time. However, in the chronic form, and when there are complicating underlying conditions, response to therapy will be slow or insignificant. Prolonged antibiotic therapy will be necessary to reduce the risk of relapse. Massive hemoptysis with lung abscess has a poor prognosis.

BIBLIOGRAPHY

Bartlett JG. Anaerobic bacterial infections of the lung. *Chest*. 1987; 91:901–909.

Bartlett JG. Lung abscess. *John Hopkins Med J*. 1982; 15:141–147.

Bryan CS, Reynolds KL. Bacteremic nosocomial pneumonia. *Am Rev Respir Dis*. 1984; 129:668–671.

Craven DE, Steger KA. Nosocomial pneumonia in the intubated patient: new concepts on pathogenesis and prevention. *Infect Dis Clin North Am*. 1989; 3:843–866.

Fang GD, Fine M, Orloff J, et al. New and emerging etiologies for community-acquired pneumonia with implications for therapy. *Medicine*. 1990; 69:307–316.

Fekety FR Jr, Caldwell J, Gump D, et al. Bacteria, viruses, and mycoplasma in acute pneumonia in adults. *Am Rev Respir Dis*. 1971; 104:499–507.

Ferstenfeld JE, Schlueter DP, Rytel MW, Molloy RP. Recognition and treatment of adult respiratory distress syndrome secondary to viral interstitial pneumonia. *Am J Med*. 1975; 58:708–718.

Finland M. Pneumonia and pneumococcal infection, with special reference to pneumococcal pneumonia. *Am Rev Respir Dis*. 1979; 120:481–502.

Huxley EJ, Viroslav J, Gray WR, Pierce AK. Pharyngeal aspiration in normal adults and patients with depressed consciousness. *Am J Med*. 1978; 64:564–568.

Lerner AM. The gram-negative bacillary pneumonias. *Dis Mon*. 1980; 27 (2):1–56.

Luby JP. Pneumonia caused by *Mycoplasma pneumoniae* infection. *Clin Chest Med*. 1991; 12:237–244.

Mansel JK, Rosenow EC, Smith TF, Martin JW. *Mycoplasma pneumoniae* pneumonia. *Chest*. 1989; 95:639–646.

Matthay RA, Greene WH. Pulmonary infections in the immunocompromised patient. *Med Clin North Am*. 1980; 64:529–551.

McIntosh K. Respiratory syncytial virus infection in infants and children: diagnosis and treatment. *Pediatr Rev*. 1987; 9:191–196.

Muder RR, Yu VL, Fang GD. Community-acquired Legionnaires' disease. *Semin Respir Infect*. 1989; 4:32–39.

Murray HW, Tuazon CU. Atypical pneumonias. *Med Clin North Am*. 1980; 64:507–527.

Nguyen MLT, Yu VL. Legionella infection. *Clin Chest Med*. 1991; 12:257–268.

Pierce AK, Sanford JP. Aerobic gram-negative bacillary pneumonias. *Am Rev Respir Dis*. 1974; 110:647–658.

Reynolds HY. Pulmonary host defenses. State of the art. *Chest*. 1989; 95 (suppl):223S–230S.

Ruben FL, Nguyen MLT. Viral pneumonitis. *Clin Chest Med*. 1991; 12:223–235.

Rytel MW. Pneumococcal pneumonia: still a serious problem. *J Respir Dis*. 1990; 11:83–95.

Segreti J, Bone RC. Overwhelming pneumonia. *Dis Mon*. 1987; 33 (1):1–59.

Stover, DE, Zaman MB, Hadju SI, et al. Bronchoalveolar lavage in the diagnosis of diffuse pulmonary infiltrates in the immunosuppressed host. *Ann Intern Med*. 1984; 101:1–7.

Verghese A, Berk SL. Bacterial pneumonia in the elderly. *Medicine*. 1983: 62:271–285.

Wohl MEB, Chernick V. Bronchiolitis. *Am Rev Respir Dis*. 1978; 118:759–781.

CHAPTER 4

Pulmonary Disease Due to Mycobacteria

Mycobacteria are rod-shaped bacteria (bacilli) with a characteristic staining property related to their unusual cell wall, which has a high lipid and wax content. Once stained, they resist decolorization by acid or alcohol, and are therefore called *acid-fast bacilli*. They cannot be classified either as gram-positive or gram-negative. These organisms require special culture media for their growth. They have a slow replication time of about 24 hours (replication time of streptococci is about 20 minutes).

Of the several groups of mycobacteria, mammalian tubercle bacilli *Mycobacterium tuberculosis* and *Mycobacterium bovis* are the agents of tuberculosis in humans and cattle. In addition, certain other mycobacteria may cause pulmonary infection in humans. They are known as *atypical mycobacteria*.

TUBERCULOSIS

Tuberculosis is one of the oldest diseases known to afflict the human race and still remains one of the most widespread maladies in the world. Many organs may be affected; however, the most common site of tuberculosis is the lung, which is also the major port of entry and primary source of dissemination of **tubercle** bacilli. Tuberculosis is usually a chronic infection with variable manifestations, depending on the stage and duration of the disease, host response, organs involved, and many other known and unknown factors.

Epidemiology. Although tuberculosis is still an important worldwide health problem, there is significant variation in its incidence and prevalence in different parts of the world. Among the factors responsible for its high prevalence in certain countries, poverty, overpopulation, inadequate nutrition, and lack of proper health care are most noticeable. In the United States, most cases occur among alcoholics, the homeless, and immigrants from endemic regions. The advent of AIDS has resulted in a significant increase in the incidence of tuberculosis among HIV-infected persons, especially in association with intravenous drug use (see Chapter 6). Improved living conditions, social awareness, early diagnosis, and appropriate treatment have been important reasons for the decline of tuberculosis in most developed countries.

In many nations, in addition to high incidence of tuberculosis due to human mycobacteria, bovine bacilli play an important role in human infection, usually through ingestion of contaminated milk from tuberculous cattle. In more developed countries, this source of infection is almost totally eradicated, and *man* remains the only source of new infections.

The transmission of tuberculosis is from infected materials, particularly sputum from a patient with untreated pulmonary tuberculosis. It is spread in the form of aerosolized droplets during coughing, sneezing, or talking. Individuals with undiagnosed and, therefore, untreated tuberculosis are particularly dangerous in disseminating the organisms and infecting the people around them. Once the patient with tuberculosis is on proper antituberculosis drugs, the infectiveness diminishes rapidly and ceases within a few weeks while taking the medications.

Pathogenesis and Pathology. The respiratory tract is the usual route of infection by tubercle bacilli, which are carried with the aerosolized droplets deep inside the distal airways, beyond the protective mucous blanket. Once the organisms are implanted in the lung of a person who has had no prior tuberculous infection, they are unopposed and multiply freely without inciting significant reaction. Within 2 to 10 weeks, however, the body's reactivity changes and specific inflammation takes place. This coincides with development

of positive tuberculin reaction (see below). In the infected area a characteristic **granuloma** develops with necrosis and production of peculiar cheesy material at the center. The draining regional lymph nodes, usually hilar, also become infected and enlarged. The infection is often confined to these areas and walled off by **fibrosis.** This stage of tuberculosis is known as *primary infection,* and the combination of the initial lung lesion and lymph node involvement is recognized as the *Ghon complex.* In a majority of individuals, the primary tuberculosis completely heals, leaving only a small scar, which may calcify later. Occasionally, primary infection progresses and causes a significant pulmonary lesion.

During the early stage of primary infection, some of the tubercle bacilli escape and are carried by the bloodstream to different organs where they settle. The areas that have high tissue oxygen tensions are particularly predisposed to secondary involvement by tubercle bacilli. They include the apexes of the lungs, kidneys, end of long bones, and brain. Among these, the most common site for secondary settlement of tubercle bacilli is the lung. With the development of immunity, infection in these foci, as well as in the primary focus, is usually brought under control. However, they may continue to harbor the organisms without evidence of disease activity except for a positive tuberculin test. Occasionally, the infection progresses either in the primary site or the metastatic foci, producing clinical tuberculosis in lungs, pleural effusion, meningitis, or other extrapulmonary lesions. A disseminated form may also develop in the occasional patient, which is referred to as miliary tuberculosis.

The patients with clinical evidence of tuberculosis are said to have *tuberculous disease.*

Tuberculous infection without disease is referred to the stage following primary infection when there is no clinical evidence of disease, except for a positive tuberculin test. It is assumed that a positive reaction to tuberculin indicates the presence of live bacilli in the body.

Postprimary or *reactivation tuberculosis* is the result of reactivation of tuberculous infection in one of the dormant foci at a later date (usually several years later). The factors responsible for reactivation are not entirely understood, but it seems that impairment of local and systemic body defense, due to old age, alcoholism, nutritional deficiency, diabetes, and other chronic debilitating disorders, plays a major role. Impairment of cellular immunity is considered to be a most important factor in the reactivation process. The pathologic hallmark of reactivation tuberculosis is the presence of characteristic granulomas or tubercles around areas of **caseous** necrosis. Healing with fibrosis is part of the pathologic picture, even while there is active disease. Cavitation, which is one of the distinctive features of pulmonary tuberculosis, is the result of lung tissue necrosis and sloughing. With the control of infection, the healing process continues, and eventually fibrosis replaces the granulomatous lesions. The involved lung becomes retracted and calcium may deposit. Distortion and dilatation of bronchi are common sequelae of pulmonary tuberculosis. *Reinfection* tuberculosis is referred to as acquisition of tuberculosis from an exogenous source by a patient known to have been infected from another source.

Clinical Manifestations. The vast majority of patients with *primary pulmonary infection* have no *clinical* evidence of disease, and in most instances conversion of tuberculin sensitivity from negative to positive takes place without any symptom whatever. When present, symptoms are generally mild: low-grade fever, listlessness, loss of appetite, and occasional cough may be noted. More severe symptoms may develop as a result of complications or progressive primary disease. Significant hilar node enlargement may cause more severe cough or signs of airway obstruction. Pleural involvement causes chest pain. In the disseminated form, systemic symptoms with high fever and prostration predominate. Extrathoracic involvement of meninges, kidneys, joints, bones, or lymph nodes will result in symptoms and signs referable to these structures. In tuberculous infection without disease, the only finding in relation to tuberculosis is a positive skin test.

In *postprimary* or *reactivation tuberculosis* of the lung, symptoms will depend on location, extent, and duration of disease. Classical presentation with **hectic** fever, drenching night sweat, cachexia, chronic cough, and hemoptysis characteristic of "**consumption**" is rarely seen nowadays in the United States. The diagnosis of tuberculosis in most cases is suggested by a chest x-ray taken in the process of case findings or for other reasons. Some patients will volunteer having certain symptoms such as lack of pep, generalized weakness, or mild to moderate cough. Some ma· seek medical advice for unremitti cough, bloody sputum, chest pain unexplained systemic symptoms, e cially fever. Rarely, pulmonary tuberculosis manifests with an acute onset suggesting pneumonia.

The *physical examination* is usually normal in patients with primary infection unless it is severe, progressive, or complicated. Signs of pleural effusion may be present in some patients. With minimal lesion in reactivation tuberculosis there are usually no significant physical findings. In more advanced cases, dullness to percussion, impaired breath sounds, and rales may be heard over the diseased area. The severity of fever and tachycardia is quite variable. Body temperature may range from normal to as high as 40°C. Fever is more pronounced in the evenings. Evidence of weight loss and debility usually indicate protracted disease. It is not uncommon to find signs of various predisposing conditions.

Radiographic Findings. Physical examination is often unreliable in screening for pulmonary tuberculosis, but radio-graphic examination of the chest is indispensable not only for its diagnosis, but also for its follow-up. Chest x-ray examination, along with tuberculin testing, has become the most important means for tuberculosis screening.

Roentgenographic changes in *primary intrathoracic tuberculosis* are due to involvement of lung parenchyma, hilar and/or mediastinal lymph nodes, and pleura (Fig. 4–1). Parenchymal lesion is a small area of airspace consolidation, usually located in the upper part of a lower lobe or lower part of an upper lobe at the lung periphery. Hilar and/or mediastinal lymph node enlargement is one of the important features of primary infection. It is more prominent in primary tuberculosis of children on the side of parenchymal lesion (primary complex). Sometimes lymph node enlargement is the only radiographic manifestation of primary infection. Certain children with significant lymph node enlargement may develop atelectasis of a segment or a lobe. Tuberculous

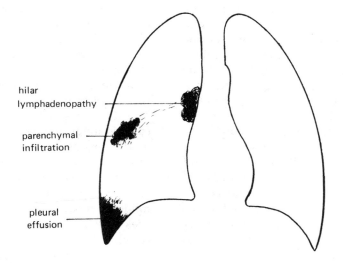

hilar
lymphadenopathy

parenchymal
infiltration

pleural
effusion

Figure 4–1. Primary intrathoracic tuberculosis.

lymphadenopathy is one of the causes of "middle-lobe syndrome," which is atelectasis of the right middle lobe.

Pleural involvement with tuberculosis usually manifests by pleural effusion. A small area of parenchymal and/or hilar calcification in adults frequently is due to healed primary tuberculosis of childhood. In many cases, particularly in adults, primary infection will have no demonstrable x-ray change.

In reactivation tuberculosis of the lungs, chest radiograph is almost always abnormal. There is a characteristic tendency for reactivation tuberculosis to involve the apical and posterior segments of the upper lobes. In the early stage, x-ray change is limited to patchy air-space density of small to moderate size. With the progression of the disease, the addition of fibrosis may result in irregularly shaped densities and retraction of the involved lobe or segment. Cavitation may be seen inside the parenchymal density. In patients whose disease has been present for a long time before being treated, the lesion may be more extensive, involving more than a lobe of the same lung or the other side (Fig. 4–2). The disease usually spreads by the bronchial route. Occasional dissemination by bloodstream will give rise to miliary tuberculosis. It is characterized on radiographic study by diffuse bilateral small nodular densities.

Tuberculosis in patients with HIV infection is discussed in Chapter 6.

LABORATORY TESTS AND DIAGNOSIS OF PULMONARY TUBERCULOSIS

Tuberculin Test

Tuberculin reaction is an example of delayed hypersensitivity mediated by

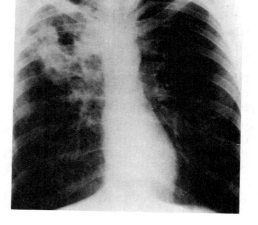

Figure 4–2. Radiograph of far-advanced cavitary pulmonary tuberculosis.

the lymphocytes. Infection with tubercle bacilli results in sensitization of lymphocytes against certain products of these organisms. Tuberculin or purified protein derivative (PPD) is a product derived from the protein fraction of the bacilli. Tuberculin skin test is the intradermal injection of a small amount of this material, which in sensitized individuals would result in a reaction manifested by an **induration** mainly from cellular infiltration. This reaction takes place within 48 to 72 hours.

As was pointed out earlier, a tuberculin test becomes positive 2 to 10 weeks following the start of tuberculous infection and remains so indefinitely, regardless of activity of the infection. Therefore, the result of a tuberculin test simply indicates whether or not an individual has been infected, presently or in the past, with tubercle bacilli. With few exceptions, a negative tuberculin test makes the diagnosis of tuberculosis unlikely.

Conventionally, 0.1 mL of PPD solution, containing 5 tuberculin units, is injected intradermally with a special tuberculin syringe making a small wheal. The injected site is inspected after 48 hours, and the size of the reaction is measured and recorded. A positive reaction is indicated by an area of induration measuring 10 mm or more in diameter. Lack of any reaction or an induration of less than 5 mm in diameter is considered to be negative. A reaction size between 5 and 9 mm is doubtful.

There are other PPD strengths, which have limited practical use.

Bacteriologic Studies

The most important laboratory study in pulmonary tuberculosis is the examination of sputum for acid-fast bacilli. Although in many instances tuberculosis is strongly suspected from clinical and radiographic data and a positive tuberculin test, its diagnosis is not certain without bacteriologic confirmation. In view of specific staining characteristics of tubercle bacilli, microscopic examination of sputum or other infected material on smear, stained by the acid-fast (Ziehl-Neelsen) technique, is most helpful for diagnosis. If not seen in a direct smear, the organisms may often be demonstrated after sputum or other suspected material is concentrated by one of several available methods. On the basis of positive smear for acid-fast bacilli, antituberculous therapy is initiated and the patient's contacts are examined.

Findings on microscopic examination should be confirmed by culture or, rarely, by animal inoculation. Culture is essential for differentiating *M tuberculosis* from other acid-fast organisms; it will also allow for drug-susceptibility studies. Furthermore, when the number of bacilli is small, the microscopic examination may fail to demonstrate them; but culture or animal inoculation will often reveal their presence.

The success of bacteriologic identification of tubercle bacilli depends on material submitted for such an examination. Sputum should be expectorated from deep in the lungs, preferable in the morning. Saliva or nasal secretions are not acceptable. Proper collection of sputum is discussed elsewhere (Chapter 2). Sometimes material obtained by gastric washing, laryngeal swab, suctioning, or bronchoscopy is submitted for bacteriologic examination. Pleural fluid, if present, should be likewise examined. In certain circumstances, as in children with hilar **lymphadenopathy,** bacteriologic proof is not required for a clinical diagnosis. Occasionally, diagnosis of tuberculosis can be made only by pathologic and bacteriologic studies of surgically resected tissue. Recent development of very sensitive assays for detection of specific antigens and antibodies is very promising for early diagnosis of tuberculosis. These tests would identify the presence of antigens derived from tubercle bacilli or would detect specific antibodies against them. Practical application of this technologic advance for diagnosis of tuberculosis remains to be defined.

Other laboratory findings are nonspecific and rarely helpful in diagnosing pulmonary tuberculosis. Pulmonary function studies are abnormal in advanced stages of tuberculosis or when there is underlying chronic pulmonary disease. Occasionally, with far-advanced disease, there may be evidence of respiratory failure with severe hypoxemia and hypercapnia.

Management. Early diagnosis and proper treatment of pulmonary tuberculosis are not only essential for the patient's complete recovery, but are also most important public health measures against tuberculosis. Unfortunately, many tuberculous patients are not detected and some are not properly treated; thus, they continue to infect others.

Once a patient with active pulmonary tuberculosis is recognized, he may be hospitalized and, during the infective stage of his disease, isolated. Fortunately, with the institution of appropriate chemotherapy, this stage is quite short. Infectivity diminishes rapidly, and within a few weeks of continuous therapy patients are considered virtually noninfectious. In the past, most patients with pulmonary tuberculosis were confined to a sanatorium for prolonged periods of time, but they are now being successfully treated as outpatients or are hospitalized only for a short time. A short hospitalization is advisable for initial management of pulmonary tuberculosis in certain patients for several reasons, including adequate diagnostic studies; observation for effect and possible side effects of drugs; isolation of the patient from family members during the infective period of disease; and teaching the patient about his illness, how to cope with it, and how to cooperate with long-term therapy.

Certain measures will reduce the infectivity of the patient with pulmonary tuberculosis. Having the patient wear a mask or at least cover the mouth and nose during coughing and sneezing should be encouraged. Expectorated sputum should be carefully handled and properly disposed. Adequate ventilation of the patient's room with 20 or more room-air changes an hour and use of ultraviolet light are very effective in reducing the number of infectious particles in the air. Extreme care should be exercised in using respiratory therapy equipment, with particular attention to decontamination procedures. Personal items such as clothes, bedding, and dishes are not causes of tuberculosis infection under usual circumstances. The most effective way of controlling the infectivity of the patient with active tuberculosis is early proper chemotherapy.

Chemotherapy is the essence of treatment of tuberculosis today. Properly selected drugs administered for an adequate length of time will virtually ensure a successful outcome in almost all patients with tuberculosis.

Isoniazid (INH) is considered to be the most effective antituberculous drug. Except for chemoprophylaxis, it should be used in combination with one or sometimes more drugs. The most commonly used companion drug is rifampin. Both INH and rifampin are **bactericidal**. This combination has been a very successful chemotherapeutic regimen, which has shortened the duration of an effective therapy from 1.5 to 2 years to only 9 months in most cases. An effective, even shorter course, chemotherapy is the addition of a third drug, pyrazinamide (PZA), to INH and rifampin for the first 2 months followed by a two-drug regimen for an additional 4 months. Ethambutol and streptomycin may be used in certain situations. Chemotherapeutic regimens that do not include the combination of INH and rifampin necessitate a longer duration of treatment, usually 18 to 24 months. There are other antituberculosis drugs that are occasionally used when tubercle bacilli show resistance to the more commonly used agents.

Preventive Measures. The cycle of perpetuation of tuberculosis among the human race can be broken by various preventive and therapeutic measures, as shown in Figure 4–3. Although the avoidance of contact and preventive therapy soon after contact are measures that would prevent development of infection, they are much less practical because most contacts remain unrecognized. Identification and treatment of infected persons to prevent them from becoming infectious, and the early diagnosis and proper therapy of individuals with infectious tuberculosis to make them noninfectious, are the most effective and practical preventive measures. If both of these objectives are achieved

in all cases, the eradication of tuberculosis from the face of the earth would become a reality. Unfortunately, socioeconomic factors in the world make this ultimate goal unrealistic at this time. These measures, however, continue to work in developed and in some developing countries as judged from the steady decline in the incidence of active cases and tuberculin converters.

Chemoprophylaxis refers to treatment of individuals who have no detectable disease, but are at risk of developing it. They include the household members and other close associates of recently diagnosed tuberculous patients; newly infected persons as manifested by recent tuberculin conversion; positive tuberculin reactors with abnormal chest x-ray, suggesting old tuberculous lesion without positive bacteriology and prior TB

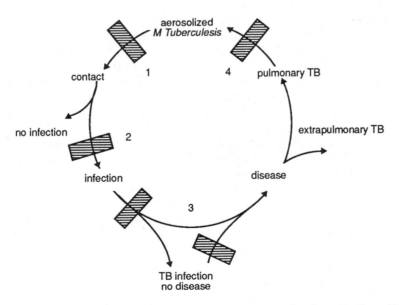

Figure 4–3. Cycle of tuberculosis (TB). Proper intervention at any sites (bars 1 to 4) would break the cycle of perpetuation of tuberculosis, but a more practical method is the treatment of infected individuals to prevent them from becoming infectious (bars 3) and of patients with pulmonary tuberculosis to make them noninfectious (bar 4).

therapy; and children with positive tuberculin test. Although every patient with a positive tuberculin test is at higher risk of developing active tuberculosis than nonreactors, the hazard of liver toxicity from isoniazid, the drug of choice for chemoprophylaxis, should be considered in deciding such therapy. Only patients at high enough risk are selected for prophylactic treatment. The usual duration of INH chemoprophylaxis is 1 year.

Vaccination with BCG (bacillus of Calmette and Guérin) derived from an attenuated strain of *M bovis,* confers cellular immunity against tuberculosis with little or no danger of reactivation as seen in naturally infected individuals. Its practical usefulness in countries like the United States where tuberculosis disease occurs mostly in persons who are already infected is very limited. It is indicated only for noninfected (negative tuberculin test) persons who cannot avoid repeated exposure, such as Peace Corps volunteers, missionaries, and State Department employees working in countries with a high prevalence of tuberculosis.

Course and Prognosis. Except for patients with severe and overwhelming disease at the time of diagnosis, prognosis of pulmonary tuberculosis is generally very good if proper treatment is instituted and continued for an adequate length of time. A majority of patients will be able to return to their usual occupation and live a normal life. The most important cause of therapeutic failure is lack of patient cooperation in taking the prescribed medications. This is more commonly seen among alcoholics, who not only are at higher risk in developing tuberculosis, but also are less compliant in continuing their

treatment. These patients not uncommonly will have recurrent disease, and some will develop resistant forms of tuberculous infection.

With early diagnosis and proper treatment, respiratory functional impairment will be unusual, whereas with advanced and destructive tuberculosis resulting from late diagnosis or improper therapy, significant pulmonary insufficiency will often ensue. Other complications of healed or inactive tuberculosis include hemoptysis from residual bronchiectasis and superinfection with aspergillus in the form of a fungus ball inside a residual cavity.

PULMONARY INFECTION SECONDARY TO ATYPICAL MYCOBACTERIA

Certain mycobacteria other than *M tuberculosis* and *M bovis* may occasionally cause pulmonary lesion in man. These organisms have certain growth and other biologic characteristics that differentiate them from *M tuberculosis.* They are generally known as atypical or "anonymous" mycobacteria. Many of them appear to be saprophytic in soil. These bacteria are occasionally isolated from sputum in the absence of demonstrable disease or from the sputum of patients with known pulmonary tuberculosis. Sometimes they are the direct cause of a tuberculosis-like lung disease. Their transmission from man to man has not been proved; therefore, patients infected with these organisms are not considered to be infective and thus need not be isolated.

Pulmonary disease caused by atypical mycobacteria has no characteristic features and is often mistaken for tuberculosis due to typical tubercle bacilli. Diagnosis is established only by repeated demonstration of organisms on culture, as their staining characteristics (acid-fastness) are similar to *M tuberculosis*.

Although there are many species of atypical mycobacteria that have been associated with pulmonary infection, the most important ones are *M kansasii, M avium-intracellulare,* and *M scrofulaceum.* The latter is an important cause of cervical lymphadenopathy in children. Pulmonary infection with *M kansasii* responds well to the usual antituberculosis drugs. But most other atypical mycobacteria are often drug resistant, and therefore susceptibility studies are necessary for selection of proper drugs. Occasionally, pulmonary lesions are treated by surgical resection, particularly when they are localized.

As we shall see in Chapter 6, patients with immunologic deficiency are prone to infection with typical as well as atypical mycobacteria that may result in disseminated and often fatal disease. Patients with acquired immunodeficiency syndrome (AIDS) are especially susceptible to infection with *M avium-intracellulare,* which often disseminates inexorably.

BIBLIOGRAPHY

American Thoracic Society. Diagnostic standards and classification of tuberculosis. *Am Rev Respir Dis.* 1990; 142:725–735.

American Thoracic Society. Treatment of tuberculosis and tuberculosis infection in adults and children. *Am Rev Respir Dis.* 1986; 134–163.

Bailey WC. Treatment of atypical mycobacterial disease. *Chest.* 1983; 84:625–628.

Dannenberg AM Jr. Immune mechanisms in the pathogenesis of pulmonary tuberculosis. *Rev Infect Dis.* 1989; 11 (suppl 2):S369–S378.

Grosset JM. Present status of chemotherapy for tuberculosis. *Rev Infect Dis.* 1989; 11 (suppl 2):S347–S352.

Johnston RF, Wildrick KH. The impact of chemotherapy on the care of patients with tuberculosis. *Am Rev Respir Dis.* 1974; 109:636–664.

Modilevsky T, Sattler FR, Barnes PF. Mycobacterial disease in patients with human immunodeficiency virus infection. *Arch Intern Med.* 1989; 149:2201–2205.

Rouillon A, Perdrizet S, Parrot R. Transmission of tubercle bacilli: the effects of chemotherapy. *Tubercle.* 1976; 57:275–299.

Snider DE Jr. The tuberculin skin test. *Am Rev Respir Dis.* 1982; 125 (no. 3: part 2):108–118.

Wolinsky E. Nontuberculous mycobacterial and associated diseases. *Am Rev Respir Dis.* 1979; 119:107–159.

CHAPTER 5

Fungus Infection of the Lung

Among the fungi causing pulmonary disease in man, *Histoplasma capsulatum,* the agent of *histoplasmosis,* and *Coccidioides immitis,* the cause of *coccidioidomycosis,* are by far the most important in the United States. In this chapter these two diseases plus blastomycosis and aspergillosis will be discussed (Fig. 5–1).

HISTOPLASMOSIS

Epidemiology and Pathogenesis. Histoplasmosis is one of the most preva-

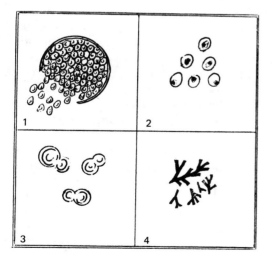

Figure 5–1. Fungi commonly causing respiratory tract infection. (1) *Coccidiodes immitis;* (2) *Histoplasma capsulatum;* (3) *Blastomyces dermatitidis;* (4) *Aspergillus fumigatus.*

lent infections in certain parts of the United States. The causative agent, *Histoplasma capsulatum,* is a common fungus in soil, particularly when it is enriched by large quantities of droppings from certain birds, such as pigeons, starlings, blackbirds, chickens, and probably many others. The birds themselves do not carry the organisms. Bats, however, whose manure also facilitates the growth of these fungi, may be infected and, thus, may carry the fungi. Chicken coops and starling roosts are some of the common sources of exposure to *H capsulatum.*

The endemic areas in the United States are predominantly in the Ohio and Mississippi River valleys, but the infection has also been demonstrated in eastern states along many other river valleys, such as the Potomac, Delaware, Hudson, and St. Lawrence valleys. In certain states such as Tennessee, Kentucky, Arkansas, and Missouri, histoplasmin skin test, which is a good indicator of prevalence of infection, is positive in as many as 90% of the adult population.

H capsulatum has two morphologic forms, **mycelial** and *yeastlike,* dependent on environmental factors. In nature and in the culture media at room temperature, it assumes the mycelial form (mold); in infected tissues, and in culture media at 37°C, it is in a yeast form. Human infection is usually the result of inhalation of spores spread in the air from the naturally occurring mycelial form.

As in tuberculosis, implantation of the organisms in the lung results in a primary infection in a previously uninfected individual, with regional lymph node involvement. Before the onset of hypersensitivity, significant spread of the fungi via the blood stream takes place. With the development of immunity through a cellular mechanism, the infected tissues react with necrosis and granuloma formation, halting the spread of the disease in both primary and metastatic sites. A positive histoplasmin skin test is an indication of cellular immunity against *H capsulatum*. These foci later become calcified. The primary infection is, therefore, similar to tuberculosis, except for the tendency for multiple pulmonary and extrapulmonary foci, which may undergo extensive calcification.

Postprimary chronic histoplasmosis is most likely due to exogenous reinfection rather than endogenous reactivation as occurs in tuberculosis. There is evidence that following primary infection the organisms do not usually survive very long, and subsequent acute infections from outside sources are common in endemic regions. In comparison with the high prevalence of acute infection, chronic disease is uncommon.

Rarely, histoplasmosis, under certain circumstances, especially when there is impaired cellular immunity, may take a highly invasive form involving many organs and resulting in death. This form is referred to as *disseminated histoplasmosis*.

Clinical Manifestations. The vast majority of adults and older children with acute or primary infection do not have recognizable clinical symptoms; the conversion of skin reactivity to histoplasmin is the only evidence of the infection. Individuals with heavy exposure, however, will have symptoms of an influenza-like illness, manifested by chills, fever, headache, and generalized aches and pains. Nonproductive cough and substernal chest discomfort may also be present. These symptoms usually subside within a few days without any therapy. In younger children, primary infection is much more serious. Radiographic changes in acute histoplasmosis show patchy parenchymal densities, which may be diffuse and scattered throughout both lung fields. Hilar lymph nodes are frequently enlarged.

Disseminated histoplasmosis is an extremely serious, but fortunately rare, infection. It occurs in young children or in a setting of deficient immunologic state. Pulmonary involvement in disseminated histoplasmosis, which is the rule in children, is usually not significant in adults, in whom clinical manifestations are predominantly extrathoracic. In association with AIDS, histoplasmosis may manifest as a rapidly progressive and severe infection, as discussed in Chapter 6.

Chronic active or *progressive pulmonary histoplasmosis* is mostly a disease of middle-aged white males; it is uncommon in females and rare in blacks. There is often evidence of underlying chronic obstructive pulmonary disease. The incident of chronic pulmonary histoplasmosis is very low in comparison with the high infection rate. Symptoms, physical findings, and radiographic changes are similar to pulmonary tuberculosis. Apical and posterior segments of upper lobes are predominantly involved. It is frequently bilateral, and cavitation is common. A less destructive form has been described as *early noncavitary histoplasmosis,* which tends to heal spontaneously. Mediastinal lymphadenopathy may cause compression of adjacent structures. Fibrosing mediastinitis is another complication in which an exaggerated fibrotic reaction to histoplasma antigen results in narrowing or obstruction of blood vessels and/or airways.

Laboratory Studies and Diagnosis.

Histoplasmin is a filtrate of culture medium in which *H capsulatum* has been growing for several months. Intradermal injection of this material, known as histoplasmin skin test, shows a delayed reaction in individuals who have been infected with histoplasma. It becomes positive with primary infection and remains so more or less indefinitely, regardless of disease activity. In certain situations, it may be negative despite the presence of active disease, such as in disseminated histoplasmosis. Histoplasmin skin test, therefore, has limited diagnostic usefulness.

A serologic test such as *complement fixation* is more helpful in the diagnosis of histoplasmosis, as it is positive mostly during the active stage of the disease. It may be negative during the early stage of infection, however. Detection of antigen in blood or urine, using a sensitive assay, is also considered to be diagnostic.

Demonstration of *H capsulatum* from the sputum or other sources is the only conclusive proof of the diagnosis; however, the result of bacteriologic studies may be unrevealing. Sometimes diagnosis of histoplasmosis is made by biopsy and pathologic examination. Bone marrow examination has a very high yield in disseminated histoplasmosis. Blood culture may also be positive.

Management. The vast majority of patients with primary infection will require no therapy. Treatment, however, is indicated in acute disseminated illness and chronic progressive pulmonary histoplasmosis. As amphotericin B, the agent most effective against histoplasmosis, is potentially toxic, patients are carefully selected for therapy with this drug. Ketoconazole is another drug that has proven to be effective, mostly in acute cases, and it has the advantage of being an oral agent and less toxic. Whether it will eventually replace amphotericin B remains to be seen. Amphotericin B, however, is still the drug of choice for treatment of disseminated disease. Rarely will surgical resection of the involved lung be necessary. Patients with active histoplasmosis need not be isolated, as human-to-human transmission of this infection does not occur under usual circumstances.

Course and Prognosis. The prognosis for acute histoplasmosis in adults and older children is excellent; spontaneous rapid recovery is the rule. With recovery from initial infection, recurrence or reinfection is very uncommon, except in severely **immunocompromised** patients, as seen with AIDS. The prognosis in infants and patients with disseminated histoplasmosis is usually grave. Chronic progressive pulmonary histoplasmosis with cavitation may result in significant pulmonary functional impairment and eventual respiratory insufficiency.

COCCIDIOIDOMYCOSIS

Coccidioidomycosis is a fungal disease, usually self-limited, which primarily involves the lungs, but may spread to the lymph nodes, skin, bone, central nervous system, and other organs.

Epidemiology and Pathogenesis. Coccidioidomycosis is endemic in the southwestern United States, particularly the desert areas of California, Arizona, Nevada, New Mexico, Texas, and Utah. In some of these areas the prevalence of positive skin tests is as high as 90%.

The causative agent, *C immitis*, is a dimorphic fungus existing in the mycelial (moldy) form in soil of semiarid regions. Its spores (**arthroconidia**), after being inhaled and settled in the lung, germinate to form characteristic **spherules.** Spherules are round and thin-walled cells that produce numerous endospores (spherule-endospore phase). The endospores, once released, make more spherules. The tissue responds to the endospores initially by nonspecific inflammation; but once immunity is developed, granulomatous reaction takes place and the infection is brought under control. The development of immunity can be demonstrated by positive reaction to the intradermal injection of *coccidioidin* (a filtrate of culture medium growing *C immitis*) or **spherulin** (a product of the spherule-endospore phase). In occasional patients who do not develop immunity, the infection spreads systemically to involve many organs in the body.

Clinical Manifestations. Over 60% of infected individuals have no symptoms, and the conversion of skin reactivity is the only indication of infection. In the majority of remaining cases, a mild flulike syndrome develops. This illness, commonly known as "desert fever," manifests by low-grade fever, malaise, headache, body aches and pains, and cough. These symptoms are self-limited and subside in several days. Only a small percentage of these symptomatic patients will have a more prolonged illness from persistent lung involvement lasting for weeks and months. *Disseminated* disease, involving extrathoracic organs, occurs in only a small fraction of the latter group. For some unknown reasons, nonwhite males are much more susceptible to developing the disseminated form, which is very rare in white females. Immunosuppression from various causes is a significant predisposing factor for widespread disease, which is being recognized in increasing numbers in patients with AIDS. Dissemination should be suspected when there is persistent fever, weight loss, or signs of extrapulmonary involvement, such as lymphadenopathy, enlarged liver or spleen, skin or bone lesions, and signs of meningitis. The latter is the most serious manifestation of disseminated coccidioidomycosis.

Radiographic Findings. Radiographic changes are variable. Localized parenchymal consolidation with or without hilar or mediastinal lymph node enlargement is the most common x-ray change during acute infection. Sometimes single or multiple nodules may be demonstrated. Cavity formation, with its characteristic thin wall, may occasionally follow the above lesions. A thin-walled cavity may be the only radiographic evidence of pulmonary coccidioidomycosis. Diffuse bilateral micronodular pattern is seen in disseminated disease. Pleural effusion may be present in some cases.

Diagnosis. The diagnosis of coccidioidomycosis is often suggested by the clinical presentation and x-ray findings in an appropriate epidemiologic setting. The coccidioidin, or spherulin, skin test becomes positive within 2 to 3 weeks of the onset of infection. It is frequently negative in the disseminated form. Serologic tests commonly performed are precipitin and complement fixation tests. Precipitin antibodies appear soon after infection; complement fixing antibodies are found later and last longer. Persistence of positive serology beyond 6 months or high complement fixation titer with negative skin test suggests dissemination. With recovery, serologic tests become negative. In certain situations and for conclusive diagnosis, isolation of organisms from the sputum or other infected materials is necessary. The laboratory should be warned if coccidioidomycosis is suspected, as the mold form of *C immitis* should be handled with utmost care to prevent accidental infection of the personnel. Occasionally, the diagnosis is made by the biopsy method.

Management and Prognosis. As was mentioned earlier, the majority of patients have self-limited and mild disease, which is often unapparent, and requires no specific therapy. All patients with pulmonary coccidioidomycosis should be closely followed, especially when there is a cavitary lesion. Lack of spontaneous improvement of lung lesions or their progression and persistence of symptoms may be an indication for specific therapy. Disseminated coccidioidomycosis should always be treated. Although ketokonazole seems to be effective in many pulmonary and extrapulmonary lesions, amphotericin B is the therapeutic agent of choice, especially for the treatment of meningitis. Occasionally, surgical resection may be indicated in persisting localized lesions or when there is recurrent hemoptysis. Disseminated disease, particularly with meningitis, has a poor prognosis.

BLASTOMYCOSIS

North American blastomycosis is a chronic fungus infection that originates in the respiratory tract and often spreads to the skin and occasionally to other organs. It is seen mostly in the central and southeastern United States. It affects predominantly middle-aged males. The causative organism, *Blastomyces dermatitidis*, is a dimorphic fungus, existing as a budding yeastlike form in the tissues and in the mycelial or moldy form in soil.

Pulmonary blastomycosis begins as a mild to moderate respiratory infection with cough, expectoration, chest pain, and sometimes hemoptysis. It may heal spontaneously or slowly progress. With progression of the disease, systemic symptoms of fever, night sweats, anorexia, and weight loss become evident. Physical signs are nonspecific and less remarkable. There may be dullness to percussion, decreased breath sounds, or rales over the involved area. The chest x-ray usually shows homogeneous mass lesion or patchy air-space density. Upper lobes are more frequently involved than lower lobes. Cavity formation is uncommon. Skin lesion is a characteristic feature of blastomycosis, which may be the only manifestation of the disease. It is a chronic, slowly progressive warty and crusting lesion located mostly on the exposed areas of the skin.

Pulmonary blastomycosis is often mistaken for other more common conditions, such as pneumonia, tuberculosis, malignancy, or other fungus infections. Definite diagnosis will depend on demonstration of typical budding yeastlike organisms on smear or culture from the diseased sources. The skin test and the serologic examination have no diagnostic value in blastomycosis.

Because of lack of significant immunity against the infection, and the danger of progression and dissemination, patients with blastomycosis should be treated with amphotericin B, the agent most effective thus far. Ketoconazole has been shown to be effective in some patients and may become an alternative agent for treatment of blastomycosis. If untreated, blastomycosis may take a protracted and progressive course, ending fatally in many cases. Treated patients generally do well.

ASPERGILLOSIS

Aspergillosis refers to various pathologic conditions resulting from infection with one of many species of *Aspergillus*. This ubiquitous fungus grows as mold on organic material: the familiar blue-green mold on bread or other food items is usually an *Aspergillus*. It seems, therefore, that exposure to the spores (conidia) of this very common fungus is inevitable. Fortunately it can cause disease only in a relatively small number of people, and then only under certain circumstances. The fungus may also live as a saprophyte in the respiratory tract, especially in patients with chronic lung disease. Among the species of *Aspergillus* known to cause disease in man, *A fumigatus* is the most important. In this section, the better-known clinical conditions that result from infection with and/or reaction to this fungus are briefly discussed.

Allergic Aspergillosis. Two types of hypersensitivity reactions are known to occur, dependent on the immunologic state of the host. In individuals without underlying asthma, heavy or repeated exposure may result in a condition known as *extrinsic allergic alveolitis*, which is discussed in Chapter 14. Malt worker's lung is an example in which exposure to moldy barley from *Aspergillus* results in this type of alveolitis. *Allergic bronchopulmonary aspergillosis*, on the other hand, is a disease that occurs in a background of long-standing asthma. It is characterized by episodic asthmatic attacks, expectoration of mucus plugs, transient irregular pulmonary infiltrates, and **atelectasis.** Peripheral blood eosinophilia, elevated immunoglobulin E (IgE), high specific antibodies against *A fumigatus*, positive skin reactivity to the fungal antigen, and positive sputum culture for the fungus are important for its diagnosis. Recurrent acute episodes may eventually result in chronic changes of pulmonary fibrosis and/or bronchiectasis. Characteristically, pulmonary fibrosis develops in the upper lobes, and bronchiectasis involves the central bronchi. Allergic bronchopulmonary aspergillosis involves both type I and type III immunologic reactions (see Chapter 14). Systemic corticosteroids are effective in its management, whereas inhaled corticosteroids have no significant role. Antifungal drugs also are ineffective. Proper bronchial toilet, with adequate humidification, use of bronchodilators, and postural drainage, is very important in the management of patients with this disease.

Aspergilloma. Also known as fungus ball, aspergilloma is usually the result of colonization of aspergillus in a preformed pulmonary cavity or **cyst.** Although a variety of cavitary or cystic lung diseases may be the site of aspergilloma, tuberculosis and sarcoidosis are the most common underlying chronic conditions. The cavity in which a fungus ball develops may occasionally result from destructive changes from other types of pulmonary aspergillosis (see below). The ball is formed by tightly matted fungal mycelia with fibrin, mucus, and cellular debris. Most patients with aspergilloma have no symptoms referable to it, although they may be symptomatic from their underlying chronic pulmonary disease. Its most significant complication is hemoptysis, which may be quite severe and life threatening. Characteristic radiographic changes are almost diagnostic (Fig. 5–2). In less obvious cases, standard or computerized **tomography** helps to delineate the intracavitary ball. In some cases, aspergilloma may resolve spontaneously. It rarely causes locally invasive aspergillosis. Unless serious complications develop, treatment of aspergilloma should be conservative. Surgical resection is considered if massive or recurrent hemoptysis occurs and the pa-

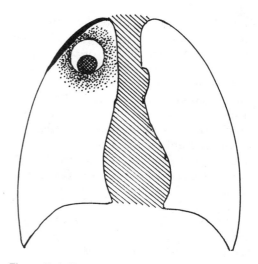

Figure 5–2. Fungus ball (aspergilloma) in a cavity.

tient is a reasonable surgical risk. Local antifungal therapy has been used in some patients with limited success. Systemic treatment may be indicated when there is evidence of local invasion.

Chronic Necrotizing Pulmonary Aspergillosis. This is a localized lung infection that has a chronic course and often mimics tuberculosis. Patients with this condition are usually middle-aged and often have underlying chronic conditions such as diabetes, malnutrition, or chronic obstructive lung disease. Radiographic film shows an infiltrative process involving predominantly one of the upper lobes with cavity formation and fibrosis. The cavity is frequently the site of a fungus ball. The disease may be present for a number of months or even years before the diagnosis is made. The clinical course, radiographic finding, repeated isolation of aspergillus from the sputum or bronchoscopically-obtained secretions, absence of other pathogenic organisms, and lack of response to antibiotics and anti-tuberculosis drugs should suggest the diagnosis of chronic necrotizing aspergillosis. It is usually confirmed by demonstration of tissue invasion by the fungus on pathologic examination or its response to antifungal drugs. Amphotericin B, with or without the addition of another antifungal drug, flucytosine, is the agent of choice for its treatment. Surgical resection may be necessary in some cases.

Invasive or Disseminated Aspergillosis.

Invasive or disseminated aspergillosis is a most serious and often fatal disease. It is almost exclusively seen in patients with severe debilitating conditions, particularly when they are treated with immunosuppressive drugs and are profoundly **granulocytopenic.** In addition to progressive pulmonary lesion, invasion of other organs is very common. Blood vessels may be invaded, causing their occlusion, which in turn results in tissue infarction and necrosis. Pulmonary manifestations may be overshadowed by severe systemic symptoms and neurologic signs. Diagnosis of invasive aspergillosis is usually made by pathologic examination of resected tissue and, not infrequently, by autopsy. Treatment is often unsuccessful because of delay in diagnosis and severity of the underlying condition.

BIBLIOGRAPHY

Ampel NM, Wieden MA, Galgiani JN. Coccidioidomycosis: Clinical update. *Rev Infect Dis.* 1989; 11:897–911.

Binder RE, Faling LJ, Pugatch RD, et al. Chronic necrotizing pulmonary aspergillosis: a discrete clinical entity. *Medicine.* 1982; 61:109–124.

Bradsher RW. Blastomycosis. *Infect Dis Clin North Am.* 1988; 2:877–898.

Goodwin RA, Loyd JE, Des Prez RM. Histoplasmosis in normal hosts. *Medicine.* 1981; 60:231–266.

Greenberger PA. Allergic bronchopulmonary aspergillosis and fungosis. *Clin Chest Med.* 1988; 9:599–608.

Herbert PA, Bayer AS. Fungal pneumonia: invasive pulmonary aspergillosis. *Chest.* 1981; 80:220–225.

Johnson PC, Sarosi GA. Histoplasmosis. *Semin Respir Med.* 1987; 9:145–151.

Levine BE. Coccidioidomycosis. *Semin Respir Med.* 1987; 9:152–158.

Levitz SM. Aspergillosis. *Infect Dis Clin North Am.* 1989; 3(1):1–18.

Sarosi GA. Management of fungal diseases. *Am Rev Respir Dis.* 1983; 127:250–253.

Wheat, LJ. Histoplasmosis. *Infect Dis Clin North Am.* 1988; 2:841–859.

CHAPTER 6

Infection with the Human Immunodeficiency Virus: Pulmonary Complications

The term *acquired immunodeficiency syndrome* (AIDS) was coined in 1981 to characterize a newly recognized fatal illness among young homosexual men, manifested by certain unusual **opportunistic** infections and/or a rare form of cancer. Without a known prior susceptibility to these uncommon diseases, it soom became apparent that these patients had somehow developed a severe deficiency of their immune system. Intense clinical and laboratory research began to produce a prolific amount of knowledge about this dreadful disease that has continued to afflict and kill an increasing number of young people. Before long, it was learned that AIDS represents only a short terminal phase of a large spectrum of disorders resulting from infection with a hitherto unrecognized virus that slowly and relentlessly destroys the body's immunologic defenses.

HUMAN IMMUNODEFICIENCY VIRUS

The causative virus finally became known as *human immunodeficiency virus* (HIV). Of two forms of this virus, HIV1 is responsible for most cases of AIDS worldwide and for almost all cases in the United States. Infection with HIV2, however, is being reported from West Africa with increasing frequency. HIV is a retrovirus, and as such has a dense core made of proteins, including the characteristic enzyme *reverse* **transcriptase,** and **genomic** RNA; and a surface envelope made of glycoproteins. Once the virus enters the target cell, the genomic RNA and reverse transcriptase are released into the host cell cytoplasm. **Proviral** DNA, produced by the viral reverse transcriptase, either remains in the cytoplasm or is integrated into the host cell's chromosomal DNA, where it may remain in a latent phase. Transcription of viral genomic RNA and formation of viral proteins result in the replication of new viruses, which are released from the cell to infect other host cells.

IMMUNOLOGIC CONSEQUENCES OF HIV INFECTION

The cells that are attacked by HIV are primarily the blood cells with special surface molecules known as CD4, which act as high-affinity receptors for the virus. T lymphocytes with helper and inducer activities have the highest expression of these molecules on their surface and, thus, are primary targets for the viral particles. These cells are known as CD4-positive cells or T4 lymphocytes. As other cell populations, such as macrophages, blood monocytes, and certain nerve cells, have such viral receptors, they may also be infected. Infection of CD4-positive lymphocytes results in their quantitative and qualitative deficiency. Normally about 65% of peripheral blood T cells are CD4-positive cells, amounting to over 1000/mm^3 of blood. This number reduces to less than 100/mm^3 in most patients with full-blown AIDS. As only a small percentage of these cells become infected, their direct killing by viral invasion does not explain their marked reduction. It is likely that other poorly understood mechanisms contribute to the depletion of this population of cells.

Infected macrophages and monocytes are not killed by the virus. They serve as viral reservoirs and as vehicles for transferring HIV to other sites, notably the central nervous sytem (CNS).

The immunologic effects of HIV infection are mostly related to the reduc-tion of the number of T helper cells, which have the central role in cell-mediated immunity. Almost all of the immunologic abnormalities in AIDS are explained by the depletion of these cells and their defective helper function, including an inadequate production of **lymphokines.** As the cells with CD8 markers, ie, the lymphocytes with suppressor and cytotoxic activities, are not directly affected by the virus, their number is not reduced; it may even increase. As a result, an imbalance develops between these cells, known as CD8-positive or T8 lymphocytes, and CD4-positive cells. A so-called T4/T8 ratio, which is normally around 2, therefore may be reduced to less than 1 (reversal of T4/T8 ratio). Infection of macrophages and monocytes by HIV may also alter their function, contributing further to the impairment of cell-mediated immunity.

In addition to the deterioration of cellular immunity, the humoral component of the immune system is also affected by HIV infection. Despite an enhanced **polyclonal** production of immunoglobulins by B lymphocytes, they are defective in making antibodies against newly acquired infections. Dysfunction of this system may also result in autoimmune disorders, among which **thrombocytopenia** is the best known. Soon after HIV infection, antibodies against viral antigens are produced. These antibodies, unlike those against most other viruses, are not protective. They are the bases for the serologic diagnosis of HIV infection.

Immunologic impairment resulting from HIV infection is a very slow but steadily progressive process. It seems that every infected person will eventually show evidence of advanced **immu-**

nodeficiency, characteristic of AIDS. It has been estimated that the average time between contracting the infection and the development of AIDS is about 8 years. This has been referred to as the "incubation period," which may be a misnomer considering the fact that HIV infection is a continuum, and AIDS is only its terminal part. As will be discussed later, it is with the occurrence of one or more of the complications that this diagnosis is made. AIDS, therefore, represents a stage of immunologic deterioration from HIV infection in which such complications become inevitable.

The currently approved and commonly used antiviral agent zidovudine (formerly called azidothymidin or AZT) reduces the viral replication by inhibiting the enzyme reverse transcriptase. It seems that in most cases of HIV infection, the progression of immunologic impairment is slowed and the risk of opportunistic infection is significantly diminished. Dideoxyinosine (DDI) and other related antiviral drugs, which also show effectiveness against HIV, are being clinically tried. As of this writing, their long-term efficacy has not been determined.

EPIDEMIOLOGY AND TRANSMISSION OF HIV INFECTION

HIV infection is occurring worldwide. As many as 130 countries have reported at least one case of AIDS. The United States has the largest number of reported cases, accounting for about two thirds of the known cases of AIDS in the world. Ever since AIDS was first recognized in 1981, over 120,000 cases of the disease have been reported in the United

States, as of July 1990. By the end of 1990, over 100,000 people in this country had died from AIDS, while an additional 1 to 1.5 million were suspected to have been infected with HIV. The incidence of AIDS has steadily increased and will continue to rise at least for the next several years. Even with the unlikely event of the elimination of new infections, there is a large enough pool of infected poeple who will keep on maintaining the very high incidence rate of AIDS. It is estimated that in 1991–1993, close to 200,000 additional cases will die from AIDS in the United States.

The main risk groups for HIV infection in the United States have continued to be homosexuals, bisexuals, intravenous (IV) drug users, and the children of infected mothers. With the proper screening of blood donors and identification of infected blood since 1985, blood and its products rarely cause HIV infection today. Yet there are still individuals infected with HIV who received such blood products prior to 1985, such as hemophiliacs. Heterosexual transmission, although potentially a serious risk for the spread of the infection, has, as of this writing, remained relatively low in the United States. Occupational exposure has engendered significant fear and anxiety among health care workers. Such exposure has caused only a few irrefutable cases of HIV infection among these workers, which has mostly occurred subsequent to contaminated needle sticks. With strict adherence to *universal precaution,* the incidence of occupational infection is expected to become even less. Infection by casual contact, as in households, schools, or workplaces, is virtually unknown.

Infectivity of individuals with HIV infection is variable, but there is a significant correlation between the severity of HIV-induced immunodeficiency and infectivity. Patients with full-blown AIDS are much more apt to infect others than are asymptomatic individuals with HIV infection. Public health measures for prevention of the spread of this dreadful infection will not succeed without an intense educational campaign. Such measures together with proper education, seem to have been effective in many homosexual communities. Unfortunately, the spread of infection among IV drug users not only remains unabated, but continues to rise.

CLINICAL SPECTRUM OF HIV INFECTION

HIV infection is often silent and remains so for an indefinite period of time before causing any clinically recognizable sign or symptom. However, a few weeks after the onset of infection, some individuals present with an acute **syndrome** characterized by fever, headache, excessive sweating, general malaise, joint and muscle pain, enlarged lymph glands, and skin rash. This infectious mononucleosis-like syndrome, which is believed to result from the direct effect of HIV infection, usually subsides spontaneously. More commonly, clinical manifestations are more protracted and develop more insidiously. Generalized lymphadenopathy, prolonged fever, fatigue, weight loss, diarrhea, oral thrush, anemia, and thrombocytopenia may occur singly or in various combinations. As none of these clinical presentations would fulfill the criteria for the diagnosis of AIDS, and patients with these various syndromes will eventually develop one or

more of the complications necessary for this diagnosis, they are considered as **prodromes** for AIDS. The terms *pre-AIDS syndromes* or *AIDS-related conditions* or complex (ARC) have been applied to these varied clinical states.

Manifestations of AIDS are the result of several processes that occur when the immunologic state has deteriorated to a critical point. They comprise infectious, neoplastic, and probably immunologic complications. Some of these processes are included in the criteria set forth by the federal Centers for Disease Control (CDC) as required for the purpose of surveillance-case definition of AIDS. The latest revision has also taken into consideration the HIV antibody status and the CD4-positive lymphocyte count. Clinically important noninfectious manifestations of AIDS are malignant diseases, notably Kaposi's sarcoma and non-Hodgkin's lymphoma, although viruses have been implicated in their causation. By far the most common manifestations or complications of AIDS are infectious in nature. Table 6–1 lists some important infections involved in clinical manifestations of AIDS. Many of these conditions would meet the CDC criteria for case definition of AIDS under appropriate circumstances. For more detailed information, the reader should consult an updated CDC publication on the subject.

PULMONARY COMPLICATIONS OF AIDS

Pulmonary disorders are the major causes of mortality and morbidity in patients with HIV infection. Normally the respiratory tract, despite its constant exposure to environmental pathogenic

TABLE 6–1. CLINICALLY IMPORTANT INFECTIOUS COMPLICATIONS OF AIDS

Causative Organism	Common Clinical Conditions
Viruses	
HIV	HIV encephalopathy (AIDS dementia), HIV wasting syndrome
Cytomegalovirus	Pneumonia, retinitis, dissemination
EB virus	B-cell lymphoma
Herpes simplex virus	Recurrent severe and protracted infection, esophagitis, pneumonia
Papovavirus	Progressive multifocal leukoencephalopathy
Protozoa	
Pneumocystis carinii	Pneumonia
Toxoplasma	Encephalitis
Cryptosporidia	Protracted diarrhea
Isospora	Protracted diarrhea
Fungi	
Candida	Mucocutaneous infection, esophagitis, tracheobronchitis, dissemination
Cryptococcus	Meningitis, dissemination
Histoplasma	Disseminated infection
Coccidioides	Disseminated infection
Mycobacteria	
M avium complex	Disseminated infection
M tuberculosis	Pulmonary and extrapulmonary tuberculosis, dissemination
Other Bacteria	
Salmonella	Recurrent sepsis
Encapsulated bacteria	Recurrent pneumonia, septicemia

agents, is well protected because of its intricate and highly effective defense system. Alveolar macrophages with their inherent phagocytic activities and their ability to recruit other immunologically competent cells, particularly T lymphocytes, play an essential role in dealing with agents eluding the mechanical defenses of the airways. It is, therefore, understandable that deficiency of cellular immunity resulting from HIV infection readily predisposes the lungs to invasion by microorganisms that would normally be held in check. Viruses, mycobacteria, fungi, and protozoa are such organisms that are often considered as opportunistic. Defective B-cell function and quantitative and qualitative abnormalities of phagocytic blood cells resulting from an advanced stage of HIV infection and/or medications facilitate respiratory infection with common bacteria. Easy recognition of respiratory symptoms and signs, ready radiographic detection of lung lesions, and their early effect on pulmonary function and blood gases make pulmonary complications quite apparent. The exact nature of them, however, may not be clinically recognized. A postmortem study of a large number of patients who had died of AIDS showed that almost all of them had pathologic evidence of pulmonary disease, many with more than one pathologic condition, although a significant number of these conditions were not diagnosed correctly before death. Severe and progressive respiratory failure as a consequence of pulmonary complications is considered to be the most common cause of death in patients with AIDS.

Pulmonary complications of AIDS in the remainder of this chapter are discussed according to their causes, which are either infectious or noninfectious, although the exact cause(s) of some of them is (are) unknown. Infectious complications are by far the most common. Clinical manifestations of these complications almost always include respiratory symptoms of cough and progressive dyspnea. Chest pain is relatively uncommon. Systemic symptoms of fever, malaise, anorexia, and weight loss are frequently present. Radiographic studies may show recognizable patterns; however, they are not by themselves diagnostic. It is the patient's history of either known HIV infection, or being in a risk group for such an infection, that makes the clinician consider not only the usual but, more often, the unusual causes of respiratory disease.

Pneumocystis Carinii Pneumonia

The most common clinically recognizable serious complication of AIDS is *Pneumocystis carinii* pneumonia (PCP). Its occurrence is the basis of the diagnosis of AIDS in about 60% of patients with this disease in the United States. An additional 20% develop PCP during the course of their illness after the diagnosis of AIDS is made based on other criteria. Moreover, many AIDS patients develop PCP more than once during their lifetime.

Pneumocystis carinii has been recognized as a protozoan, although its exact **taxonomy** has been questioned, as it also has certain characteristics of a fastidious fungus. Identification is by its distinctive morphologic and staining features. It is believed that most healthy persons become infected without developing the disease. It seems that the reactivation of a dormant infection in AIDS or other severely immunocompromised states is the cause of PCP. Lungs are the primary, and often the only site, of active disease. Rarely, other organs have been shown to become infected. The onset of PCP signifies an advanced deficiency of cell-mediated immunity, and there is a strong correlation between its occurrence and the number of CD4-positive lymphocytes; AIDS patients with PCP have a CD4$^+$ lymphocyte count of under 200/mm^3 and at times fewer than 100/mm^3.

The organisms, unopposed by lung defenses, occupy the surface of alveolar epithelial lining, going through continual cycles of **trophozoite** stage and cyst formation, and in the process multiply rapidly, filling the alveolar spaces. The number of organisms in PCP secondary to AIDS is much larger than in PCP due to other immunosuppressed states. Increased alveolar capillary permeability, exudation of fluid, infiltration with inflammatory cells, and loss of surfactant are the pathologic changes that, together with an abundant number of organisms, result in severe impairment of gas transport. Clinical manifestations of PCP in AIDS patients usually begin insidiously and progress slowly. Fever, cough, and increasing dyspnea are typical presenting symptoms. Cough is nonproductive and dyspnea may only be noted with exertion. Chest pain is very uncommon. Most patients do not seek medical advice for several weeks from the onset of symptoms. By the time that they consult a physician, most have significant dyspnea.

Physical examination of a patient with PCP usually indicates fever with evidence of associated conditions seen in most AIDS patients, such as oral thrush, wasting, and generalized lymphadenopathy. Signs of respiratory difficulty, such as tachypnea, are often apparent. Examination of the lungs may be normal despite significant abnormalities in radiographic film. The latter usually shows a diffuse interstitial and sometimes an alveolar pattern of density throughout the lungs. If the study is done earlier, it may show only minimal or no changes. Atypical patterns, such as focal consolidation, perihilar density, or cystic changes, may also be seen. Hilar lymphadenopathy and pleural effusions are rarely ever seen with PCP alone. Their presence should suggest other diagnoses. A helpful study, when chest radiograph is normal or shows questionable changes, is gallium-67 scan. Significant pulmonary uptake of this radioisotope with normal chest x-ray film is highly suggestive of PCP. Pulmonary function tests indicate restrictive impairment with reduced diffusion capacity. The latter is very sensitive in detecting early disease. It should be noted, however, that reduced diffusion capacity may be secondary to long-standing IV drug use. Blood-gas abnormalities may also be noted early in the course of PCP. Low PO_2 usually with low PCO_2 is common.

Although PCP is often suspected from the clinical presentation on a background of HIV infection or high-risk behavior, its definitive diagnosis necessitates demonstration of organisms from a specimen of lung secretion or tissue. As patients with PCP usually do not produce sputum spontaneously, it should be induced by hypertonic saline nebulized by an ultrasonic device. Adequate cleansing of the mouth and throat before the sputum induction, and proper collection, processing, and staining of sputum, are both essential for a successful result. Diagnostic sensitivity of such a study, if properly done, is close to 70%. Bronchoscopy is usually performed when sputum induction is not possible or its result is not diagnostic. Bronchoalveolar lavage is preferred to brushing and **transbronchial** biopsy, unless other diagnostic

possibilities are also seriously considered. Samples obtained bronchoscopically or by sputum induction should always be studied for other organisms, especially for mycobacteria.

Figure 6–1 shows an algorithm that is used in diagnostic planning for AIDS or suspected AIDS patients presenting with significant respiratory symptoms. Therapeutic management of PCP in AIDS patients consists of treatment with an agent effective against pneumocystis and supportive care. Most patients, being hypoxemic, require oxygen therapy and may even need intubation and mechanical ventilatory support. Approved drug regimen, at the time of this writing, is either a combination of trimethoprim and sulfamethoxazole (TMP-SMX) or pentamidine, which is given for a 2- to 3-week period. Although both regimens are quite effective, they have significant side effects in AIDS patients, which may necessitate the discontinuation of one regimen and starting the other. Other experimental treatment modalities show promise based on preliminary studies. They include aerosolized pentamidine, trimethoprim-dapsone combination, and trimetrexate. As an adjunctive therapy, corticosteroid administration seems to improve survival in patients with AIDS complicated by moderately severe to severe PCP. It may prevent the occurrence of respiratory failure in these patients.

Prophylaxis with TMP-SMX is effective, but its significant side effects preclude its use in many instances. Recently approved aerosolized pentamidine for prophylaxis is devoid of serious side effects, but cough is a frequent complaint with this treatment and wheezing is occasionally noted. These side effects are much more common in smokers and

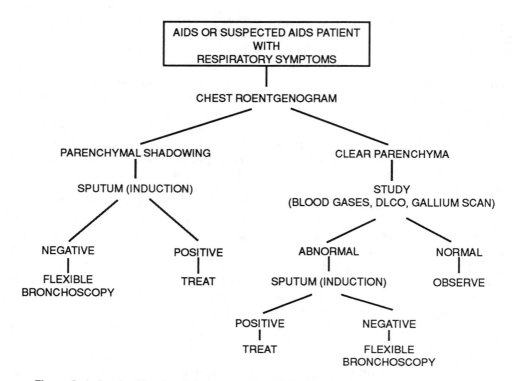

```
            ┌─────────────────────────────────┐
            │  AIDS OR SUSPECTED AIDS PATIENT  │
            │              WITH               │
            │      RESPIRATORY SYMPTOMS       │
            └─────────────────────────────────┘

                   CHEST ROENTGENOGRAM

   PARENCHYMAL SHADOWING              CLEAR PARENCHYMA

     SPUTUM (INDUCTION)                    STUDY
                              (BLOOD GASES, DLCO, GALLIUM SCAN)

 NEGATIVE        POSITIVE       ABNORMAL            NORMAL

 FLEXIBLE        TREAT      SPUTUM (INDUCTION)      OBSERVE
BRONCHOSCOPY

                       POSITIVE        NEGATIVE

                        TREAT          FLEXIBLE
                                     BRONCHOSCOPY
```

Figure 6–1. An algorithm for clinical approach to HIV-infected patients with respiratory symptoms.

asthmatics. Pretreatment with a bronchodilator is effective in reducing these side effects. Pentamidine aerosol is approved by the Food and Drug Administration (FDA) for both primary and secondary prophylaxis against PCP. Primary prophylaxis is for individuals infected with HIV whose absolute CD4-positive lymphocyte count is under 200/mm³ or when less than 20% of blood lymphocytes are CD4-positive. The most commonly used regimen is inhalation of 300 milligrams (mgm) of pentamidine dissolved in 6 mL of sterile water and aerosolized by a compressed-air nebulizer, given once every 4 weeks. Respirgard II, which has a filter designed to remove most of pentamidine from

exhaled air, is recommended by the FDA for this purpose. Other nebulizers and different dose regimens are also being evaluated for the prophylactic administration of pentamidine aerosol. Therapists or other health care providers administering aerosolized pentamidine should be aware of the possibility of patients having active tuberculosis and should take appropriate measures to prevent exposure. This precaution should also be taken when sputum induction is carried out.

Tuberculosis

As discussed in Chapter 4, infection with *Mycobacterium tuberculosis* in most instances remains dormant and suppressed by the body's defense system, positive reaction to tuberculin skin test being the only evidence for such an infection. Reactivation of this latent infection is usually the result of alteration of defense mechanisms, especially weakening of the cell-mediated immunity. The epidemic of HIV infection has caused an extraordinary increase in the population of immunedeficient individuals, predisposing them to active tuberculosis. This disease is emerging as a very important complication of HIV infection, particularly among IV drug users who generally have a high prevalence of preexisting tuberculous infection. As in every case of active tuberculosis, the importance of its early recognition in HIV-infected patients cannot be overemphasized. Among the numerous infectious diseases complicating AIDS, tuberculosis is the only readily transmittable disease that can infect others, regardless of their immunologic state. Health workers should always be on the alert for tuberculosis whenever they are taking care of AIDS patients. Moreover, tuberculosis is an easily treatable disease, even in patients with AIDS, and its infectivity diminishes rapidly with the institution of an appropriate chemotherapeutic regimen. Prophylactic treatment also seems to be effective in preventing the reactivation of tuberculosis in HIV-infected individuals.

As in the general population, the most common pathogenetic mechanism of tuberculous disease in HIV-infected patients is the reactivation of a latent tuberculous focus. It usually develops before, rather than after, the diagnosis of AIDS. Probably because of higher virulence and pathogenecity of *M tuberculosis* than other truly opportunistic organisms such as *Pneumocystic carinii,* active tuber-

culosis develops with a lesser degree of immunodeficiency. It has been shown that the number of CD4-positive lymphocytes (an excellent indicator of immunologic state in HIV infection) is only moderately reduced when active tuberculosis is diagnosed. It seems, therefore, that it may be an early clinical manifestation of HIV infection, especially in individuals and populations known to have higher rates of tuberculous infection. The incidence of tuberculosis in patients meeting the criteria for the diagnosis of AIDS may be as high as 10%. When young patients with recently developed tuberculosis are checked for HIV antibody, a significant percentage of them prove to be positive, indicating that the incidence of HIV-related tuberculosis could be even higher. In one study when tuberculin-positive IV drug users with known HIV status were prospectively followed, there was a significant difference in the incidence of active tuberculosis between groups with and without HIV infection.

Clinical and radiographic features of tuberculosis occurring in HIV-infected patients vary significantly in relation to the stage of immunologic deficiency. When it develops in the early stage of HIV infection, it tends to have the features of tuberculosis in the general population with an apparently normal immunologic state. However, if it occurs when other manifestations of AIDS have developed, the clinical and radiographic characteristics may be quite different. In this setting, extrapulmonary and disseminated forms are much more common, and pulmonary lesions may be atypical in their locations and other radiographic features. Hilar and mediastinal lymphadenopathy, predominant involvement of lower lung fields, the diffuse nature of infiltration, and lack of cavitation result in diagnostic difficulty. Concurrent presence of other opportunistic infections or malignancy in AIDS patients confounds the clinical picture.

Diagnosis of tuberculosis in HIV-infected patients necessitates a high index of suspicion. Intravenous drug users and other population groups with a history of tuberculosis exposure and/or with positive tuberculin test are primary suspects for active tuberculosis when presenting with respiratory or systemic symptoms. Tuberculin reaction, being a cellular hypersensitivity, may be negative in the late stage of HIV infection despite active tuberculosis. However, in its earlier stages when cellular immunity is still functional, a tuberculin test is useful in detecting tuberculous infection, and its result would be helpful for additional diagnostic and therapeutic planning. With increasing deterioration of immunologic state with HIV infection, reactivity to tuberculin progressively diminishes. To increase the diagnostic sensitivity of the tuberculin test, it has been recommended that a reaction size of >5 mm of induration (instead of > 10 mm) at the site of intradermal injection of 5 tuberculin units of PPD, to be considered as positive when applied to patients with HIV infection. Frequently, negative test results in AIDS patients with active tuberculosis indicate that additional diagnostic studies, such as bacteriologic examination of sputum and other available specimens, should be pursued whenever the diagnosis of tuberculosis is suspected, regardless of the result of the tuberculin test. As most patients with HIV infection and respiratory symptoms are studied for PCP, material obtained for this purpose should also be examined for tubercle bacilli. Common occurrence of atypical mycobacterial disease in AIDS (see below) makes cultural identification of acid-fast organisms mandatory. Antituberculosis therapy, however, should be initiated whenever acid-fast bacilli are seen in sputum or other specimens while awaiting its definitive identification by culture.

A three-drug regimen is the currently recommended therapy for patients with HIV infection including AIDS, which should contain isoniazid and rifampin. Pyrazinamide is the preferred third drug, which is given for the first 2 months. Total duration of treatment should be at least 9 months. Isoniazid prophylaxis should be given to all HIV-infected individuals with a positive tuberculin test if active tuberculosis is excluded.

Atypical Mycobacterial Disease

Although other atypical mycobacteria may infect patients with AIDS, *Mycobacterium avium* complex (MAC) is by far the most significant. Infection with this organism in these patients usually presents as a widely disseminated disease involving many organs as well as the bloodstream. The lung is the most likely primary site of infection, which in normal hosts rarely ever spreads elsewhere. In some patients with an underlying chronic lung disease but normal immunologic state, MAC may cause local lesions. In severe deficiency of cell-mediated immunity, as in full-blown AIDS, it readily disseminates from its primary site. Pulmonary lesions may or may not be radiographically apparent. Disseminated atypical mycobacterial disease meets the criteria for the diagnosis of AIDS according to the CDC surveillance-case definition. Therefore, disseminated disease with these organisms almost always denotes an advanced stage of HIV infection. This explains the lack of pathologic reaction in the form of granuloma formation, despite the presence of extremely large numbers of bacteria in involved organs.

Clinical manifestations of MAC disease in patients with AIDS is often obscured by the concurrent presence of other complications. Systemic signs and symptoms of chills, fever, and weight loss are usually explained by other infectious or noninfectious conditions. Respiratory manifestations, if present, are nonspecific. Chest radiograph may be normal despite demonstration of acid-fast organisms in sputum. In many instances the diagnosis is made on postmortem examination. As most patients with AIDS die from other infectious causes, the clinical importance and prognostic significance of MAC infection, even when it is widely disseminated, often remain unclear.

Presently available therapeutic agents are disappointingly ineffective in the treatment of disseminated MAC infection. As the differentiation from *M tuberculosis* is not possible on morphologic or straining characteristics of the organisms, most patients with positive smear of sputum or other pathologic material are treated with antituberculosis drugs until proper identification of causative bacteria is made by culture.

Viral Pneumonia

Three prevalent herpesviruses, namely cytomegalovirus (CMV), herpes simplex virus (HSV), and varicella-zoster virus (VZV), may infect the lungs in AIDS patients. After infection earlier in life, under normal conditions these viruses live in a dormant state, contained by the body's cell-mediated immunity. Reactivation of this latent infection occurs when this important defense system weakens. Cytomegalovirus infection is by far the most common, and pulmonary involvement is a frequent occurrence in AIDS. It also infects other organs such as the eye, liver, and gastrointestinal tract. Although CMV is often isolated from respiratory-tract secretions or lung tissue from AIDS patients with pneumonic infiltration, its role is usually uncertain. Its association with *Pneumocystic carinii* pneumonia is very common. However, as most such patients improve after treatment for PCP, it appears that CMV has no clinically significant part in this situation. Uncommonly, CMV may be the sole agent responsible for pneumonia. Dyspnea and nonproductive cough are the usual symptoms in patients with CMV pneumonia. Isolation of the virus from pulmonary secretions is not diagnostic of CMP pneumonia. Its definitive diagnosis requires histologic and/or cytologic evidence of infection with this virus. There is no satisfactory treatment for CMV pneumonia. The antiviral agent *ganciclovir*, although less effective against CMV pneumonia than against CMV retinitis and colitis, may be tried.

Both HSV and VZV behave as opportunistic infections in AIDS patients; in addition to causing recurrent skin lesions, they may disseminate and involve other organs. Pulmonary involvement, although uncommon, may be the cause of severe hypoxemic respiratory failure. In view of the treatable nature of these infections, their early diagnosis is important. Acyclovir is effective against infection by both of these viruses.

Among other viruses implicated in causing pulmonary complications in AIDS patients, Epstein-Barr virus (EBV) is noteworthy. B-cell lymphoma in these patients is considered to be related to infection with EBV. Its role in causing interstitial pneumonia has also been suggested.

Pulmonary Mycoses

Infection with *Candida albicans*, the most common fungal infection in AIDS, is the cause of oral thrush and may result in painful esophagitis. It uncommonly affects the tracheobronchial tree and rarely results in pneumonia. Clinically more significant mycotic diseases involving the lungs are histoplasmosis, coccidioidomycosis, and cryptococcosis, which may occur in patients with AIDS. As was mentioned in Chapter 5, both histoplasmosis and coccidioidomycosis may manifest as widespread disease in immunocompromised patients. The disseminated form of either of these **mycoses** when it occurs in patients known to be HIV-positive fulfills the criteria for the diagnosis of AIDS. However, extrapulmonary cryptococcosis in individuals without other known causes of immunosuppression is enough for such diagnosis, even when the HIV status is unknown.

Cases of disseminated histoplasmosis in AIDS patients are being reported mostly from the **endemic** areas, although some have occurred in patients from nonendemic regions, most likely as a result of activation of an earlier infection. Its clinical manifestations are nonspecific and difficult to differentiate from those of other conditions occurring in AIDS. Pulmonary involvement may mimic PCP or tuberculosis and may progress to respiratory failure. Diagnosis of

disseminated histoplasmosis can only be made by demonstration and identification of its causative fungus, *Histoplasma capsulatum,* from involved tissues or blood. The clinical course of histoplasmosis is more severe and its response to amphotericin B is less satisfactory in AIDS than in other immunosuppressed states.

Disseminated coccidioidomycosis in AIDS patients has been reported only from endemic areas. Whether it is the result of reactivation of a dormant infection or progression of a recent infection is not known. It seems that either mechanism may cause dissemination in severely immunocompromised persons. The lungs are almost always involved and pleural effusion is common. Both systemic and pulmonary manifestations are nonspecific. Central nervous system (CNS) signs and skin lesions are not uncommon. The diagnosis is made by identification of the fungus *Coccidioides immitis* from sputum, bronchoscopically obtained material, pleural effusion, or other tissues. Serologic tests are less useful for the diagnosis of coccidioidomycosis in AIDS. Treatment, although less effective, is the administration of amphotericin B as in patients without AIDS.

Cryptococcal disease in AIDS patients is predominantly a CNS disorder in the form of meningitis or cerebral infection. The primary infection, however, occurs in the lungs in a more or less silent manner, from which it disseminates to other organs, especially the CNS. Clinically apparent pulmonary disease from *Cryptococcus neoformans* often coexists with CNS infection. It may cause pneumonic consolidation, interstitial infiltration, or pleural effusion. Diagnosis is usually made by the examination of bronchoscopically obtained material. In patients suspected to have cryptococcal infection, cerebrospinal fluid should always be examined. Amphotericin B, with or without flucytosine, is the drug of choice. A new antifungal agent, fluconazole, seems to be equally effective in cryptococcal meningitis. It is available in oral and intravenous forms. Because of frequent relapses, lifelong treatment is often recommended.

Bacterial Pneumonia

Although most serious infections occurring in patients with AIDS are opportunistic, common pathogenic bacteria are the cause of pneumonia in a significant number of these patients. In view of its high mortality and, at the same time, good response to proper antibiotics, bacterial pneumonia should always be considered in the differential diagnosis of pulmonary manifestations of AIDS. *Streptococcus pneumoniae* and *Haemophilus influenzae* are the organisms most commonly involved. Infection with these bacteria is more prevalent in HIV-infected individuals than in an age-matched control group. As was mentioned earlier in this chapter, a higher incidence of infection with bacteria, especially encapsulated organisms, is mainly related to the abnormality of humoral immunity that occurs in patients with HIV infection. Deficiency of antibody production in response to new infections is compounded by impaired phagocytic activity of macrophages and, perhaps, granulocytes. Bacterial pneumonia occurs more frequently in IV drug users than other risk groups with HIV infection. Other bacteria that are known to cause pneumonia in this population include *Branhamella catarrhalis*, beta-hemolytic *streptococcus*, *Staphylococcus aureus*, and *Legionella pneumophila*.

Clinical manifestations of bacterial pneumonia in HIV-infected or AIDS patients are not much different from those seen in **immunocompetent** hosts. The onset of symptoms of chills, fever, and cough is abrupt and more acute than those due to PCP. Other distinguishing features are sputum production and pleuritic chest pain, which are usually lacking in PCP. Chest x-ray film may show lobar, segmental, or diffuse infiltrations. Bacterial pneumonia may co-exist with an opportunistic pulmonary infection, such as PCP. Both the rate of recurrence and frequency of bacteremia are higher when the pneumonia occurs in HIV-infected patients than in the general population.

Diagnosis of bacterial pneumonia is based on clinical presentation and the result of sputum examination. Blood cultures should always be obtained. Empirical therapy with the trimethoprim-sulfamethoxazole combination is an accepted treatment, which is effective against most organisms causing community-acquired pneumonia. A more specific antibiotic, however, should be selected whenever bacteriologic information is available. In adults, active immunization with pneumococcal vaccine is not usually effective. In patients with recurrent pneumonia, antibiotic prophylaxis may be tried.

Malignant Disease Involving the Lungs

Although immunologic deficiency as a contributing factor in the pathogenesis of the malignant process has been known for a long time, AIDS has added a new dimension to this intriguing oncological phenomenon. Among **neoplastic** diseases, Kaposi's sarcoma (KS) stands alone as a highly prevalent malignancy in AIDS. There is also a relatively increased incidence of non-Hodgkin's lymphomas.

Although recognized for over a century before the AIDS epidemic, KS in the Western world occurred only rarely as a slow-growing malignancy in older individuals. In association with HIV infection, it behaves as a highly aggressive multicentric cancer whose onset signifies an advanced stage of immunodeficiency. When it occurs in a young person, KS by itself fulfills the criteria for the diagnosis of AIDS, even when the HIV status is unknown. For no apparent reason, it is more prevalent among homosexuals than IV drug users or hemophiliacs. This marked difference in its incidence and other epidemiologic data suggest that KS is related to infection with an as yet unidentified virus that is transmitted mainly through homosexual activity along with or in proximity to HIV infection. In recent years its incidence has been declining, but its prognosis is becoming worse. Earlier in AIDS epidemics, almost 60% of homosexuals with AIDS developed KS in the course of their illness; recently, it occurs in about 20%. Skin and mucous membranes are the most common sites of Kaposi's lesions, which appear as purplish to bluish nodules or plaques of various sizes. The gastrointestinal tract and lungs are often involved, usually following skin lesions, but they may occur without them. From autopsy studies, about 60% of patients with KS show evidence of pulmonary involvement, which may not have been clinically recognized. Tumors may develop in the lung parenchyma, bronchi, lymph nodes, and pleura. Although uncommon, bronchoscopically demonstrable changes appear as discrete, bright red mucosal lesions at the branching points of the bronchi, which are highly characteristic of pulmonary KS.

Clinically, pulmonary KS has no characteristic manifestations. Diagnosis is usually suspected when unexplained radiographic changes are seen in patients with cutaneous or mucosal KS. This cancer is responsible for about a third of the episodes of pulmonary lesions in patients with known KS elsewhere in the body. Radiographic changes are more suggestive of KS when focal parenchymal or perihilar densities are seen with pleural effusion and intrathoracic lymph node enlargement. Pathologic diagnosis from bronchoscopically obtained material is not usually successful, even when apparent endobronchial lesions are biopsied. As thoracotomy is rarely performed for the evaluation of lung lesions in AIDS, the diagnosis of pulmonary KS remains uncertain in most incidences. Although pulmonary KS denotes a poor prognosis, most patients succumb to other, mostly infectious, complications of AIDS. Various treatment modalities are under investigation. **Alpha interferon** seems to be promising.

The AIDS-associated lymphomas constitute the second most common malignant complication. They are mostly B-cell tumors, probably caused by EBV infection. They behave differently from histologically similar tumors in immunocompetent patients. Extranodal lesions are common, which occur in the CNS, gastrointestinal tract, and intrathoracic organs. These lymphomas are high-grade malignancies, progress rapidly, and often terminate fatally. Intrathoracic lesions may appear as pulmonary **nodules,** masses, interstitial infiltrates, pleural effusion, and/or mediastinal lymphadenopathy. The response of these lymphomas to chemotherapy is poor.

Other Noninfectious Pulmonary Complications

Diffuse interstitial pattern is the most common radiographic change due to pulmonary complications of AIDS. The vast majority of cases are infectious in nature and occasionally are due to a malignancy. In association with HIV infection, however, other interstitial lung diseases develop whose etiology and pathogenesis are poorly understood. One such pathologic condition known as lymphoid interstitial pneumonia (LIP) occurs frequently in children with HIV infection and meets the criteria for the diagnosis of AIDS if the patient is younger than 13 years of age. LIP has been reported in adults only sporadically. It occurs more commonly in blacks than in whites. Diffuse infiltration of the lungs by mononuclear cells, especially lymphocytes, is the main pathologic finding. Lymphocytes have CD8 markers. Frequent association with peripheral blood lymphocytosis with an increased number of CD8-positive T cells suggests that these cells have a pathogenetic role in this disease. A closely related condition known as *pulmonary lymphoid hyperplasia* is characterized by focal and nodular accumulation of lymphocytes in lung tissue.

Although LIP occurs much less commonly in adults than children, it should be included in the differential diagnosis of interstitial lung disease in HIV-infected patients. LIP develops earlier in the course of HIV infection, before the diagnosis of AIDS is made.

Clinical manifestations of cough and dyspnea have an insidious onset. Chest radiograph shows bilateral reticulonodular densities predominantly involving the lower lung fields, often mimicking PCP. Because of its uncommon occurrence in adults, LIP is less often suspected. Although transbronchial biopsy may suggest the diagnosis, it can only be proven by open lung biopsy. As spontaneous improvement may take place, a period of observation is recommended before deciding for treatment with corticosteroids.

Another form of interstitial lung disease in adults with HIV infection has been described with nonspecific pathologic changes of mononuclear cell infiltration, but also associated with **edema,** alveolar cell **hyperplasia,** and fibrous deposition. Symptoms are usually mild and consist of cough and exertional dyspnea. Both chest x-ray findings of bilateral diffuse interstitial density and clinical symptoms often stabilize, or even resolve, spontaneously.

BIBLIOGRAPHY

Baskin MI, Abd AG, Ilowite JS. Regional deposition of aerosolized petamidine: effects of body position and breathing pattern. *Ann Intern Med.* 1990; 113:677–683.

Beck JM, Shellito J. Effects of human immunodeficiency virus on pulmonary host defenses. *Semin Respir Infect.* 1989; 4:75–84.

Braun MM, Byers RH, Heyward WL, et al. Acquired immunodeficiency syndrome and extrapulmonary tuberculosis in the United States. *Arch Intern Med.* 1990; 150:1913–1916.

Centers for Disease Control. Guidelines for prophylaxis against *Pneumocystis carinii* pneumonia for persons infected with human immunodeficiency virus. *MMWR*. 1989; 38 (suppl 5):1–9.

Chaisson RE. Bacterial pneumonia in patients with human immunodeficiency virus infection. *Semin Respir Infect*. 1989; 4:133–138.

Chaisson RE, Slutkin G. Tuberculosis and human immunodeficiency virus infection. *J Infect Dis*. 1989; 159:96–100.

Conte JE Jr, Chernoff D, Feigal DW, et al. Intravenous or inhaled pentamidine for treating *Pneumocystis carinii* pneumonia in AIDS. *Ann Intern Med*. 1990; 113:203–209.

Davey RT Jr, Lane HC. Laboratory methods in the diagnosis and prognostic staging of infection with human immunodeficiency virus type 1. *Rev Infect Dis*. 1990; 12:912–930.

DeLorenzo LJ, Huang CT, Maguire GP, Stone DJ. Roentgenographic patterns of *Pneumocystis carinii* pneumonia in 104 patients with AIDS. *Chest*. 1987; 91:323–327.

Drugs for HIV infection. *Med Lett Drugs Ther*. 1990; 31:11–13.

Fauci AS. The human immunodeficiency virus: infectivity and mechanisms of pathogenesis. *Science*. 1988; 239:617–622.

Fish DG, Ampel NM, Galgiani JN, et al. Coccidioidomycosis during human immunodeficiency virus infection. Medicine. 1990;69:384–391.

Gagnon S, Boota AM, Fischl MA, et al. Corticosteroids as adjunctive therapy for severe *Pneumocystis carinii* pneumonia in the acquired immunodeficiency syndrome. *N Engl J Med*. 1990; 323:1444–1450.

Glatt AE, Chirgwin K. *Pneumocystis carinii* pneumonia in human immunodeficiency virus-infected patients. *Arch Intern Med*. 1990; 150:271–279.

Godwin CR, Brown DT, Masur H, et al. Sputum induction: a quick and sensitive technique for diagnosing *Pneumocystis carinii* pneumonia in immunosuppressed patients. *Respir Care*. 1991; 36:33–39.

Graybill JR. Histoplasmosis and AIDS. *J Infect Dis*. 1988; 158:623–626.

Hopewell PC. Tuberculosis and human immunodeficiency virus infection. *Semin Respir Infect*. 1989; 4:111–122.

Horsburgh CR Jr. *Mycobacterium avium* complex infection in the acquired immunodeficiency syndrome. *N Eng J Med*. 1991; 324:1332–1338.

Hoth DF Jr, Myers MW. Current status of HIV therapy. *Hosp Pract*. 1991; 26(1):94–117.

Jules-Elysee KM, Stover DE, Zaman MB, et al. Aerosalized pentamidine: effect on diagnosis and prevention of *Pneumocystis carinii* pneumonia. *Ann Intern Med*. 1990; 112:750–757.

Kramer EL, Sanger JH, Garay SM, et al. Diagnostic implications of Ga-67 chest scan patterns in human immunodeficiency virus-seropositive patients. *Radiology*. 1989; 170:671–676.

Leoung GS, Feigal DW, Montgomery AB, et al. Aerosolized pentamidine for prophylaxis against *Pneumocystis carinii* pneumonia. *N Engl J Med*. 1990; 323:769–775.

MacDonell KB, Glassroth J. *Mycobacterium avium* complex and other nontuberculous mycobacteria in patients with HIV infection. *Semin Respir Infect*. 1989; 4:123–132.

Macher AM, DeVinatea ML, Turr SM, Angritt P. AIDS and the mycoses. *Infect Dis Clin North Am*. 1988; 2:827–839.

Masur H, Ognibene FP, Yarchoan R, et al. CD4 counts as predictors of opportunistic pneumonias in human immunodeficiency virus (HIV) infection. *Ann Intern Med*. 1989; 111:223–231.

Miller RF, Semple SJG. Glucocorticoid therapy for severe *Pneumocystis carinii* pneumonia. *J Infect*. 1990; 21:131–137.

Montaner JSG, Lawson LM, Gervais A, et al. Aerosol pentamidine for secondary prophylaxis of AIDS-related *Pneumocystis carinii* pneumonia. *Ann Intern Med*. 1991; 114:948–953.

Mortality atributable to HIV infection/AIDS—United States, 1981–1990. *MMWR*. 1991; 40:41–44.

Murphy RL, Lavelle JP, Allan JD, et al. Aerosol pentamidine prophylaxis following *Pneumocystis carinii* pneumonia in AIDS patients. *AM J Med*. 1991; 90:418–426.

Murray JF, Mills J. Pulmonary infectious complications of human immunodeficiency virus infection. *Am Rev Respir Dis*. 1990; 141:1356–1372, 1582–1598.

Polish LB, Cohn DL, Ryder JW, et al. Pulmonary non-Hodgkin's lymphoma in AIDS. *Chest*. 1989; 96:1321–1326.

Polsky B, Gold JWM, Whimbey E, et al. Bacterial pneumonia in patients with the acquired immunodeficiency syndrome. *Ann Intern Med*. 1986; 104:38–41.

Schooley RT. Cytomegalovirus in the setting of infection with human immunodeficiency virus. *Rev Infect Dis*. 1990; 12 (suppl 7):S811–S819.

Selwyn PA, Hartel D, Lewis VA, et al. A prospective study of the risk for tuberculosis among intravenous drug users with human immunodeficiency virus infection. *N Engl J Med*. 1989; 320:545–550.

Soo Hoo GW, Mohsenifar Z, Meyer RD. Inhaled or intravenous pentamidine therapy for *Pneumocystis carinii* pneumonia in AIDS. *Ann Intern Med*. 1990; 113:195–202.

Tindall B, Cooper DA. Primary HIV infection: host responses and intervention strategies. *AIDS*.1991; 5:1–14.

Toronto Aerosolized Pentamidine Study (TAPS) Group. Acute pulmonary effects of aerosolized pentamidine. *Chest*. 1990; 98:907–910.

Wachter RM, Russi MB, Bloch DA, et al. *Pneumocystis carinii* pneumonia and respiratory failure in AIDS: improved outcomes and increased use of intensive care units. *Am Rev Respir Dis*. 1991; 143:251–256.

Wallace JM. Pulmonary infection in human immunodeficiency disease: viral pulmonary infections. *Semin Respir Infect*. 1989; 4:147–154.

Wallace JM, Hannah J. Cytomegalovirus pneumonitis in patients with AIDS. *Chest*. 1987; 92:198–203.

Wasser L, Talavera W. Pulmonary cryptococcosis in AIDS. *Chest*. 1987; 92:692–695.

Wheat LJ, Connolly-Stringfield PA, Baker RL, et al. Disseminated histoplasmosis in the acquired immunodeficiency: clinical findings, diagnosis, and treatment, and review of the literature. *Medicine* 1990; 69: 361–374.

White DA, Matthay RA. Noninfectious pulmonary complications of infection with the human immunodeficiency virus. *Am Rev Respir Dis*. 1989; 140:1763–1787.

Obstructive Airways Diseases

CHAPTER 7

Diseases of the Upper Respiratory Tract: Upper Airway Obstruction

The upper respiratory tract includes the nose, paranasal sinuses, pharnyx, larynx, and trachea. The pharynx is divided into three continuous components: **nasopharynx,** the section above the soft palate; **oropharynx,** the part that can be seen when the mouth is wide open and the tongue is depressed; and **hypopharynx** or **laryngopharynx,** the part below the level of the epiglottis to the level of the cricoid cartilage. The latter two parts make a common pathway for both food and air. The nasopharynx above and the larynx below are protected by the proper function of the soft palate and the epiglottis, which close them respectively with the act of **deglutition** and/or vomiting. The larynx is also divided into three regions: supraglottic, glottic, and subglottic. (Fig. 7–1). The trachea is divided into extrathoracic and in trathoracic portions.

In the course of their physiologic functions of warming, humidifying, and cleansing inspired air, the upper airways are exposed to a variety of irritants, allergens, and infectious agents. Upper respiratory infections, which include the common cold, are the most prevalent disorders of the respiratory tract. There are several noninfectious pathologic conditions that may also involve the upper respiratory tract. As some of these disorders may result in clinically significant respiratory complications by impeding airflow, they will be briefly discussed in this chapter.

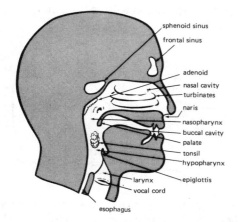

Figure 7–1. Upper respiratory tract.

sphenoid sinus
frontal sinus
adenoid
nasal cavity
turbinates
naris
nasopharynx
buccal cavity
palate
tonsil
hypopharynx
larynx
epiglottis
vocal cord
esophagus

NASAL AND NASOPHARYNGEAL OBSTRUCTION

Because of the presence of dual pathways to the pharynx, through the nose and the mouth, obstruction of the nose and the nasopharynx usually does not result in ventilatory impairment. The long-held belief that newborn infants are obligate nasal breathers has recently been refuted. It has been demonstrated that infants become able to mouth-breathe after a short but variable interval following nasal obstruction. Chronic obstructive lesions in these locations, as seen in individuals with chronically enlarged adenoids, have been implicated in sleep-related breathing disorders (see Chapter 24). Obstruction in these areas may be the cause of some difficulties encountered during oxygen administration by the nasal route, nasopharyngeal or nasotracheal intubation, and suctioning. Moreover, with mouth breathing, inspired air may not be properly warmed or humidified, resulting in dryness and irritation of the upper air passages.

OROPHARYNGEAL AND HYPOPHARYNGEAL OBSTRUCTION

As a common pathway for both food and respired air, this part of the pharynx is endowed with several deglutitory muscles, not the least of which is the tongue. It has recently been demonstrated that the respiratory control system also regulates the tone of muscles in this area, preventing their relaxation and their tendency to collapse during inspiration. As the weight of the tongue tends to displace it backward in the supine position, the importance of ade-

quate muscle tone in this position is obvious. A common problem in unconscious patients is the obstruction of the airway resulting from total relaxation of the muscles of the jaw, the tongue, and the pharyngeal wall (Fig. 7–2).

In the obstructive form of sleep apnea, as discussed elsewhere in this book, the obstruction to airflow during inspiration most commonly occurs in the oropharynx. It results from periodic loss of tone of muscles of the tongue and the pharynx during certain stages of sleep. During apnea, the tongue is displaced backward, touching the soft palate and the uvula; and the relaxed pharyngeal wall at this level is sucked toward the base of the tongue with inspiratory effort, thus completing the obstruction.

Sudden upper airway obstruction may develop from the impaction of a large piece of food in the hypopharynx (Fig. 7–3). This may occur as a result of poor eating habits, particularly when the victim attempts to swallow an improperly chewed, excessively large bite of meat. This catastrophic event, known since antiquity, has been highly publicized and its on-the-site emergency

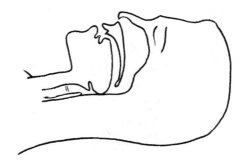

Figure 7–2. Hypopharyngeal obstruction in comatose patient in supine position. Obstruction results from relaxation of muscles of the jaw, tongue, and pharyngeal wall, causing backward displacement of the base of the tongue.

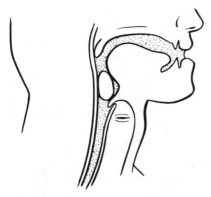

Figure 7–3. Hypopharyngeal obstruction by a bolus of food.

treatment effectively popularized in recent years, thanks to J. J. Heimlich's innovative effort.

Other causes of pharyngeal obstruction include neoplastic lesions, traumatic injury, and marked inflammatory swelling and/or abscess of the pharyngeal wall.

LARYNGEAL OBSTRUCTION

Because of peculiarities of structure and anatomic position of the larynx, this organ is a frequent site for upper airway obstruction from a variety of causes. The small size of the larynx in young children especially predisposes them to laryngeal obstruction. The most common cause in this age group is inflammation of laryngeal structures due to infection.

Supraglottic obstruction is commonly due to *epiglottitis*, which is one of the most serious infectious diseases in young children. It is usually caused by *Hemophilus influenzae*, although other bacteria and viruses may be involved. The onset of the disease is sudden, with sore throat, high fever, and **prostration.**

Inspiratory dyspnea develops rapidly, manifested by *stridor* and inspiratory retraction of intercostal and supraclavicular spaces. Because of the rapidity of progression of airway obstruction, early recognition of this condition is essential for institution of proper and life-saving measures. Epiglottitis in adults is less dramatic but may at times cause significant airway obstruction.

Glottic obstruction may occur from a tumor, a foreign body, or bilateral paralysis of vocal cords.

The most common cause of *subglottic* obstruction in children is croup, which includes several infectious conditions involving the larynx, trachea, and bronchi (laryngotracheobronchitis). It is characterized by a barking or "croupy" cough, which may or may not be associated with hoarseness and signs of upper airway obstruction. It has almost always a viral etiology, parainfluenza virus being involved in most cases.

Laryngeal obstruction may occur as a result of other conditions, which include congenital defects, allergic laryngeal edema, neoplastic lesions, and traumatic injury. The latter may result from endotracheal intubation. Diphtheria used to be one of the most common causes of laryngeal obstruction in the past. Fortunately, it is rarely encountered nowadays in the United States thanks to preventive vaccination.

TRACHEAL OBSTRUCTION

Tracheal lesions are uncommon causes of upper airway obstruction. Well-recognized conditions resulting in tracheal obstruction are tracheal stenosis (following tracheostomy, prolonged tracheal intubation, or trauma) and tumors.

The latter may be an intralumenal growth such as tracheal carcinoma or an extralumenal mass lesion compressing the trachea, particularly its intrathoracic portion.

DIAGNOSIS OF UPPER AIRWAY OBSTRUCTION

Prompt and accurate diagnosis of upper airway obstruction, its location, and its cause is the key for its proper management. Complete obstruction with no airflow should be diagnosed and treated on the scene immediately. In confronting an unconscious patient, who may or may not be breathing, the possibility of airway obstruction should always be considered, and the establishment and maintenance of an adequate airway should be given the highest priority. In a situation in which there is no airflow, obstructed airway will be recognized in the process of resuscitation when the lungs cannot be inflated by artificial means or by mouth-to-mouth respiration. The diagnosis of complete airway obstruction from food lodged in the hypopharynx is often made by individuals witnessing the incident. The victim, while eating, suddenly stops breathing and is unable to make any sound or cough, becoming pale and agitated. If he knows the "universal distress sign for choking," he may grab his neck over the larynx with his thumb and index finger (Fig. 7–4).

Partial upper airway obstruction is usually suspected, and diagnosed, from a history and a physical examination. History of aspiration of a foreign object; traumatic injury or infection in or around the upper airways; alteration of

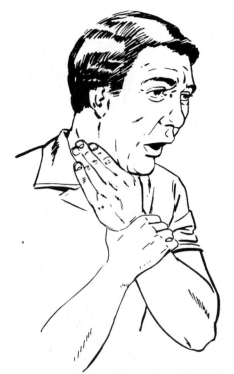

Figure 7–4. Universal distress signal for choking.

voice; and respiratory symptoms of dyspnea, cough, wheezing, and stridor should alert one to the possibility of partial obstruction. Physical findings of hoarseness or aphonia, inspiratory stridor, inspiratory and expiratory wheezes originating from the upper airway, inspiratory retraction of intercostal spaces and supraclavicular regions, and mass lesions in the pharynx are helpful diagnostic clues.

As epiglottitis is a most serious cause of upper airway obstruction, particularly in children, it should be suspected when a sudden onset of fever is associated with sore throat, difficulty in swallowing, and drooling. Signs of upper airway obstruction may supervene in a dramatic fashion, usually within 12 hours of the first clinical manifestation. An attempt at direct visualization of the epiglottis should not be made in suspected epiglottitis unless it is done by an otolaryngologist in a well-equipped area. A lateral x-ray of the neck is diagnostic, but should be done only when the diagnosis is in doubt and there is no imminent danger of airway obstruction.

Croup is usually diagnosed in a young child by its characteristic sudden onset of harsh barking cough with varying degrees of inspiratory stridor, occurring after a few days of upper respiratory tract symptoms. It has a fluctuating course, usually with nocturnal worsening, which lasts several days followed by full recovery in most pa-

tients. Only an occasional child may progress to life-threatening upper airway obstruction.

The diagnosis of less acute or chronic airway obstruction from other causes, suspected from a history or a physical examination, is made by direct visualization or by endoscopy of the suspected area and appropriate radiologic studies, including computerized tomographic (CT) scanning. These studies also help in estimating the severity of the obstruction and selecting as well as timing of necessary therapeutic measures.

Partial upper airway obstruction is sometimes mistaken for disease of the lower respiratory tract, particularly asthma. Vocal cord dysfunction without

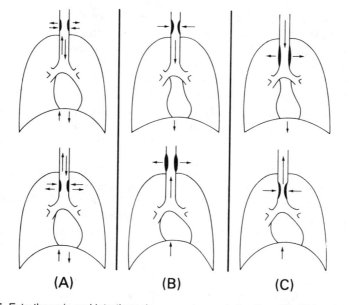

(A) **(B)** **(C)**

Figure 7–5. Extrathoracic and intrathoracic upper airway obstruction. (A), With a fixed obstruction, either extrathoracic (top) or intrathoracic (bottom), the obstruction size does not change with forced inspiration or expiration. (B), With variable extrathoracic obstruction, the obstruction is increased during forced inspiration (top) and is decreased during forced expiration. (C), With variable intrathoracic obstruction, the obstruction is diminished with forced inspiration (top) and increased with forced expiration (bottom).

an organic cause may sometimes result in significant respiratory difficulty, which is often erroneously diagnosed as asthma. Long-standing upper airway obstruction may also mimic chronic obstructive lung disease by its respiratory symptoms and complications, including hypoxemia, hypercapnia, and cor pulmonale. It also may manifest itself as sleep apnea syndrome (see Chapter 24).

Pulmonary Function Studies in Upper Airway Obstruction

Routine spirometry of a forced expiratory vital capacity may suggest the presence of partial upper airway obstruction. The maximum expiratory-inspiratory flow-volume loop, however, is most informative. Airways are subjected to changes in their lumen during a respiratory cycle according to the location of the airway inside or outside the thorax. Intrathoracic airways will tend to widen during inspiration and narrow during expiration. The reverse is true with extrathoracic airways. This is because of changes in transmural pressure (the difference between the intraluminal and external pressure) during the respiratory cycle. If an obstructing lesion is pliable and thus influenced by the transmural pressure, it is called variable; if stiff and unyielding to pressure changes, it is termed fixed (Fig. 7–5). Therefore, in upper airway obstruction, a fixed lesion, regardless of its intrathoracic or extrathoracic location, will limit the airflow during both expiration and inspiration. A flow-volume loop obtained in a patient with this type of obstruction will show flattening of both the inspiratory and expiratory curves (Fig. 7–6B).

With an extrathoracic variable obstruction, the inspiratory half of the loop is mostly affected and thus flattened (Fig. 7–6C); whereas with intrathoracic variable obstruction, the expiratory curve is flat (Fig. 7–6D).

MANAGEMENT OF UPPER AIRWAY OBSTRUCTION

The therapeutic strategy in upper airway obstruction will depend on several factors, which include the degree of obstruction; its progression, nature, and location; and associated conditions. However, the immediate therapeutic goal is the same, ie, establishing and maintaining adequate airflow.

In the management of unconscious patients with an obstruction resulting from backward displacement of the jaw and tongue, extending the neck and moving the mandible forward by chin lift will usually correct the pharyngeal obstruction. Extending the neck separates the posterior wall of the pharynx from the base of the tongue, while displacing the mandible forward by chin lift widens the pharynx further (Figs. 7–7 and 7–8). It should, be emphasized, however, that whenever a traumatic cause for unconsciousness is suspected, the possibility of concomitant injury to the cervical spine should be considered and necessary precautions undertaken. Any foreign material or secretion should be removed by suctioning or other means. Insertion of an oropharyngeal or nasopharyngeal airway will help to maintain airway patency in unconscious patients.

The principle of management of complete airway obstruction occurring as the result of impaction of food in the hypopharynx is the dislodgement of the obstructing material. As this should be

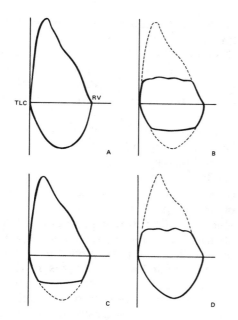

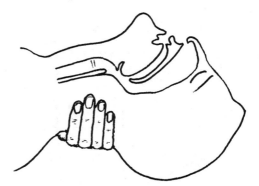

Figure 7–7. Extension of the neck results in opening of the obstructed airway from loss of consciousness.

Figure 7–6. Maximum expiratory-inspiratory flow-volume loop. (A), normal; (B), fixed (extrathoracic or intrathoracic) obstruction; (C), variable extrathoracic obstruction; and (D), variable intrathoracic obstruction.

done immediately and at the scene by a lay person, the maneuvers used are indirect and are based on exerting sudden pressure over the chest or below the diaphragm. An increase in intrathoracic pressure by its transmission to the upper airway jolts the occluding material loose, and it is subsequently ejected. These maneuvers include the well-known *Heimlich maneuver* (abdominal thrust, as in Fig. 7–9), chest thrust, and back blows. As they are abundantly popularized in lay publications and graphically displayed in restaurants, they will not be discussed in this book. Readers interested in further information should consult the publications on the subject, some of which appear in the references at the end of this chapter.

Patients with **epiglottitis** should be immediately hospitalized and closely observed, preferably in a respiratory care unit. Securing an adequate airway is the most important aspect of its management. Early endotracheal intubation is considered by many experts to be the method of choice in these patients, although some still prefer tracheostomy. As most cases are due to infection with *H influenzae,* an effective antibiotic against this organism should be administered. A short-course treatment with corticosteroids is also recommended.

Children with **croup** should be hos-

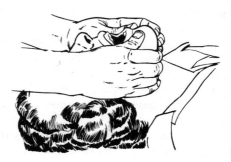

Figure 7–8. Maneuver for backward tilting of the head, forward displacement of the mandible, and opening of the mouth.

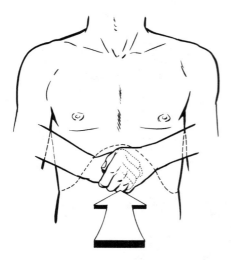

Figure 7–9. Position of hands and direction of pressure in Heimlich maneuver.

pitalized if there is any evidence of an impaired airway or if **supraglottitis** cannot be excluded. Otherwise, most patients are managed symptomatically at home with proper instruction to the parents. As croup is a viral illness, antibiotics have no role in its treatment unless there is a bacterial superinfection. Adequate humidification and oxygenation with or without the use of inhalational therapy (eg, racemic epinephrine) are all that is needed in the management of croup when there is no significant airway obstruction.

Allergic swelling of the upper airway (angioedema of the larynx) is treated with systemic epinephrine, antihistamines, and corticosteroids. Rarely, mechanical airway restoration will be needed.

Most causes of less acute or chronic upper airway obstruction are due to lesions treatable only by surgical intervention. Tracheostomy for lesions located in the larnyx or proximal to it will

often be necessary. For unresectable tracheal cancer, laser therapy has shown excellent short-term success.

A temporizing measure useful in some instances of upper airway obstruction is the administration of a low-density gas mixture, which reduces the resistance due to obstruction in the large airways. One such mixture is helium-oxygen, which is given in a ratio of 80/20, unless a higher oxygen concentration is desired. Although restoration of an adequate airway is the primary objective of treatment in upper airway obstruction, sometimes because of technical difficulty or patient refusal, administration of a low-density gas mixture may provide rapid relief. If the obstruction is nonprogressive and reversible, it may obviate the necessity for surgery. This method can also improve a marginal airflow to one that would allow adequate time for changing an emergency bedside procedure to one that can be done in an operating room.

BIBLIOGRAPHY

Acres JC, Kryger MH. Clinical significance of pulmonary function tests: upper airway obstruction. *Chest.* 1981; 80:207–211.

Christopher KL, Wood RP, Echert RC, et al. Vocal cord dysfunction presenting as asthma. *N Engl J Med.* 1983; 308:1566–1570.

Davis HW, Gartner JC, Galvis AG, et al. Acute upper airway obstruction: croup and epiglottitis. *Pediatr Clin North Am.* 1981; 28:859–880.

Heimlich HJ, Uhley MH. The Heimlich maneuver. *Clin Symposia.* 1979; 31(3):3–32.

Hoffman JR. Treatment of foreign body obstruction of the upper airway. *West J Med.* 1982; 136:11–22.

Levin DL, Muster AJ, Pachman LM, et al.

Cor pulmonale secondary to upper airway obstruction. *Chest*. 1975; 68:166–171.

Mandel EM, Reynolds CF. Sleep disorders associated with upper airway obstruction in children. *Pediatr Clin North Am*. 1981; 28(4):897–903.

O'Hollaren MT. Masqueraders in clinical allergy: laryngeal dysfunction causing dyspnea. *Ann Allergy*. 1990; 65:351–356.

Olsen KD, Kern EB, Westbrook PR. Sleep and breathing disturbance secondary to nasal obstruction. *Otolaryngol Head Neck Surg*. 1981; 89:804–810.

Rodenstein DO, Stanescu DC. The soft palate and breathing. *Am Rev Respir Dis*. 1986; 134:311–325.

Sheikh KH, Mostow SR. Epiglottitis—An increasing problem for adults. *West J Med*. 1989; 151:520–524.

Skrinskas GJ, Hyland RH, Hutcheon MA. Using helium-oxygen mixtures in the management of acute upper airway obstruction. *Can Med Assoc J*. 1983; 128:555–558.

Standards and guidelines for cardiopulmonary resuscitation (CPR) and emergency cardiac care (ECC). *JAMA*. 1986; 255: 2905–2984.

Stretton M, Newth CJL. Croup and epiglottitis: key to successful therapy. *J Respir Dis*. 1991; 12:86–94.

Thompson DS. Emergency airway management. *Am Fam Physician*. 1975; 11(5):146–153.

Zulliger JJ, Schuller DE, Beach TP, et al. Assessment of intubation in croup and epiglottitis. *Ann Otol Rhinol Laryngol*. 1982; 91:403–406.

CHAPTER 8

Chronic Obstructive Pulmonary Disease

Chronic obstructive pulmonary disease (COPD) is a clinical term used to include groups of conditions associated with chronic obstruction to air flow within the lungs. These conditions consist of chronic bronchitis, emphysema, and asthma, although bronchiectasis and cystic fibrosis are also sometimes included.

Chronic obstructive lung disease, also known as chronic airflow obstruction (CAO), is by far the most common chronic pulmonary disorder. It has been estimated that over 15 million Americans have the disease. Disability from COPD is second only to that from heart disease.

Despite development of a vast body of knowledge in this area, there is still a great deal of controversy over definitions and terminology. Those relating to early stages have not yet been universally accepted and the role of small airway disease as a forerunner of chronic bronchitis and emphysema has not been conclusively established. Emphysema is defined in anatomic terms, whereas chronic bronchitis and asthma are defined in clinical terms. Frequent overlapping of these three conditions adds to the complexity. Because of coexistence of two or more of these conditions and frequent difficulty in differentiating them clinically, the designation of "chronic obstructive pulmonary disease" is a useful one in clinical medicine. For descriptive purposes, however, we shall discuss them separately.

CHRONIC BRONCHITIS

Chronic bronchitis is defined as chronic excessive production of mucus from the bronchi not due to known specific disease such as tuberculosis or bronchiectasis. It manifests clinically by cough and increased sputum for at least 3 consecutive months each year for 2 successive years. The anatomical correlate is an increase in size and number of the mucus-producing elements in the bronchi.

Etiology. The major factors associated with chronic bronchitis are tobacco smoking and age. There is also a significant difference in its incidence between males and females; middle-aged males are most commonly afflicted. By far, the most important etiologic factor is *cigarette smoking*. A direct relationship exists between the amount and the duration of cigarette smoking and the severity of bronchitis, although significant individual variation occurs in the effect of smoking on the respiratory tract. The etiologic role of other factors, without the effect of smoking, appears to be much less important.

Severe and recurrent respiratory infection in childhood has been implicated as a cause of increased susceptibility to the harmful effects of smoking later in life and, therefore, may have an ancillary role. A direct role for infection, however, has not been definitely established in the etiology of chronic bronchitis. The role of infection is more significant in exacerbation of symptoms and progressive deterioration of the clinical course. Earlier in the course of chronic bronchitis, the sputum consists only of mucus, indicating lack of infection. A change, however, in the sputum to a more purulent state in the course of the disease is indicative of intercurrent bacterial infection. Thus, the role of bacterial infection in chronic bronchitis is mainly a secondary one. Infection with respiratory viruses is probably a common precipitating cause of acute exacerbations, but there is no evidence to implicate viruses as a primary factor in the etiology of chronic bronchitis. Recurrent acute bronchitis in nonsmokers with otherwise normal lungs does not seem to proceed to chronic bronchitis.

Compared with cigarette smoking, the significance of air pollution as an etiologic factor in chronic bronchitis is much less important. Chronic bronchitis is a rare disease among the nonsmoking population. Heavy atmospheric pollution with sulfur dioxide (SO_2) and particulate matter is an important factor in exacerbation of this condition.

Pathology and Pathogenesis. There has been no general agreement on morphologic criteria for pathologic diagnosis of chronic bronchitis. The increased mucus production is due to enlargement of bronchial *mucous glands* and an increase in the number of *goblet cells*. They are the most consistent pathologic changes. Other pathologic findings include the presence of mucous plugs in the peripheral airways, inflammation of bronchial and bronchiolar walls, loss of **cilia,** and other changes due to complicating factors, particularly infection. In advanced stages of chronic bronchitis, emphysematous changes are also present. The bronchial secretion in chronic bronchitis has a somewhat different composition, resulting in alteration of the consistency of sputum and difficulty in its removal.

The pathogenic mechanism of chronic bronchitis is not entirely clear. There is ample evidence, however, that chronic and protracted irritation of bronchial mucosa is the major factor in causing hypertrophy and hyperplasia of mucus-producing glands and cells, as well as in perpetuating the mucosal inflammation. Decrease in ciliary function and alteration in physicochemical characteristics of bronchial secretions impair their clearance, predisposing to recurrent respiratory infection. Damaged and inflamed mucosa enhances the sensitivity of the irritant receptors which, in turn, causes bronchial hyperreactivity.

Pathophysiology. Physiologic changes in chronic bronchitis are related to narrowing of the airways. Most patients with chronic bronchitis however, have normal airway resistance. In this so-called *simple bronchitis,* maximal expiratory flow rates are normal, although more sensitive tests for determining obstruction of small airways are frequently abnormal. This apparent discrepancy is due to the fact that the contribution by the small airways (with a diameter of less than 2 mm) to the total flow resistance is relatively small and not readily detectable. The term *obstructive bronchitis* is used when there is a significant and easily identifiable increase in airway resistance. The latter is the result of obstructive changes in larger airways from narrowing of their lumen and increased secretions. In addition to the alteration of lung mechanics due to airflow obstruction, maldistribution of ventilation is almost always present. Mismatching of ventilation with perfusion of blood causes abnormality of gas exchange as reflected in the alteration of blood gases. With advancing disease and increasing airway obstruction, progressive hypoxemia and hypercapnia (respiratory failure) develop. Increased pulmonary vascular resistance, right-side heart failure, and sometimes polycythemia are other late complications.

Clinical Manifestations. The majority of patients with chronic bronchitis are so accustomed to the symptoms of cough and expectoration that they will not be disturbed by them and, therefore, will not seek medical care. Many will deny any symptoms, and only upon careful and repeated questioning will they admit having cough and sputum production. The patients whose symptoms consist of only cough and expectoration of mucus for many years

are considered to have *simple uncomplicated chronic bronchitis.* Other patients will give a history of frequent "chest colds" with exacerbation of symptoms: cough becoming more severe and sputum more abundant and often purulent. The onset of dyspnea, which indicates the development of significant airway obstruction, is usually insidious, but may show abrupt exacerbations with bouts of respiratory infection. These patients are considered to have *obstructive* chronic bronchitis. Dyspnea is at first mild and brought about only by exertion. Some patients will adjust their way of life and activities in order to avoid this symptom. With the progression of disease, the patients will become more and more dyspneic with less and less effort, eventually remaining dyspneic all the time. At this stage, other symptoms of respiratory failure will be evident.

The physical examination usually reveals no significant abnormal findings in patients with the *simple* form of chronic bronchitis. In the *obstructive* form, there may be evidence of prolonged expiration and wheezing. Rales, which usually clear with coughing, are due to presence of secretions in the airways. In the more advanced stage of chronic bronchitis, patients are dyspneic at rest, and features of emphysema may be present (see below). Signs of respiratory failure are discussed elsewhere. (Chapter 25)

Radiographic Study. The radiographic changes in uncomplicated chronic bronchitis are not significant. Abnormalities such as hyperinflation and increased lung markings are usually due to concomitant emphysema or other complicating causes.

Pulmonary Function Tests. In the early stage and in uncomplicated chronic bronchitis, routine pulmonary function studies with a spirometer are usually normal. However, with more sensitive tests that identify obstruction of small airways, it is possible to demonstrate this abnormality in most cases. Measurement of the closing volume is one of the useful tests for this purpose. Increased residual volume may be the first detectable physiologic abnormality in the natural history of chronic obstructive bronchitis. In more advanced stages of the disease, flow rates, as demonstrated by spirometric tests, or flow-volume studies, are abnormal. In addition to expiratory flow limitation (as in emphysema), inspiratory flow rates are also reduced in obstructive chronic bronchitis. The total lung capacity is usually normal.

Management. As therapeutic measures in chronic bronchitis are also applicable to pulmonary emphysema, to avoid repetition, they will be discussed under the heading of Management of Chronic Obstructive Pulmonary Disease at the end of this chapter.

Course and Prognosis. As was indicated earlier, the course of chronic bronchitis is quite variable. Most patients will have symptoms of chronic cough and expectoration for many years without developing any disability or complication and have a normal life span. On the other hand, some patients will progress to a more symptomatic stage with increasing airway obstruction and deterioration of pulmonary function, with or without frequent respiratory tract infections. They may reach the stage of severe respiratory insufficiency and failure. Pulmonary emphysema is a common complication of chronic bron-

chitis. In the early stage of the disease, it is almost impossible to predict the course of chronic bronchitis. Once the patient shows evidence of pulmonary functional abnormality, the prognosis becomes much less favorable. Obviously, factors such as cessation of smoking and proper therapy will influence the outcome.

PULMONARY EMPHYSEMA

Definition and Classification. Pulmonary emphysema is defined in anatomical terms as permanent abnormal enlargement of air spaces distal to terminal bronchioles associated with destructive changes of alveolar walls.

The terminal bronchiole is a purely conducting structure, but the generations of airways distal to it have increasingly more alveoli in their walls (Fig. 8–1). The portion of the lung distal to the

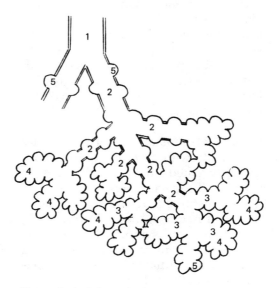

Figure 8–1. Schematic drawing of normal distal airways and air spaces (acinus). (1) Terminal bronchiole; (2) respiratory bronchiole; (3) alveolar duct; (4) alveolar sac; (5) alveoli.

terminal bronchiole is called **acinus,** which is considered by some to be the anatomic unit of the lung. There are some 25,000 such units, which make up about 300 million total alveoli of the lungs.

Simple overdistension of the air spaces without destructive lesions, seen in an asthmatic attack, old age, or compensatory overdistension of remaining lung after pneumonectomy, should not be considered as emphysema (Fig. 8–2).

Depending on the site of involvement in the acinus, emphysema has been divided into several forms. The most common ones are **centrilobular** and **panlobular.** In centrilobular or centriacinar emphysema, the lesion is in the center of the lobules, which corresponds to enlargement and destructive changes in the respiratory bronchioles (Fig. 8–3). This form of emphysema often involves the upper lung fields and is almost always associated with chronic bronchitis. It rarely occurs in nonsmokers.

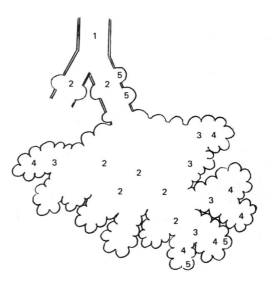

Figure 8–3. Centrilobular emphysema.

In panlobular or **panacinar** emphysema (Fig. 8–4), which is less common than the centrilobular variety, the entire acinus is more or less involved. The normal architecture of the alveoli and other air spaces is lost. They are enlarged and their septa are destroyed, resulting in significant loss of pulmonary parenchyma. Many bullae of various sizes are often present. Panlobular emphysema occurs throughout the lung, but lower and anterior lung fields are more predominantly involved. Its correlation with cigarette smoking is less than in centrilobular emphysema. Emphysema in association with familial alpha$_1$-antiprotease deficiency (see below) is usually panlobular.

Bullous emphysema or bullous disease of the lung usually refers to a pulmonary condition in which there are isolated emphysematous changes with development of bullae, in the apparent absence of underlying generalized emphysema. A **bulla** is defined as an air space that measures more than 1 cm in diameter in

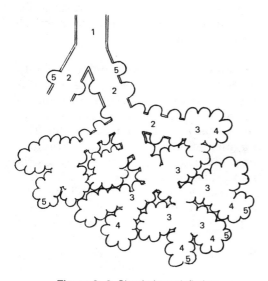

Figure 8–2. Simple hyperinflation.

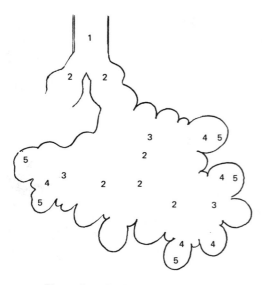

Figure 8–4. Panlobular emphysema.

its distended state. Superficial subpleural collection of air is referred to as a **bleb.** The sizes of bullous lesions vary considerably; sometimes a single or several bullae may occupy a large portion of the hemithorax (giant bulla), compressing the adjacent lung tissue. Bullous changes are not uncommonly seen with generalized emphysema.

Etiology and Pathogenesis. Because of a definite relationship between cigarette smoking and chronic bronchitis, which is frequently associated with emphysema, it is inevitable to conclude that smoking is the major known etiologic factor in pulmonary emphysema. Emphysema, however, is known to occur in individuals who have never smoked, and many patients with long-standing chronic bronchitis do not develop clinically significant emphysema. Therefore, it seems that other factors, some genetic and familial, are involved in the pathogenesis of emphysema.

A small minority of patients with emphysema are known to have a genetically determined deficiency of a serum compound that normally inhibits the effect of **proteases** (enzymes that digest proteins). This compound, referred to as alpha$_1$-**antiprotease** (antitrypsin), also blocks the enzymatic effect of proteases on elastin and collagen, the major protein components of the lung structure. Proteases, including **elastase,** which are present in the polymorphonuclear leukocytes and macrophages, may be released from them during an inflammatory process. Based on this information and experimental studies of papain-induced emphysema in animals, the "protease-antiprotease" hypothesis of pathogenesis of emphysema has developed. According to this theory, the major factor resulting in alveolar disruption in emphysema is the elastin-attacking enzyme (elastase) released from the phagocytic cells, unopposed by its inhibitor. Protease/antiprotease imbalance, best exemplified by alpha$_1$-antiprotease deficiency, may result from factors such as infection, respiratory irritants (cigarette smoke), and inactivation of inhibitors.

Pathophysiology. Although commonly associated chronic bronchitis contributes to airway obstruction in emphysema, *airflow limitation* in pure emphysema has a different mechanism. The fragmentation and disruption of pulmonary elastic tissue, which also supports noncartilagenous distal airways, cause reduced *elastic recoil* of the lung. Increased intrathoracic pressure during expiration results in the collapse and the premature closure of the airways that lack the support of radial traction by the elastic parenchyma. As this is the major mechanism of increased flow resistance in pure emphysema, flow rates are affected only during expiration; unless there is associated obstructive bronchitis, inspiratory flow rates are normal. *Large residual volume,* another characteristic feature of emphysema, is due to early closure of airways (air trapping) as well as overdistended air spaces. Lung capacities that include residual volume (FRC, TLC) are also increased. The area of gas-exchanging surface of the alveolar-capillary membrane is reduced as a result of disruption and destruction of alveolar walls. This pathologic change is responsible for the *reduction of diffusing capacity* in emphysema. Airway resistance and compliance in different regions of the lung in emphysema are quite variable due to nonuniformity of pathologic changes. This is the cause of *uneven ventilation* and *mismatching of ventilation with blood flow,* which, in turn, explain the *increased physiologic dead space* and *abnormal blood gases* demonstrated in emphysema.

Clinical Manifestations. The symptoms of pulmonary emphysema are variable and by no means specific. Patients with localized emphysema usually have no symptoms. Frequently, the symptoms of chronic bronchitis with cough and expectoration predominate the clinical picture, at least in the early stage. **Dyspnea,** which initially occurs only with exertion, gradually increases in its intensity. It is almost impossible to be certain in patients with chronic bronchitis if or when emphysema has occurred. Patients without preceding or complicating bronchitis may develop exertional dyspnea as the only symptom, cough and expectoration being

absent. The rate of progression of dyspnea is variable. Some patients will have a very slow and imperceptible increase in their shortness of breath; others will have a more rapid progression of dyspnea and onset of disability. Most patients will adjust their physical activities in order to avoid or minimize their symptoms. Nevertheless, dyspnea will occur with less and less effort until the patients remain short of breath even at rest.

Severity of dyspnea does not always correlate with the degree of pathologic or physiologic abnormalities. Although some patients with chronic airway obstruction will increase their ventilation in order to maintain relatively normal blood gases, others, with the same amount of disease, will show less, if any, change in their ventilatory effort. The patients in the first group will have more dyspnea than the patients in the latter group. This difference in response is probably due to a difference in sensitivity of the respiratory centers or their chemoreceptors.

As in chronic bronchitis, the course of pulmonary emphysema is frequently interspersed by periods of exacerbation of symptoms, usually related to intercurrent infections or other complications. The onset of respiratory failure is also usually precipitated by such events.

Physical findings may be normal in mild or localized emphysema. In more advanced cases, there is evidence of an enlarged thoracic volume with an increase in the anteroposterior diameter of the chest. Dorsal kyphosis, prominent anterior chest, elevated ribs, flaring of costal margin, and widening of costal angle give the chest the appearance of a barrel (Fig. 8–5). The patient may appear dyspneic, using his accessory respira-

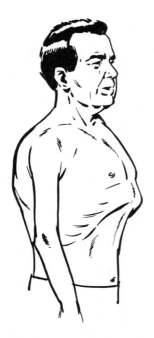

Figure 8–5. Barrel chest of emphysema.

tory muscles. To facilitate their use, some patients assume a sitting position, bend over, and rest the elbows on their thighs. The expiratory phase of respiration is prolonged, and the patient may be breathing against pursed lips. Overdistension of the lungs manifests by increased resonance to percussion, which may include areas that are normally dull (eg, over the heart or liver). Breath sounds are reduced in intensity and may be difficult to hear. Sometimes, expiratory wheezes may be heard. Heart sounds appear distant. Other physical findings, such as cyanosis and other signs of respiratory failure, may be present in the advanced stage of emphysema. (Chapter 25)

Radiographic Changes. Changes in the chest x-ray of patients with emphysema are variable and depend on type,

extent, and severity of the disease. Several radiographic changes correlate with the presence of emphysema. These include depression and flattening of the diaphragm, **hyperlucency,** reduced vascular markings, widened space between the sternum and the heart, and increased anteroposterior diameter of the chest (Figs. 8–6 and 8–7). Most of these

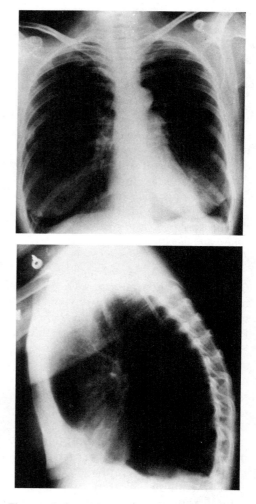

Figures 8–6 and 8–7. Posteroanterior and lateral radiographs of the chest in a patient with severe emphysema.

changes are indicative of overinflation. Demonstration of bullous lesions, however, is an unequivocal x-ray sign of emphysema. Sometimes chest radiograph may show increased markings without x-ray evidence of hyperinflation. Thus, although chest x-ray films may show characteristic and even diagnostic radiographic changes, their absence does not exclude the diagnosis of pulmonary emphysema.

Pulmonary Function Tests. In emphysema, hyperinflation is due to *increased* residual volume, which may be as high as several times normal (Fig. 8–8). Therefore, FRC is also increased. Body plethysmography will give a more accurate determination of these parameters than the gas equilibration method because of the presence of poorly communicating regions of the lung. Despite *reduction* of *vital capacity* in emphysema, *total lung capacity* is generally increased.

The ratio of residual volume to the total lung capacity is greatly increased. Expiratory flow rates are good indicators of the severity of emphysema. The forced spirogram is usually characteristic (Fig. 8–9). FEV_1 and MMFR are useful parameters in evaluating the severity and progression of the disease. Maximal expiratory flow-volume (MEFV) curve is a sensitive test for detection of early emphysema. Reduction of diffusing capacity in emphysema usually differentiates it from other forms of COPD (ie, chronic bronchitis and asthma). Nitrogen washout is prolonged, and other tests of intrapulmonary gas mixing are abnormal.

Arterial blood studies may show normal findings in mild, even moderate, emphysema, but they are abnormal in more advanced cases. Reduced arterial PO_2 is the most common abnormality, particularly during exacerbations. Although often normal, arterial PCO_2 may

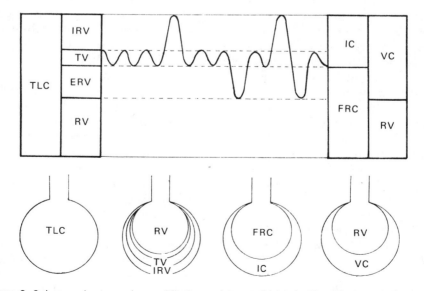

Figure 8–8. Lung volumes and capacities in emphysema. Note significant increase in residual volume.

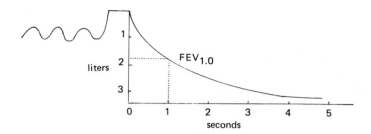

Figure 8–9. Forced spirogram in emphysema. $FEV_{1.0}$ is less than 50% of vital capacity, which is also reduced.

be chronically elevated and/or may show an acute rise during an intercurrent infection or other complications.

Course and Prognosis. The natural course of pulmonary emphysema is variable; some patients will show rapid progression of their disease with early onset of disability; others will have a much slower rate of change in their respiratory function. It appears, however, that most patients will have a fairly predictable slow decline in their pulmonary functions, as judged from yearly deterioration of expiratory flow rates. It has been estimated that the average time from the onset of the disease to the stage of severe respiratory impairment is about 20 to 25 years. There is a good correlation between the severity of airway obstruction, as judged by FEV_1, and mortality from emphysema. With an FEV_1 below 750 mL, very few patients will survive 5 years. This is also the case once respiratory failure develops.

MANAGEMENT OF CHRONIC OBSTRUCTIVE PULMONARY DISEASE

In view of the well-establish role of smoking in the pathogenesis of chronic

bronchitis, complete cessation of smoking is the most effective preventive measure against this disease and the only certain means of favorably affecting its course. Early changes of chronic bronchitis, when the obstruction is limited to the small airways, are more or less reversible when the inciting factors are eliminated. With the prevailing uncertainty about the pathogenesis of emphysema, it is almost impossible to predict (except in individuals with alpha 1-antiprotease deficiency) who will develop the disease under the influence of environmental factors such as cigarette smoking. It is, therefore, important to avoid factors that are known or suspected to play a major role in the pathogenesis of emphysema. Unfortunately, the structural changes in well-established disease, particularly with emphysema, are irreversible; thus, prevention, or slowing of the progression of disease by avoiding further insults, should be one of the main objectives of its management.

Preliminary results of treatment of patients with alpha 1-antiprotease deficiency with the recently marketed drug Prolastin are promising in slowing the progression of their emphysema. The drug, also known as alpha 1-proteinase inhibitor, has to be administered intravenously throughout the patient's life. Its long-term effectiveness remains to be determined.

The most important phase of treatment of established COPD is *outpatient management,* which should include measures to control the progression of the disease, to prevent complications and the need for frequent hospitalizations, to control or at least alleviate the symptoms, and to teach the patient how to cope with his illness and disability. Although the individual patient's needs are variable, these general measures are applicable to almost all patients with COPD.

In addition to cigarette smoke, other respiratory irritants should be avoided as much as possible. Patients should be instructed about proper bronchial hygiene by adequate hydration, humidification of inspired air, postural drainage, and other respiratory physiotherapeutic maneuvers. These simple and inexpensive measures would be adequate for treatment of the majority of patients with uncomplicated chronic bronchitis, and should also be considered as an important part of the therapeutic regimen in more advanced disease.

Expectorants and mucolytic agents have shown no significant therapeutic benefit in COPD. Although bronchodilators are often used in management of COPD, their therapeutic effectiveness has been demonstrated objectively in only a limited number of patients, especially in those with significant bronchospastic component to their airway obstruction. Drugs such as one of inhaled beta-adrenergic agents or a theophylline preparation may be used. Ipratropium bromide, an **anticholinergic** bronchodilator, seems to be more effective in COPD and has no significant side effects. Responders to inhaled bronchodi-

lators are also likely to respond to corticosteroids. The latter drugs should be administered after careful consideration because their prolonged use results in significant untoward effects.

Infection, bacterial as well as viral, plays a major role in the exacerbation of COPD and contributes significantly to the disability from this condition. It seems to be partly responsible for progressive deterioration of respiratory function in these patients. Preventive measures, such as immunization against pneumococcal infection and influenza, should be undertaken. In patients with frequent *bacterial* respiratory infections, antibiotic prophylaxis sometimes is considered. Most pulmonary specialists, however, prefer prompt use of antibiotics when there is evidence of bacterial infection, often judged by change in cough and characteristics of sputum to a more purulent form and sometimes supported by bacteriologic studies. The choice of antibiotic is based on the frequent isolation of pneumococci and/or *H influenzae* from the sputum of such patients. Two of the most commonly used antibiotics are ampicillin and one of the synthetic tetracyclines. A combination of trimethoprim with sulfamethoxazole (Septra or Bactrim) and some of the oral cephalosporins are excellent alternatives.

One of the most important aspects of outpatient management of COPD is the proper education of the patients, and/or their families, about their disease and adequate explanation of the therapeutic regimen. Success in their cooperation and compliance with treatment often depends on their understanding of their illness and measures directed toward it. Proper reconditioning exercise programs, breathing retraining, adequate nutrition, psychosocial support, and vocational counseling are essential for comprehensive care and rehabilitation of these patients.

When indicated, bronchodilators and sometimes corticosteroids are preferably administered in aerosolized form by hand nebulizers or metered dose inhalers. There is no significant advantage of IPPB therapy over simpler inhalation therapy in COPD patients, as was concluded in a recent multicenter trial. The use of IPPB for home management is not recommended.

Exercise programs are intended to help more efficient use of the respiratory muscles and to improve endurance. Although not resulting in any significant improvement in pulmonary function as determined by the usual tests, these programs are known to increase exercise tolerance and enhance the sense of well-being.

Patients with advanced disease remain in a state of chronic respiratory failure manifested by severe hypoxemia with or without hypercapnia. Such patients should be considered for continuous oxygen therapy if their arterial PO_2 is chronically lower than 55 torr or if there is evidence of cor pulmonale or secondary polycythemia with a P_aO_2 of less than 60 torr. It should be documented that hypoxemia persists despite optimal medical management. Some patients with COPD develop severe hypoxemia, sometimes to an alarmingly low level, during sleep, while they have only mild to moderate hypoxemia during wakefulness. These patients are candidates for nocturnal oxygen therapy.

Hospitalized patients with COPD usually have serious complications, including pneumonia and respiratory failure; or they are hospitalized for unrelated conditions. The management of patients with respiratory failure due to COPD is discussed in Chapter 25. Patients with COPD undergoing major thoracic or abdominal surgery are at much higher risk in developing respiratory complications. Proper preoperative and postoperative respiratory care will minimize these complications.

BIBLIOGRAPHY

Alpha$_1$-proteinase inhibitor for alpha$_1$-antitrypsin deficiency. *Med Lett Drugs Ther.* 1988; 30:29–30.

Anthonisen NR. Long-term oxygen therapy. *Ann Intern Med.* 1983; 99:519–527.

Bégin P, Grassino A. Inspiratory muscle dysfuncion and chronic hypercapnia in chronic obstructive pulmonary disease. *Am Rev Respir Dis.* 1991; 143:905–912.

Burrows B. Airways obstructive diseases: pathogenetic mechanisms and natural histories of the disorders. *Med Clin North Am.* 1990; 74:547–559.

Crofton J, Masironi R. Chronic airways disease: the smoking component. *Chest.* 1989; 96(suppl):349S–355S.

Crystal RG. α_1-antitrypsin deficiency: pathogenesis and treatment. Hosp Pract. 1991; 26(2):73–86.

Goldstein RS, Ramcharan V, Bowes G, et al. Effect of supplemental nocturnal oxygen on gas exchange in patients with severe obstructive lung disease. *N Engl J Med.* 1984; 310:425–429.

Griffith DE, Garcia JGN. Tobacco cigarettes, smoking, smoking cessation, and chronic obstructive pulmonary disease. *Semin Respir Med.* 1989; 10:356–371.

Gross NJ. The use of anticholinergic agents in the treatment of airways disease. *Clin Chest Med.* 1988; 9:591–598.

Gump DW, Phillips CA, Forsyth BR, et al. Role of infection in chronic bronchitis. *Am Rev Respir Dis.* 1976; 113:465–474.

Hodgkin JE. Prognosis in chronic obstructive pulmonary disease. *Clin Chest Med.* 1990; 11:555–569.

Idell S, Garcia JGN. Mechanisms of smoking-induced lung injury. *Semin Respir Med.* 1989; 10:345–355.

Intermittent positive pressure breathing therapy of chronic obstructive pulmonary disease: a clinical trial. *Ann Intern Med.* 1983; 99:612–620.

Janoff A. Elastases and emphysema: current assessment of the protease-antiprotease hypothesis. *Am Rev Respir Dis.* 1985; 132:417–433.

Kronenberg RS, Girard WM. Sleep disordered breathing in chronic obstructive pulmonary disease. *Semin Respir Med.* 1986; 8:171–176.

Murciano D, Aubier M, Lecocguic Y, Pariente R. Effects of theophylline on diaphragmatic strength and fatigue in patients with COPD. *N Engl J Med.* 1984; 311:349–353.

O'Connor GT, Sparrow D, Weiss ST. The role of allergy and nonspecific airway hyperresponsiveness in the pathogenesis of chronic pulmonary disease. *Am Rev Respir Dis.* 1989; 140:225–252.

Owens GR, Rogers RM, Pennock BE, Levin D. The diffusing capacity as a predictor of arterial oxygen desaturation during exercise in patients with chronic obstructive pulmonary disease. *N Engl J Med.* 1984; 310:1218–1221.

Pardy RL, Rivington RN, Despas PJ, Macklem PT. Inspiratory muscle training compared with physiotherapy in patients with chronic airflow limitation. *Am Rev Respir Dis.* 1981; 123:421–425.

Petty TL. Home oxygen—a revolution in the care of advanced COPD. *Med Clin North Am.* 1990; 74:715–729.

Phillipson EA, Goldstein RS. Breathing during sleep in chronic obstructive pulmonary disease. *Chest.* 1984; 85 (6, suppl):24S–30S.

Ramsdell JW, Nachtwey FJ, Moser KM. Bronchial hyperreactivity in chronic obstructive bronchitis. *Am Rev Respir Dis.* 1982; 126:829–832.

Rosen RL, Bone RC. Treatment of acute exacerbations in chronic obstructive pulmonary disease. *Med Clin North Am.* 1990; 74:691–700.

Samet JM, Tager IB, Speizer FE. The relationship between respiratory illness in childhood and chronic air-flow obstruction in adulthood. *Am Rev Respir Dis.* 1983; 127:508–523.

Silverman EK, Pierce JA, Province MA, et al. Variability of pulmonary function in alpha-1-antitrypsine deficiency: clinical correlates. *Ann Intern Med.* 1989; 111:982–991.

Snider GL. Chronic obstructive pulmonary disease: risk factors, pathophysiology, and pathogenesis. *Am Rev Med.* 1989; 40:411–429.

Stubbing DG, Mathur PN, Roberts RS, Campbell EJM. Some physical signs in patients with chronic airflow obstruction. *Am Rev Respir Dis.* 1982; 125:549–552.

Sweer L, Zwillich CW. Dyspnea in the patient with chronic obstructive pulmonary disease. *Clin Chest Med.* 1990; 11:417–445.

Swinburn CR, Mould H, Stone TN, et al. Symptomatic benefit of supplemental oxygen in hypoxemic patients with chronic lung disease. *Am Rev Respir Dis.* 1991; 143:913–915.

Ziment I. Pharmacologic therapy of obstructive airway disease. *Clin Chest Med.* 1990; 11:461–486.

CHAPTER 9

Asthma

Asthma is a respiratory disease characterized by an increased reactivity of the airways to various stimuli. It is manifested by periodic wheezing and dyspnea that improves either spontaneously or consequent to therapy. Clinical manifestations are the result of the widespread narrowing of the bronchi from bronchospasm, mucosal swelling, and increased secretions.

ETIOLOGY, PATHOGENESIS, AND CLASSIFICATION

Asthma is a common respiratory disease that may begin at any age. In about half of the cases, however, the onset is before age 10. In over one-third of the patients, there is a history of asthma in members of the immediate family. It is estimated that about 4% to 5% of the population in the United States has asthma.

Hyperreactivity of the airways, the central feature of asthma, is a condition in which the trachea and bronchi show an exaggerated sensitivity to the bronchoconstrictive effect of a variety of physical, pharmacologic, and biologic agents. As discussed on page 57, it can be verified by the inhalation of a small quantity of an agent, such as methacholine, which at that dose has little effect on normal individuals. Although the exact mechanism of airway hyperresponsiveness is unknown, several factors, including genetic predisposition, autonomous nervous imbalance, and the alteration of **adrenergic** receptors have been implicated in its development. There is increasing evidence, however, that inflammation of the airways, and their **epithelial** damage resulting from various factors, plays a major role in causing, augmenting, and sustaining bronchial hyperreactivity. Despite advancement in the understanding of the pathogenesis of asthma and the mechanisms of airway narrowing resulting from a variety of triggering factors, it has not been possible to develop a unifying etiologic concept for such a heterogenous clinical condition as asthma.

Depending on whether a *specific* external cause for asthma can be demonstrated or not, asthma is classified into extrinsic and intrinsic categories. As *nonspecific* stimuli may result in asthmatic reaction in both of these categories, they have no discriminating role in this classification. Because extrinsic asthma is most frequently the result of an **allergy,** the terms *allergic asthma* and *extrinsic asthma* are often used interchangeably. However, there are other causes of extrinsic asthma besides allergies, in which case it is known as *extrinsic nonallergic asthma*. Most cases of occupational asthma are considered to be nonallergic, but related to exposure to specific agents. In *intrinsic asthma*, no specific cause can be identified; there is no personal or family history of allergy; and it is most common in individuals whose asthma begins later in life. Despite this apparent distinction, a significant overlap exists between extrinsic and intrinsic asthma. Different factors in various combinations may be responsible in many cases, and thus it may be impossible to categorize them.

Regardless of the underlying causes of asthma, many factors trigger an asthma attack as nonspecific stimuli. Specific stimuli may also act as triggers, but only in sensitized asthmatics. In addition, airway reactivity is enhanced by some of the nonspecific, and almost all of the specific, factors when they cause airway inflammation and/or mucosal epithelial damage. Important factors that may precipitate or exacerbate an asthma attack are listed in Table 9–1. It

TABLE 9–1. PRECIPITATING OR EXACERBATING FACTORS IN ASTHMA

Allergens*
Viral infection of respiratory tract
Irritating dusts, fumes, or gases
Exercise—cold air
Occupational exposure to certain substances*
Aspirin and related anti-inflammatory drugs
Certain food additives and preservatives
Emotions
Esophageal reflux
Sleep

*Denotes specific factors; the rest are nonspecific.

should be noted, however, that in many instances the provoking cause of the asthma attack remains undetermined. Bronchial narrowing during an attack is from a varying combination of several changes. They include contraction of smooth muscles, increased secretions by mucous glands and goblet cells, edema of the bronchial wall, cellular infiltration, and the dilation of small blood vessels. The mechanism of production of these changes under diverse provoking factors may differ. The role of these factors and some of the well-recognized categories of asthma are briefly discussed below. Understanding their various pathogenetic mechanisms is very important in making rational therapeutic decisions.

Allergic Asthma

Allergic asthma, which commonly begins early in life, is an *immediate* or *type 1* hypersensitivity reaction that requires the presence of specific immunoglobulin E (IgE) class of antibodies. This type of reaction occurs in individuals who have **atopy,** which is a hypersensitivity state with a genetic predisposition characterized by the production of an excessive amount of IgE antibodies against a variety of antigens. About 10% to 20% of the general population are atopic and have the tendency to develop hay fever, asthma, eczema, and other IgE-mediated allergic reactions. These types of hypersensitivity reactions result from the interaction of antigens (allergens) with their specific IgE antibodies, which tend to attach to the mast cells, basophilic granulocytes, and perhaps other cells. Mast cells have the highest concentration of IgE molecules on their surface. The cross-linking of two IgE antibody molecules by specific antigen signals the initiation of a series of intracellular biochemical events, resulting in the release of several mediators. Some of these mediators are preformed and stored as specially stainable granules, and many others are rapidly synthesized as a result of the signal from the antigen-antibody interaction.

Among the many chemical mediators identified thus far, important ones are *histamine, eosinophil chemotactic factor of anaphylaxis* (*ECF-A*), *neutrophil chemotactic factor* (*NCF*), **leukotrienes** (formerly known as slow-reacting substance of **anaphylaxis,** or SRS-A), **prostaglandins,** and *platelet-activating factor*. The first three substances are preformed, while the last three are freshly synthesized from arachidonic acid, which is a phospholipid constituent. The respiratory tract is one of the few sites in which there is a large number of mast cells. In allergic asthma, the target organ for the mediators from these cells is the tracheobronchial tree. Their effects are on smooth muscles, microvasculature, mucous glands, and the migration of inflammatory cells. In addition, some of these mediators also stimulate sensory nerve endings in the airway epithelium leading to a reflex **bronchoconstriction** through the cholinergic effect of the **vagus nerve.** The common allergenic substances often incriminated in allergic asthma include pollens of trees, grass, and weeds; antigens of molds; house dust; house mites; and animal feather or dander.

There are certain patterns of asthmatic response to allergenic exposure. *Early response* occurs within several minutes of exposure to an inhaled antigen and resolves within about an hour. *Late asthmatic response* begins several hours after exposure and lasts much longer. A late asthmatic reaction may or may not follow an early response; it may also occur without an early reaction. When an immediate response is followed by a late one, it is called a *dual asthmatic response*. In addition to the difference in the time of occurrence and duration of these two basic responses, they are very dissimilar in their effect on the airway reactivity: while the immediate allergic response has little effect on the baseline bronchial hyperreactivity, late response enhances it significantly. As a result of a late asthmatic reaction, airways become even more susceptible to the bronchoconstrictive effect of both specific and nonspecific stimuli. This increased hyperresponsiveness that may persist long after antigenic exposure has stopped has been considered to be one of the reasons of the self-perpetuating state that is seen in some of the cases of untreated asthma.

Inflammation of the airways with an influx of certain blood cells, especially eosinophilic and neutrophilic granulocytes, has been implicated as the major cause of the late asthmatic response and the subsequent increase in airway hyperreactivity. Inflammatory cells, particularly eosinophils, are able to synthesize and release certain mediators that contribute to airway reaction either directly, or by stimulating mast cells. A mediator known as *histamine releasing factor* has been considered to play a major role. In addition, *major basic protein*, an important factor in eosinophilic granules, is known for its destructive effect on respiratory epithelium, which further enhances airway reactivity.

The increased production and release of various substances by mast cells are not limited to IgE-mediated allergic response. Many nonallergic causes of asthma may also operate through these mediators and share the same mechanism of airway obstruction, with the exception of the involvement of IgE antibodies (see Fig. 9–1). In many clinical situations, the distinction between allergic and nonallergic asthma is almost impossible.

Cholinergic response is a mechanism of bronchospasm in which the vagus nerve is involved. The airways are richly innervated by both the sensory and motor fibers of this nerve. Irritant receptors on the tracheobronchial mucosa are the sensory nerve endings, and the smooth muscles of the airways are innervated by its motor fibers. Stimulation of the vagus, either directly or indirectly, causes bronchospasm and increases mucosal secretions. It seems that mediators released from the mast cells and inflammatory cells interact with the action of the vagus nerve. Histamine, in addition to its direct effect on smooth muscles, may cause reflex bronchoconstriction by stimulating the sensory nerve endings of the vagus. Some of the mediators may sensitize the smooth muscles, making

them more susceptible to the bronchoconstrictive effect of vagal stimulation. On the other hand, stimulation of the vagus nerve facilitates mediator release by the mast cells. This interaction may create another positive feedback loop that sustains inflammation and bronchial narrowing (Fig. 9–1).

Occupational Asthma

Common atmospheric pollutants, including sulfur dioxide, nitrous oxide, ozone, and a variey of other noxious gases and aerosolized particulate matters are known to provoke or exacerbate bronchospasm in asthmatics, which can occur in various environments, including workplaces. The term *occupational asthma*, however, should be applied only to asthma of new onset resulting from prolonged exposure to specific inhaled substances in the work environment. Although an allergy may be the underlying mechanism in some workers, most patients with occupational asthma are not atopic and there is no evidence of an IgE-mediated

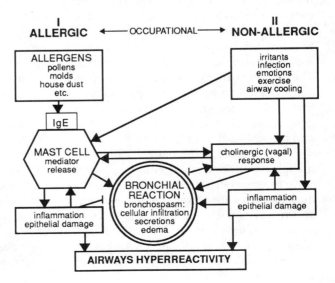

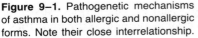

Figure 9–1. Pathogenetic mechanisms of asthma in both allergic and nonallergic forms. Note their close interrelationship.

hypersensitivity reaction. Chemical effects of some of the causative agents, other types of immunologic processes, and resultant inflammation have been considered in its pathogenesis. The percentage of workers who develop occupational asthma depends on the agent involved. For example, among workers exposed to toluene diisocyanate, an important cause of occupational asthma, about 10% develop asthma. As in allergic asthma, exposure to the specific inhaled substances in the workplace not only results in asthma attacks but also increases airway responsiveness to the same agents and to nonspecific asthma-provoking factors.

Numerous substances have been recognized to cause occupational asthma. The more common and important causes are isocyanates in workers involved with polyurethane, plastics, and varnish and car spray painters; trimellitic anhydride among workers with epoxy resins; organic dusts from various woods, plants, and grain flours in sawmill operators, tea workers, and bakers; animal products in laboratory workers or other animal handlers; enzymes among detergent and pharmaceutical manufacturers; and a variety of other chemicals in different workplaces.

Infection and Asthma

Respiratory tract infection is often suspected in acute asthmatic attacks. Although bacterial infection may occasionally be a complicating condition of asthma, viral upper respiratory tract infection is a much more frequent preceding event. Because of a lack of an obvious precipitating cause of nonallergic asthma, infection is considered to play a more important role. It seems,

however, that common viral respiratory tract infection also acts as a nonspecific factor in provoking bronchospasm in allergic asthma. Asthmatic episodes in children, whose asthma is most often allergy-related, are frequently precipitated by a viral respiratory tract infection. It has been demonstrated that infection with certain viruses, such as respiratory syncytial virus, rhinovirus, and influenza virus can cause transient airway hyperreactivity in normal subjects. In asthmatics, infection with such viruses may not only precipitate an asthma attack, but they may also increase airway responsiveness to other nonspecific provoking factors and, if sensitized, to certain specific agents. Inflammatory changes and epithelial injury are suggested to be the cause of increased airway responsiveness, as in allergic asthma. The relationship of aspergillus infection and asthma is discussed in Chapter 5.

Exercise-Induced Asthma

It is well-known that many asthmatic subjects, especially children and young adults, develop bronchospasm following exercise. This may be the first manifestation of asthma. Exercise usually has to be vigorous (eg, running fast for several minutes) to have a clinically significant effect on the airways, as it is the high minute ventilation that is essential for provoking a bronchospastic attack. It occurs *after*, rather than during exercise. The maximal bronchoconstriction occurs 5 to 10 minutes after the completion of exercise. Both the cooling and drying of the airway mucosa occur with the increased ventilation of exercise. The inspired air, before reaching the alveoli, is conditioned to be saturated with water vapor and to have a temperature of 37°C. This is accomplished by heat exchange with, and evaporation of water from, the airway mucosa. Although both heat exchange with inspired air and evaporation cause mucosal cooling, the latter is more important, which also causes water loss. With a high minute ventilation, the cooling and drying effect is increased. Exercise in cold dry air, such as cross-country skiing, is more likely to provoke a bronchoconstrictor response than exercise in a warm and humid environment, as swimming in a heated pool. Because the cooling and drying of the airways occur simultaneously, it is almost impossible to determine which of these mechanisms causes bronchospasm in exercise-induced asthma. As it has been shown that hypertonicity of the periciliary fluid in the bronchi can by itself cause bronchospasm, it seems that the water loss from the airways during vigorous exercise, especially in cold dry air, is a more important factor in causing bronchoconstriction. In exercise-induced asthma, both the cholinergic reaction as a result of the stimulation of irritant receptors of the airways, and mediator release from the mast cells, are most likely involved.

Asthma Related to the Intake of Aspirin, Food Additives, and Food Preservatives

Aspirin and other nonsteroidal anti-inflammatory drugs (NSAIDs) are known to precipitate or exacerbate asthma. About 10% to 20% of asthmatics have an associated sensitivity to aspirin or related drugs. Nasal polyps are often present in these patients, who are usually adults and have a more chronic and unremitting asthma. It is postulated that the mechanism of action of these drugs is through their effect on arachidonic acid metabolism, which results in the formation of an additional amount of leukotrienes. Sensitivity to aspirin and other NSAIDs has no definable immunologic basis and is considered to be an idiosyncratic reaction. There is a significant cross-reactivity between these agents.

Beta-adrenergic blocking agents, commonly used for the treatment of hypertension and some cardiac and noncardiac diseases, are known to cause or enhance an asthmatic attack. Most of these agents are nonselective—that is, they block both beta-1 (predominantly cardiac) and beta-2 (predominantly bronchial) adrenergic receptors. Even beta-1-selective drugs may have some bronchospastic effect.

Among the food additives, tartrazine, a yellow food coloring agent, is known to provoke an asthma attack. Patients sensitive to aspirin usually react to this agent. **Bisulfites** and metabisulfites are used in the food-processing industry as preservatives and antioxidants. Restaurant food, especially from salad bars, contains significant amounts of these agents. They are also used in certain wines, beers, dried fruits, and many other preserved food items. Asthmatic reactions occur in about 5% of patients with asthma following the intake of sulfited food or drink. The mechanism of sulfite sensitivity is not clearly understood.

Nocturnal Asthma

Many asthmatic patients are known to have more difficulty with their asthma in the late night and early morning hours. The worsening of asthma may be associated with sleep at any time of the day, as the factors considered in its pathogenesis are mostly sleep-related. The contributing factors include gastroesophageal reflux; retained airway secretions from a suppressed cough reflex during sleep; late asthmatic reactions from daytime exposure to irritants or allergens in the bedroom; sleep-related changes in the function of the autonomic nervous system; and **circadian** variation in circulating factors such as epinephrine, cortisol, and histamine. It seems that patients who have more severe asthma and higher degree of bronchial hyperreactivity are also more prone to nocturnal exacerbation of their bronchospasm. The prolonged dosing interval of medications in patients who are on certain antiasthmatic drugs may be another important cause of the nocturnal exacerbation of asthma.

Clinical studies strongly suggest that in subjects with hyperreactive airways, gastroesophageal reflux, which occurs more commonly in the supine position, may result in nocturnal asthma independent of other factors. It seems that the incidence of reflux is higher in asthmatics than in the general population. Bronchodilators, such as theophylline preparations and beta-adrenergic agonists, are known to reduce the lower esophageal sphincter tone, further increasing the likelihood of regurgitation of gastric juice. Bronchospasm resulting from gastroesophageal reflux is mostly a cholinergic reflex mediated by the vagus nerve. Rarely, aspiration of regurgitated material may occur and incite an asthmatic response.

Pathologic Changes. Pathologic examination of the lungs of patients dying from asthma, which represents the most severe form of the disease, shows evidence of a widespread obstruction of the airways from mucous plugs and inflammation of the airway walls. Lungs are hyperinflated from trapped air. The infiltration of the bronchial walls with various inflammatory cells, especially eosinophils and neutrophils, thickening of airway walls, prominent bronchial smooth muscles, **hypertrophy** of mucous glands, increased number of goblet cells, and epithelial damage are usually seen. Some of these changes, to a lesser extent, can be seen in less severe asthma attacks. A limited number of bronchoalveolar lavage studies in asthma following exposure to inhaled antigens shows a predominance of eosinophils and neutrophils, indicating that inflammation is a part of the asthmatic reaction in many patients.

Pathophysiology. The pathophysiologic changes during an asthma attack are based on narrowing of the airways caused by contraction of smooth muscles, mucosal and submucosal edema, and increased secretions. Increased airway resistance results in decreased forced expiratory flows and hyperinflation. Increased respiratory work load is related to both airflow resistance and hyperinflation. In addition to mechanical disadvantage during an asthma attack, abnormal distribution of both ventilation and blood flow with their mismatching results in the alteration of arterial blood gases, particularly hypoxemia. More severe and prolonged asthma attacks may culminate in hypercapnia from worsening of ventilation-perfusion mismatching and respiratory muscle fatigue.

Clinical Manifestations. The history is often the key to the diagnosis of bronchial asthma. A history of episodic attacks of wheezing and shortness of breath with symptom-free intervals is characteristic. Many patients give a history of frequent emergency room visits and hospital admissions for their asthma attacks. Some patients have a less clear-cut history and may be seen during their first attack. Many asthmatics, mostly adults, have a more chronic form of the disease without entirely symptom-free intervals. One remarkable feature of asthma is the tremendous variation in the severity and the duration of attacks. Even in the same patient, each attack may be quite different from the others. Asthma attacks are commonly more frequent and more severe late at night or the early morning hours.

The onset of an asthmatic attack is usually insidious; mild initial wheezing and cough progress to increasingly severe dyspnea. In a fully developed attack, the patient has a sense of pressure in the chest and sometimes a feeling of suffocation. He will sit upright or lean forward to obtain maximum use of the accessory respiratory muscles. Cough, which frequently accompanies the dyspnea, is at first nonproductive, but becomes more and more productive of stringy and mucoid sputum near the end of the attack. Duration of an untreated asthma attack varies considerably, but usually is more than 1 hour, often several hours, and sometimes even several days. The history of the precipitating event, such as an upper respiratory infection or exposure to allergens or respiratory irritants, may be elicited. Frequently, however, such a history is lacking. Occupational asthma is suggested by a history of prolonged exposure to a specific agent in the workplace and typical temporal relationship of symptoms to reexposure following a weekend off work.

Physical examination will show evidence of varying degrees of respiratory difficulty, from no apparent distress to a most severe respiratory struggle. Wheezing may be audible at a distance. The chest is usually held in an expanded position, indicating hyperinflation of the lungs. Intercostal and supraclavicular retraction with inspiration may be evident, particularly in children. The patient often uses the accessory respiratory muscles. Perspiration is common, and cyanosis is sometimes observed. On auscultation of the chest, rhonchi with variable pitch and tone are heard throughout the lung fields. They are mostly expiratory, but may be inspiratory as well in more severe attacks. Sometimes, with severe airway obstruction, breath sounds may be markedly diminished or absent in certain lung regions. A valuable physical finding during an asthma attack is variation of systolic blood pressure with phases of respiration. A positive sign, known as *paradoxical pulse,* is present when the systolic blood pressure during expiration is 10 mm Hg or more higher than during inspiration. A paradoxical pulse over 20 mm Hg is often associated with a severe asthma attack. Marked **tachycardia** (pulse rate over 120/min), a respiratory rate over 30/min, and use of accessory muscles of respiration are other clinical indicators of severity.

Although symptoms of a typical asthma attack consist of the triad of dyspnea, cough, and wheezing, in some patients cough may be the only manifestation. Asthma, therefore, should be considered in the differential diagnosis of unexplained chronic or recurrent cough.

Radiographic Study. Roentgenographic examination of the chest during an asthmatic attack usually shows evidence of hyperinflation, manifested by increased lung volumes with hyperlucency of the lung fields. Less commonly, chest x-ray may reveal areas of atelectasis, peribronchial infiltration, or other densities due to bronchial obstruction with mucous plug or concomitant infection. Radiographic study should be done sparingly and only when there is question of complications, such as pneumothorax, or if the diagnosis of asthma is uncertain.

Sputum Examination. Sputum examination may provide information on the nature of the asthmatic attack and, therefore, guide the therapeutic approach. Presence of respiratory tract infection is usually judged by this examination. Purulent-appearing sputum may be misleading, as large numbers of eosinophils, which are frequently present during an asthma attack, will give the sputum this appearance. Sputum, therefore, should be examined microscopically. Significant numbers of neutrophilic white blood cells and organisms in the sputum smear indicate bacterial infection.

Pulmonary Function Tests. The abnormalities of pulmonary function tests in asthma vary appreciably from patient to patient and in the same patient, depending on activity of the disease at the time of study and severity of the attack. The most consistent changes detected by pulmonary function testing in asthmatics are indicative of increased airway resistance, which is demonstrated by expiratory flow studies. These studies will help to evaluate the severity of airway obstruction, progression of disease, and response to therapy.

Some patients, between their attacks, may be in complete remission, having entirely normal pulmonary function. Most asthmatic patients, however, will show evidence of small airway obstruction during their symptom-free intervals. This abnormality can be detected by more sensitive tests, such as closing volume determination. Some asthmatics will continue to show significant airway resistance identifiable by usual spirographic study, even after they are over their acute attacks. When physical examination and routine spirometric studies are inconclusive, a bronchial provocation test (Chapter 2) may be performed. Such a test is often considered in patients whose asthma may manifest as chronic or recurrent cough.

During the asthmatic attack, there is marked reduction in flow rates. The forced vital capacity and its derivatives are severely reduced. A simple, practical method for evaluating the severity of asthma and assessing its response to therapy is the use of a peak expiratory flowmeter. A characteristic spirographic tracing can be seen in Fig. 9–2. The flow abnormalities will be corrected, at least partially, by administration of a bronchodilator (eg, inhalation of isoproterenol).

Lung volumes and capacities are significantly affected by the asthmatic attack. Hyperinflation, a characteristic finding, is indicative of increased residual volume and FRC at the expense of vital capacity and inspiratory reserve volume, which are reduced (Fig. 9–3). Variation in airway obstruction in different lung regions results in nonuniformity of distribution of ventilation and abnormality of ventilation-perfusion ratio.

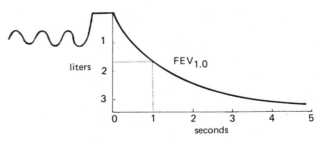

Figure 9–2. Forced spirogram during an asthma attack.

The result of these various pulmonary function tests seems to be similar to their result in pulmonary emphysema, except for the reversibility of the abnormalities in asthma. Furthermore, diffusion capacity is often normal and even increased in asthma, whereas it is significantly reduced in emphysema.

Arterial blood gas analysis has had a tremendous impact in understanding the problem of gas transport abnormalities in asthmatics and in proper management of patients with severe and intractable asthma. This test helps to identify the patients who will require hospitalization and more intensive and aggressive treatment. It is essential for monitoring the progress of patients and their response to the therapeutic measures, particularly when they are supported by mechanical ventilation.

Abnormal arterial blood gases during an asthma attack are almost the rule. The most common finding is mild to moderate hypoxemia, usually with some degree of hypocapnia. Hyperventilation may be partly due to increased hypoxemic stimulation, but frequently it is the result of neurogenic reflexes from irritant and stretch receptors and the patient's anxiety and apprehension. With more severe attacks, hypoxemia may be more pronounced. Low arterial PO_2 is due to ventilation-perfusion mismatching, which is a most common physiologic disturbance in asthma. With further clinical deterioration, arterial PCO_2 rises, reaching hypercapnic levels. This is a potentially life-threatening situation and should be considered as a medical emergency. Rapidity of the onset of ventilatory

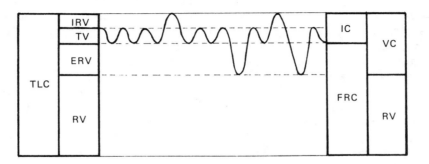

Figure 9–3. Lung volumes and capacities during an asthmatic attack. Note marked increase in RV and FRC.

failure (CO_2 retention) is not only related to the severity of airway obstruction, but may also be due to other factors, such as oversedation with drugs, uncontrolled oxygen administration, and patient exhaustion. There is also individual variation of responsiveness of the respiratory center and/or chemoreceptors, which may explain earlier CO_2 retention in some patients.

Differential Diagnosis. Because there are many other causes of dyspnea and wheezing, and asthma may manifest in atypical ways, several conditions are considered in its differential diagnosis. Chronic obstructive lung disease with its exacerbations and remissions, especially chronic obstructive bronchitis, is sometimes difficult to be differentiated from asthma. Congestive heart failure and pulmonary **embolism** among cardiovascular diseases may mimic asthma. Respiratory symptoms in the early stage of bronchiolitis in young children are often suggestive of asthma.

Disorders most likely to be mistaken for asthma and treated as such long before their exact nature is recognized are some of the conditions that result in obstruction of upper airways, including the trachea (see Chapter 7). The symptoms from these disorders may be chronic, unremitting, and unresponsive to bronchodilators; or they may be intermittent and even responsive to antiasthmatic medications. Vocal cord dysfunction without an identifiable organic cause is another condition that simulates asthmatic attacks. A high index of suspicion together with information from adequate history taking, proper physical examination, and radiographic study will help to reach an accurate diagnosis in most cases. When upper airway obstruction is suspected, a study of inspiratory and expiratory flow-volume loop is most helpful. Computerized tomographic (CT) scan of the upper airways and endoscopic studies may also be needed for a proper diagnosis.

MANAGEMENT OF ASTHMA

Proper management of asthma begins with its accurate diagnosis, determination of its severity and its effect on patient's daily function, identification of the underlying pathogenetic mechanism, and recognition of provoking and exacerbating factors.

As in any chronic disease, patients with asthma should have a thorough understanding of their disease and therapeutic measures. The importance of the role of health professionals in this regard cannot be overemphasized. The treatment plan, its objectives, and implementation should be properly explained to patients and/or their families for assuring their cooperation and compliance with the therapeutic decisions. Because asthma is a heterogeneous disease, its management should be tailored to meet individual therapeutic needs of each patient. As self-administration of metered-dose inhalers have become the mainstay of asthma therapy in outpatient settings, and their efficacy depends on their proper use, thorough instruction of patients about their correct application is the responsibility of physicians, therapists, and nurses. They should be able to demonstrate and verify the optimal method of their use. Spacer devices and special reservoir systems may be necessary to help self-administration of these inhalers, especially when the patients have difficulty with hand-breath coordination.

Adjunctive measures such as proper hydration by adequate fluid intake and humidification of rooms during the cold months should be emphasized. Some patients may have underlying emotional problems that may be at least partly responsible for their asthma attacks. Proper psychiatric counseling should be recommended for these patients. Patients should be encouraged to lead as normal a life as possible. They should not be restrained from physical activities. On the contrary, asthmatics should be encouraged to participate in regular graded exercises. Children, in particular, should not be discouraged from sports activities. With proper medical management, the majority of asthmatic children will be able to partake in physical education programs at school. There are good indications that exercise-induced bronchospasm diminishes with more training; furthermore, it can be prevented by proper medications.

Prevention of Asthma Attacks

Preventive measures play an essential part in management of patients with asthma. As asthma attacks are usually the result of interaction between a predisposed individual and provoking factors that are predominantly environmental, the elimination or avoidance of these factors and alteration of the patient's reactivity constitute the basic principle in asthma prevention. Exposure to allergenic substances, particularly the ones known to be associated with the patient's asthma; respiratory irritants such as dust, chemicals, fumes, cigarette smoke, and cold air; and infectious agents should be avoided as much as possible. As discussed earlier in this chapter, basic pathogenetic abnormality, namely hyperreactivity of airways, can also be altered by reducing exposure to allergens, asthma-producing agents in the workplace, and other factors known to cause airway inflammation.

Skin testing with various allergens is being extensively used in evaluation of patients with asthma. The majority of these patients show positive skin reaction to the commonly used test materials. Although skin testing is helpful in identifying the causative allergens and for planning of preventive and therapeutic regimen in some asthmatics, it may be misleading. Skin tests do not provide an accurate measurement of sensitivity and hyperreactivity of the bronchi in most patients. Many asthmatics with positive reaction to a known allergen may have no difficulty upon repeated or continuous exposure to that agent. Basing the patient management decision solely on the results of these tests may cause unnecessary burden and suffering to the patients and their families without a significant benefit. Bronchial inhalation challenge tests with antigen extracts, which are not yet readily available, seem to be more specific in demonstrating the causative roles of airborne allergens in asthma.

Changing the allergenic reactivity in patients with allergic asthma by **immunotherapy** may be beneficial in selected subjects. This treatment consists of regular injections of minute but gradually increasing amounts of the extracts of antigens recognized as specifically responsible for asthma attacks.

Antiasthmatic Drugs. Most of the drugs effective in the treatment of asthma attacks are also useful for their prevention. The five major categories of drugs used in the management of asthma are:

1. sympathomimetics
2. theophylline and its salts
3. anticholinergics
4. corticosteroids
5. cromolyn

Drugs in the first three categories are bronchodilators through their relaxing effect on bronchial smooth muscles; corticosteroids and cromolyn, with no bronchodilatory effect, have more complex modes of action.

Sympathomimetics. The sympathomimetics used in asthma are beta-adrenergic agonists. Commonly used agents in this category have marked similarity in their chemical structure. However, they vary in the selectivity of their effect on beta-2-adrenergic receptors located in bronchial smooth muscles, and in their duration of action. In addition to their direct bronchodilating effect, they inhibit mediator release from the mast cells. *Epinephrine* or adrenaline, which also has an alpha-receptor effect (vasoconstriction), is commonly used in an injectable form. Its beta effect is nonselective and, therefore, is both a bronchodilator and cardiac stimulator. *Isoproterenol* is a pure beta stimulator, but it is one of the least selective in its beta effect and it has the shortest duration of action. In the treatment of asthma it is almost exclusively used in aerosol form. *Metaproterenol, terbutaline, albuterol, bitolterol,* and *pirbuterol* exert a preferential effect on beta 2-adrenergic receptors and have a longer duration of action. The selectivity of *isoetharine* and its duration of action are intermediate, and it is used only by inhalational route. Metaproterenol (Alupent, Metaprel), albuterol (Proventil, Ventolin), terbutaline (Brethaire), bitolterol (Tornalate), and pirbuterol (Maxair) are equally effective aerosol bronchodilators, which are marketed in convenient metered-dose inhalers. Metaproterenol and albuterol are also available in solution form for inhalation in handheld nebulizers and other mechanical devices. Metaproterenol, terbutaline, and albuterol also have oral preparations. Terbutaline is the only drug in this group that is available in ampules for subcutaneous injection. Side effects of these beta-2 agonists are more troublesome when they are administered systemically, which include tremor, palpitation, and nervousness. Fenoterol, carbuterol, and formoterol are other effective bronchodilators that have yet to be approved for their routine clinical use.

Theophylline. Theophylline and its salts are among the most commonly used agents for the prevention and treatment of asthma attacks. Aminophylline is the only preparation in this category that is available for IV use. Theophylline is better known for its potent smooth-muscle relaxing property, although the exact mechanism of its action is not fully understood. It has other pharmacologic effects besides its bronchodilatory action. Because of the narrow margin between the therapeutic and toxic levels of theophylline, the determination of its plasma concentration is frequently needed. Slow-release oral preparations have facilitated its clinical use. Many asthmatics with frequent attacks benefit from chronic theophylline therapy for preventive purpose. With the development of safe and effective topical bronchodilators, the use of theophylline in treatment of acute asthma is waning.

Anticholinergics. Anticholinergic agents have long been known to have a bronchodilating effect in asthma; however, because of their significant systemic side effects, their use had been limited until the availability of new poorly absorbable anticholinergic aerosols. *Ipratropium bromide,* available in metered-dose inhalers, is the most commonly used drug in this category. It may be used in asthma for its additive bronchodilator effect in conjunction with other antiasthmatic agents. Because of its negligible cardiac stimulatory effect, it may be used in place of adrenergic drugs in patients with certain heart conditions. Although its bronchodilatory effect is less than that of beta-2 agonists in asthma, it is somewhat more effective in chronic obstructive bronchitis.

Corticosteroids. Corticosteroid preparations are playing an increasingly important role in the management of asthma. The exact mechanism of their action in asthma is not known, but several of their interrelated effects have been ascertained. The most important one is reduction as well as prevention of inflammation through the inhibition of various mediators of inflammation. With the increasing knowledge on the importance of inflammation in pathogenesis of asthma and with the recognition of its role in late asthmatic response and airway hyperreactivity, the anti-inflammatory effect of corticosteroids has proven to be the key to their effectiveness. These agents also enhance and potentiate the effects of beta-adrenergic drugs and also reduce mucus secretion. As their prolonged systemic administration is known to cause many significant side effects, a decision for such therapy should be made with a great deal of circumspection. Fortunately, topical preparations for inhalational use result in fewer and much less serious undesired effects. The most commonly reported problem of oral *candida* infection can be prevented, at least partly, by rinsing the mouth and throat after each treatment. The aerosol preparations are excellent substitutes for more hazardous oral corticosteroids in the long-term management of steroid-dependent asthmatics. These inhalational drugs are assuming increasingly more prominent role in outpatient management of asthma, especially when there is a heightened airway hyperreactivity. Three different types of inhaled corticosteroid preparations are presently available in the United States. They are *beclomethasone* (Beclovent, Vanceril); *triamcinolone* (Azmacort); and *flunisolide* (AeroBid), which have fairly comparable effectiveness.

Cromolyn. Cromolyn sodium (Intal) is a compound that has been shown to be effective as a prophylactic agent in management of asthma, but it has no role in treatment of an acute attack. It acts mainly through inhibition of the release of histamine and other mediators from the mast cells. Asthmatic attacks triggered by inhalation of specific agents, exercise, or by some occupational exposures can be prevented to varying degrees by prior treatment with cromolyn. It may block both early and late asthmatic responses. Cromolyn is available both as micronized powder in capsules and as solution in metered-dose inhaler. To use the powder form, the content of each capsule is inhaled into the lungs, using a special breath-activated device known as turbo-inhaler

(Spinhaler). With the availability of more convenient inhaler, the powdered form is used less frequently. Side effect of cromolyn is mainly its irritating effect on upper airways.

Treatment of an Asthma Attack

The therapeutic approach to the patient with asthma attacks depends on severity of the episode. Mild attacks without complicating factors, such as a bacterial infection, usually can be successfully treated with a bronchodilating agent taken from a metered-dose inhaler. Most patients are familiar with these episodes and are or should be properly instructed in their management. They should be alerted against abuse of their medications, particularly nebulizers. Patients requiring frequent use of inhaled bronchodilators are usually candidates for preventive regimen with cromolyn or inhaled corticosteroids.

More severe attacks and lack of response to initial self-treatment are an indication for seeking further medical help and institution of more vigorous therapy; otherwise, the asthmatic attack may become self-perpetuating and reach the intractable stage (status asthmaticus). The attacks of patients who are seen in emergency rooms usually have begun a few hours before, if not longer. A thorough objective evaluation, including the determination of arterial blood gases and the measurement of peak expiratory flow, will help in the management plan and the decision for hospitalization. Most such patients, at least for the first few hours, are treated in the emergency room. As dehydration is common at this stage, intravenous fluid therapy should be started. Oxygen therapy by the nasal route is often indicated. An adrenergic

bronchodilator, by inhalation or sometimes by injection, is given as the first drug. Some recommend intravenous aminophylline as the drug of first choice, followed by adrenergic drugs as indicated. A short course of an oral corticosteroid preparation with rapidly tapering dose is sometimes recommended. The efficacy of treatment should be closely monitored clinically and by repeat measurements of peak expiratory flow rate. Most patients will improve and may be discharged after a few hours of close observation. They should be instructed on the proper use of their maintenance medications and about their outpatient follow-up.

Some patients will be refractory to this treatment and continue to have significant airway obstruction and increasing respiratory difficulty. By definition, this is an *intractable asthma,* which is also known as *status asthmaticus.*

Status Asthmaticus and Its Treatment.
Status asthmaticus has been defined as a severe asthmatic attack that does not respond to treatment with an adequate amount of commonly used bronchodilators, that is, beta-adrenergic stimulant and aminophylline, within a few hours. This condition should not be confused with *chronic asthma,* which may also respond poorly to bronchodilators. Chronic asthma is fairly stable and tolerated by the patient despite significant functional impairment, whereas status asthmaticus is an acute progressive and life-threatening event that will rapidly lead to acute respiratory failure if not treated properly. The intractability of asthma usually is related to inflammation and mucus plugging of the airways. Mucosal damage and inflammation increase the airway hy-

perreactivity and contribute to perpetuation of bronchospasm. Hypoxemia, acidosis, and probably other factors may result in refractoriness to the bronchodilators.

Patients with status asthmaticus should be hospitalized immediately. Intravenous aminophylline drip, after the initial loading dose, should be continued. Adequate hydration cannot be overstressed. A systemic corticosteroid, given intravenously, is the mainstay of management of severe intractable asthma. Hypoxemia without CO_2 retention should be treated with oxygen-enriched air with frequent monitoring of arterial blood gases and pH. Bronchodilators will become more effective with adequate hydration, correction of hypoxemia, and administration of corticosteroids. Continuation of intravenous aminophylline with maintenance of a therapeutic blood level is usually recommended. Adrenergic agents may be administered by nebulizers, or by systemic route. Intermittent positive pressure breathing (IPPB) for this purpose provides no signficant additional benefit and may even be harmful.

Sedatives are contraindicated in patients with severe asthma. The use of mucolytic agents, because of their irritating and, hence, aggravating effect, is not recommended for asthmatics. Chest physical therapy, if tolerated, may be of some benefit in removing bronchial secretions and mucous plugs. It is more effective with proper hydration, humidification, and bronchodilatation. In patients with evidence of bacterial infection, proper antibiotics should be given without delay.

Some patients upon arrival at the hospital or shortly thereafter will be desperately ill from their severe asthma

and will fail to respond to optimal therapy. They show evidence of exhaustion, decreasing alertness, and worsening hypoxemia and hypercapnia. This is the stage of asthma attack in which intubation and mechanical ventilation will become necessary. The management of this stage of the disease is discussed in Chapter 25.

As patients with severe and **intractable** asthma may have similar episodes in the future, they should be on an appropriate regimen of antiasthmatic medications after their discharge from the hospital. Such patients would benefit from chronic corticosteroid therapy, preferably in topical form if possible.

Course and Prognosis of Asthma.
Asthma is a chronic disease with periodic recurrences over many years, if not for the patient's life. There is no actual curative treatment for it, although spontaneous recovery is not uncommon, mostly in childhood asthma. Approximately one-third of cases beginning in early childhood will recover by their adult age. Beyond that age, tendency to spontaneous recovery is much less. Appropriate therapeutic measures, however, have significant impact on the course and prognosis of asthma. Inadequately treated patients will continue to be vexed by it throughout their existence. The attacks may become progressively worse and more frequent, and remissions less complete. Nonspecific provoking factors such as respiratory infections will assume more importance. Some patients may have more chronic and continuous airways obstruction interspersed by acute exacerbations, which may be mistaken for chronic bronchitis. Actually, there are reasons to believe that chronic bronchi-

tis and even changes of emphysema may take place in many of these patients later in the course of their disease. Although pure allergic asthma does not predispose to emphysema, many intrinsic asthmatics may show the pathologic changes of emphysema.

The fatality rate from asthmatic attacks is relatively small, but patients with severe status asthmaticus and respiratory failure have considerable mortality, which has increased in recent years.

BIBLIOGRAPHY

Barnes PJ. A new approach to the treatment of asthma. *N Engl J Med.* 1989; 321:1517–1527.

Bousquet J, Hejjaoui A, Michel FB. Specific immunotherapy in asthma. *J Allergy Clin Immunol.* 1990; 86:292–305.

Busse WW. Respiratory infection: their role in airway hyperresponsiveness and pathogenesis of asthma. *J Allergy Clin Immunol.* 1990; 85:671–683.

Chapman KR, Verbeek PR, White JG, Rebuck AS. Effect of a short course of prednisone in the prevention of early relapse after the emergency room treatment of acute asthma. *N Engl J Med.* 1991; 324:788–794.

Check WA, Kaliner MA. Pharmacology and pharmacokinetics of topical corticosteroid derivatives used for asthma therapy. *Am Rev Respir Dis.* 1990; 141 (2, part 2):44–51.

Christopher KL, Wood RP, Eckert RC, et al. Vocal cord dysfunction presenting as asthma. *N Engl J Med.* 1983; 308:1566–1570.

Cockcroft DW. Occupational asthma. *Ann Allergy.* 1990; 65:169–175.

Cockroft DW. Therapy for airway inflammation in asthma. *J Allergy Clin Immunol.* 1991; 87:914–919.

Djukanović R, Roche WR, Wilson JW, et al. Mucosal inflammation in asthma. *Am Rev Respir Dis.* 1990;142:434–457.

Dolen WK, Weber RW. Assessment and management of acute asthma. *Ann Allergy.* 1989; 63:86–95.

Durham SR. Late asthmatic responses. *Respir Med.* 1990; 84:263–268.

George RB, Owens MW. Bronchial asthma. *Dis Mon.* 1991; 37:142–196.

Gleich GJ. The eosinophil and bronchial asthma: current understanding. *J Allergy Clin Immunol.* 1990; 85:422–436.

Hall JB, Wood DH. Management of the critically ill asthmatic patient. *Med Clin North Am.* 1990; 74:779–795.

Hogg JC, James AL, Paré PD. Evidence for inflammation in asthma. *Am Rev Respir Dis.* 1991; 143:S39–S42.

Hopp RJ, Townley RG, Biven RE, et al. The presence of airway reactivity before the development of asthma. *Am Rev Respir Dis.* 1990; 141:2–8.

James AL, Paré PD, Hogg JC. The mechanics of airway narrowing in asthma. *Am Rev Respir Dis.* 1989; 139:242–246.

Kay AB. Asthma and inflammation. *J Allergy Clin Immunol.* 1991; 87:893–910.

Lawrence ID, Patterson R. Topical respiratory therapy. *Adv Intern Med.* 1990; 35:27–43.

Leff AR. Endogenous regulation of bronchomotor tone. *Am Rev Respir Dis.* 1988; 137:1198–1216.

Li JTC, Reed CE. Proper use of aerosol corticosteroids to control asthma. *Mayo Clin Proc.* 1989; 64:205–210.

Macklem PT. A hypothesis linking bronchial hyperreactivity and airway inflammation: implications for therapy. *Ann Allergy.* 1990; 64:113–116.

Martin RJ, Cicutto LC, Smith HR, et al. Airways inflammation in nocturnal asthma. *Am Rev Respir Dis.* 1991; 143:351–357.

Meeker DP, Wiedemann HP. Drug-induced bronchospasm. *Clin Chest Med.* 1990; 11:163–175.

O'Connell EJ, Rojas AR, Sachs MI. Cough-type asthma: a review. *Ann Allergy.* 1991; 66:278–285.

O'Neil CE. Mechanics of occupational airways diseases induced by exposure to organic and inorganic chemicals. *Am J Med Sci.* 1990; 299:265–275.

Parker SR, Mellins RB, Sogn DD. Asthma education: a national strategy. *Am Rev Respir Dis.* 1989; 140:848–853.

Pierson WE. Exercised-induced bronchospasm in clinical practice. *Clin Rev Allergy.* 1988; 6:443–452.

Reed CE. Aerosol glucocorticoid treatment of asthma. *Am Rev Respir Dis.* 1990; 141 (2, part 2):S82–S88.

Sly RM. Mortality from asthma. *J Allergy Clin Immunol.* 1989; 84:421–434.

Woolcock AJ, Jenkins CR. Assessment of bronchial responsiveness as a guide to prognosis and therapy in asthma. *Med Clin North Am.* 1990; 74:753–765.

Zoratti E, Busse WW. Nighttime asthma symptoms: no idle threat. *J Respir Dis.* 1990; 11:137–154.

CHAPTER *10*

Bronchiectasis

Bronchiectasis is a chronic disease of bronchi and bronchioles characterized by abnormal dilatation of their lumen and associated with inflammation and destruction of their walls. Because of the impairment of bronchial clearance, increased bronchial secretion becomes stagnant and secondarily infected. This in turn causes further destruction of bronchial structure and dilatation and therefore results in a self-sustaining, sometimes progressively advancing, pathologic process.

Etiology and Pathogenesis. Although bronchiectasis is seen in all ages, its onset in the majority of patients is in childhood. The exact basic abnormality that sets the stage for the pathologic changes of bronchiectasis is not always known. The destructive process of bronchial walls, however, seems to be a bacterial infection. Among the various conditions predisposing to bronchiectasis, congenital or familial factors are most common (Table 10–1). Nearly half the cases are associated with cystic fibrosis, which is discussed in the next chapter. Congenital immunodeficiency states, particularly **agammaglobuline-mia,** because of recurrent respiratory tract infections are important predispos-

ing conditions. A newly described congenital disorder of motility of the cilia has added significantly to our understanding of the pathogenesis of recurrent airway infection and bronchiectasis. Known as ciliary **dyskinesia** or *immotile cilia syndrome,* it not only affects the cilia of the respiratory epithelial cells, but also the other ciliated cells, as well as sperm tails. Several different ultrastructural changes in cilia have been demonstrated to be the cause of their abnormal motility. The impairment of mucociliary transport leads to recurrent infections of the respiratory tract, including the nasal sinuses. Abnormal motility of sperm tails causes sterility in male patients. Well-defined and best-recognized among congenital ciliary dyskinesias is Kartagener's syndrome, which is characterized by bronchiectasis, chronic sinusitis, and **situs inversus** (transposition of the internal organs from one side to the other).

Acquired changes in the structure of the lung and the bronchi as seen following tuberculosis or other necrotizing infections are known to result in bronchiectasis. Complete or partial bronchial obstruction, which results in stasis of bronchial secretions and secondary infection, is one important cause of necrosis

TABLE 10–1. SOME OF THE KNOWN OR SUSPECTED CAUSES OF BRONCHIECTASIS

1. Cystic fibrosis
2. Ciliary dyskinesia, including Kartagener's syndrome
3. Agammaglobulinemia
4. Bronchial obstruction
5. Foreign body
6. Aspiration and inhalation injury
7. Allergic bronchopulmonary aspergillosis
8. Childhood pulmonary infection (complication of pertussis or measles)
9. Healed tuberculosis and other necrotizing lung infection

and dilatation of the bronchial walls. Moreover, collapsing of the lung tissue distal to obstruction exerts a negative pressure on bronchial walls, causing further dilatation. The aspiration of a foreign body, if not removed, is often followed by the development of bronchiectasis. Allergic bronchopulmonary aspergillosis, which affects some asthmatics, is frequently associated with bronchiectasis. This results from recurrent bouts of mucous plugging.

In many patients, however, it is more difficult to explain the sequence of events. A history of pulmonary infection developing as a complication of measles, whooping cough (**pertussis**), or other childhood diseases is frequently obtained. With routine immunization against measles and pertussis, the incidence of pneumonia as their complication has markedly diminished. The role of most of these conditions in the pathogenesis of bronchiectasis remains conjectural.

Pathology. Bronchiectasis usually affects the segmental and subsegmental bronchi and may involve one or more segments of a lobe or several lobes. It is

frequently bilateral, with a predilection for basilar segments of the lower lobes, mostly the posterior ones. Right middle lobe and lingular segments are next as common sites for bronchiectasis. Upper lobe bronchiectasis is likely to be secondary to destructive tuberculosis.

Dilatation of bronchi may have a different configuration, which is the basis for the classification of bronchiectasis into various morphologic types: cystic or **saccular, varicose** or **fusiform,** and cylindrical (Fig. 10–1).

Pathologic examination shows that the normal structure of bronchial wall is destroyed, the mucosa is atrophied, the ciliated columnar epithelium is lost or replaced by flattened squamous epithelium, the dilated lumen is often filled with purulent material, and the bronchi and bronchioles distal to ectatic areas are obstructed by secretions, inflammation, and fibrosis.

Clinical Manifestations. The most common symptoms of bronchiectasis are *cough* and *expectoration* of a large amount

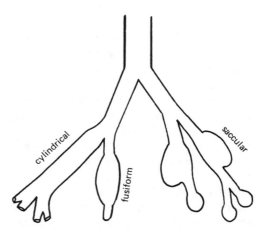

Figure 10–1. Various morphologic types of bronchiectasis.

of sputum. The latter symptom, dating back to childhood, is characteristic of bronchiectasis. Other common manifestations are hemoptysis and recurrent localized pneumonias. The amount of expectoration is variable. Some patients have copious amounts of sputum exceeding several hundred milliliters daily; others have much less or, occasionally, no expectoration at all. Bronchiectasis without increased sputum production is referred to as *dry* bronchiectasis. Generally, the amount of expectoration is largest in bronchiectasis involving the dependent bronchi; upper lobe disease is more often "dry."

Sputum is usually **mucopurulent.** The purulent component will vary with and depend on the associated infection, which may be intermittent or continuous. In some cases, the presence of anaerobic infection gives the sputum a foul odor.

Hemoptysis is a common occurrence with bronchiectasis, which may be the only presenting symptom in the "dry" form, as seen following tuberculous scarring. The amount of expectorated blood and frequency of bleeding are very variable and unpredictable. Occasionally, hemoptysis may be massive and life threatening.

Besides chronic **indolent** infection in bronchiectasis, recurrent acute respiratory infection, especially pneumonia, is common. Pneumonia in bronchiectasis tends to recur at the same location. With the progression of bronchiectasis and the development of airway obstruction, patients will have increasing dyspnea and may eventually develop respiratory failure. Chronic sinusitis is a frequent associated condition.

Physical findings in bronchiectasis vary with the degree of pathologic changes. In mild forms without complicating events, physical examination may be entirely normal. In more severe forms, rales and rhonchi may be heard over the involved area where breath sounds may be diminished. Clubbing of the fingers and toes is a common extrapulmonary manifestation of long-standing bronchiectasis. Fever is usually absent unless acute pulmonary infection supervenes.

Radiographic Examination. Standard chest x-rays may show certain abnormalities that suggest bronchiectasis. They include increased lung markings due to peribronchial fibrosis, segmental atelectasis, and occasional multiple air-fluid levels. These changes are more frequent in the lower lung fields. Computed tomography (CT) of the chest may show the structural changes to better advantage.

The diagnosis of bronchiectasis, although strongly suspected from the history, physical examination, and chest radiographs without contrast, can only be made with certainty by bronchography. Ever since the advant of CT scanners, the need for bronchography has steadily declined. It is now limited mainly to cases in which more accurate definition of bronchiectatic lesions, and their extent, is essential for considering and selecting surgical resection. This examination should be performed following treatment of recent infection and adequate bronchial toilet. Bronchography will outline the walls of the bronchi and, therefore, will easily identify the bronchiectatic areas. As in pathologic examination, bronchograms may show various forms, that is, **saccular, varicose,** and **cylindrical** changes (Fig. 10–2).

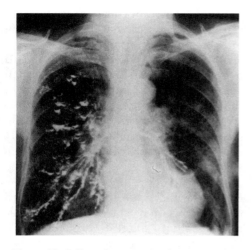

Figure 10–2. Bronchogram showing severe saccular bronchiectasis.

Sputum Examination. On sputum examination, large numbers of white blood cells and bacteria are usually seen. Most of the organisms are oropharyngeal flora, including **anaerobic** bacteria. Sometimes, other gram-positive and gram-negative organisms may be demonstrated in sputum culture. The decision on choice of antibiotic in the treatment of the intercurrent infection will depend on the result of culture and sensitivity studies of sputum.

Pulmonary Function Studies. Many patients with mild to moderate bronchiectasis will have no abnormality detectable by routine spirometry and arterial blood gas analysis. On the other hand, with advanced disease, patients may show marked derangement in lung volumes, ventilatory mechanics, distribution of ventilation, and gas exchange. Therefore, in severe bronchiectasis, both obstructive and restrictive ventilatory impairments are demonstrated. Associated chronic bronchitis and emphysema

are the major causes of obstructive components; atelectasis and fibrosis result in restrictive changes. Arterial blood gas abnormalities will depend on severity of the disease and other complicating factors. Hypoxemia is the most frequent blood gas abnormality.

Management. The principles of nonsurgical management of patients with bronchiectasis are effective removal and reduction of bronchial secretions and prevention as well as treatment of infectious complications. In patients with cylindrical bronchiectasis, cough is usually effective in clearing the airways, as the caliber of bronchi reduces normally, and there is no collapse of the outflow tract of these bronchi with the forced expiration of coughing. In contrast, saccular and varicose bronchiectasis show disproportionate collapse of the lobar bronchi on coughing without change in the bronchiectatic spaces (Fig. 10–3). The cough in patients with the latter forms of bronchiectasis will, therefore, be ineffective in emptying the dilated bronchi of their contents. Expectoration in these patients is usually the result of overflow or gravitational flow of secretions to more proximal bronchi, from where they are expulsed by coughing. Thus the bronchiectatic spaces, mostly the ones in dependent portions of the lungs, retain their secretions, facilitating infection and resulting in further bronchopulmonary damage.

The importance of emptying the dilated bronchi of the accumulated secretions cannot be overemphasized. This is done by *postural drainage* using gravitational force. The anatomical distribution and location of the involved bronchi should be known. The therapist should have adequate knowledge

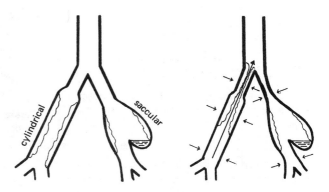

Figure 10–3. Effectiveness of cough in clearing bronchial secretions in two forms of bronchiectasis. Although cough is usually effective in clearing the secretions in cylindrical bronchiectasis, it is ineffective in emptying the content of saccular bronchiectasis.

of bronchopulmonary segmental anatomy for selection of the optimal position of the patient for maximal drainage of the involved bronchi (Figs. 10–4 through 10–10). The patient or his family should be instructed by demonstration of the proper positionings for effective drainage, which he should follow regularly. The frequency and duration of drainage sessions will depend on severity of disease and the amount of secretions; however, every patient with bronchiectasis should follow this simple, inexpensive, but important measure *at least* twice daily, on arising in the morning and at bedtime. The evacuation of secretions is facilitated by intermittent deep breathing and coughing. The use of humidification and bronchodilators may be helpful. The addition of chest percussion by cupping or mechanical devices is recom-

mended for dislodging the thick and tenacious secretions. During an acute respiratory infection, the need for more vigorous and frequent postural drainage is increased.

Although with adequate postural drainage the frequency of respiratory infection is diminished, sometimes antimicrobial drugs will be necessary. There is no question of their usefulness in treating an acute intercurrent bacterial infection; however, continuous antibiotic "prophylaxis," advocated by some, is controversial. Nevertheless, patients who show episodic change in the quantity and the characteristics of their sputum, particularly when it becomes grossly purulent, usually benefit from a short course of antibiotic therapy. Bronchoscopy is indicated when an obstructing process, especially by a foreign body, is suspected to be the cause of bronchiectasis

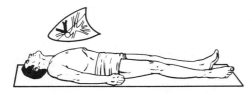

Figure 10–4. Postural drainage. Optimal position for drainage of anterior and superior segments of the upper lobes.

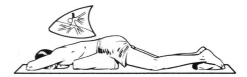

Figure 10–5. Postural drainage. Optimal position for drainage of superior segments of lower lobes.

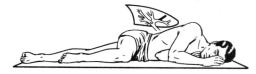

Figure 10–6. Postural drainage. Optimal position for drainage of posterior segment of the right upper lobe.

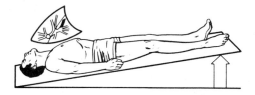

Figure 10–8. Postural drainage. Optimal position for drainage of the anterior basilar segments.

Patients with bronchiectasis, as with other chronic obstructive pulmonary diseases, should avoid smoking and exposure to dust, noxious fumes, and other respiratory irritants. Adequate humidification of their rooms during the cold months is important. Sinusitis, a frequently associated condition with bronchiectasis, should be properly treated.

The decision for surgical treatment of bronchiectasis should not be made without a trial of intensive medical management as discussed above. The condition then should be assessed in regard to the response to therapy, clinical severity, distribution of disease, form of bronchiectasis, associated pulmonary and extrapulmonary conditions, respiratory function, and other factors. Surgical resection is usually indicated when there are significant symptoms or complications in patients who fail to respond to conservative therapy, who have anatomically limited disease, and who have adequate cardiopulmonary

reserve. Significant symptoms and complications include copious and foul-smelling sputum production, recurrent hemoptysis, and frequent pneumonias. Saccular bronchiectasis is often localized and more suitable for surgery. Cylindrical bronchiectasis, on the other hand, is usually not localized and thus is not amenable to surgical therapy.

The result of surgery in proper candidates is generally good. Although some patients may develop bronchiectasis in certain parts of the remaining lungs that were judged to be free of disease before surgery, the removal of the involved area may prevent spread of disease to the remaining lungs. When surgery is contemplated, intensive preoperative medical management is important in preparing these patients and preventing operative and postoperative complications.

Course and Prognosis. Variation in the severity and the extent of the disease and other associated factors affect the

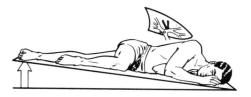

Figure 10–7. Postural drainage. Optimal position for drainage of the right middle lobe.

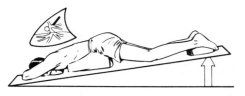

Figure 10–9. Postural drainage. Optimal position for drainage of the posterior basilar segments.

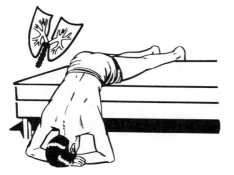

Figure 10–10. Postural drainage. Optimal position for drainage of the trachea.

prognosis to a great degree. Patients with mild bronchiectasis may have a normal life span; patients with extensive bilateral disease usually succumb within several years to respiratory and/or infectious complications. Except for a certain degree of natural improvement during adolescence in children with bronchiectasis, the course of this disease is usually one of slow deterioration interspersed by episodes of exacerbation. The progression, however, is quite variable. Obviously, proper management will have significant effect on the course and prognosis of bronchiectasis.

BIBLIOGRAPHY

Afzelius BA. A human syndrome caused by immotile cilia. *Science.* 1976; 193:317–319.

Annest LS, Kratz JM, Crawford FA Jr. Current results of treatment of bronchiectasis. *Thorac Cardiovasc Surg.* 1982; 83: 546–550.

Barker AF, Bardana EJ Jr. Bronchiectasis: update of an orphan disease. *Am Rev Respir Dis.* 1988; 137:969–978.

Cooke JC, Currie DC, Morgan AD, et al. Role of computed tomography in diagnosis of bronchiectasis. *Thorax.* 1987; 42:272–277.

Currie DC, Pavia D, Agnew JE, et al. Impaired tracheobronchial clearance in bronchiectasis. *Thorax.* 1987; 42:126–130.

Rubin BK. Immotile cilia syndrome (primary ciliary dyskinesia) and inflammatory lung disease. *Clin Chest Med.* 1988; 9:657–668.

Stanford W, Galvin JR. The diagnosis of bronchiectasis. *Clin Chest Med.* 1988; 9: 691–699.

Stockley RA. Bronchiectasis: new therapeutic approaches based on pathogenesis. *Clin Chest Med.* 1987; 8:481–494.

Wasserman SJ. Ciliary function and disease. *J Allergy Clin Immunol.* 1984; 73:17–19.

Wilson JF, Decker AM. The surgical management of childhood bronchiectasis. *Ann Surg.* 1982; 195:354–363.

CHAPTER 11

Cystic Fibrosis (Mucoviscidosis)

Cystic fibrosis or **mucoviscidosis** is a hereditary disease characterized by dysfunction of **exocrine** glands and manifested by chronic pulmonary disease, pancreatic insufficiency, abnormally high electrolyte concentration in sweat, and sometimes abnormalities of other organs. Although characteristically a disease of early childhood, cystic fibrosis is seen more and more in adolescents and young adults because of improvement in early diagnosis and management.

With early recognition and institution of proper treatment, pancreatic insufficiency rarely constitutes a serious problem nowadays, whereas the pulmonary complications of cystic fibrosis remain very grave despite great progress in this area. Rarely does a patient with cystic fibrosis escape pulmonary involvement, and most patients eventually succumb to it.

Etiology and Incidence. Cystic fibrosis is a hereditary disease transmitted as a *Mendelian recessive* trait. As a most significant breakthrough in cystic fibrosis research, the location of its gene in chromosome 7 was recently accomplished, which accounts for about 75% of cases of cystic fibrosis. The single-gene carriers (heterozygotes) have no clinically demonstrable disease. If both parents are carriers, their children, regardless of their sex, will have a 25% chance of having cystic fibrosis and a 50% chance of being carriers (Fig. 11–1). Thus, both parents of a child with cystic fibrosis are carriers.

Cystic fibrosis is much more common in whites than in blacks. Its incidence has been estimated to be 1 in 2,000 live births in Caucasians and 1 in 17,000 live births in blacks. About 5% of Caucasians are **heterozygous** for cystic

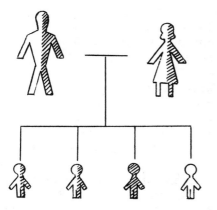

Figure 11–1. Mode of inheritance in cystic fibrosis. Both parents are carriers; one out of four children has cystic fibrosis and half of the children are carriers.

fibrosis. It is the most frequent lethal hereditary disease in this population.

Pathogenesis and Pathology. An increased concentration of sweat electrolytes and an abnormality of mucus secretion and elimination are the two distinct and well-recognized pathologic conditions in cystic fibrosis. There is increasing evidence that these apparently separate disorders have a common basic pathogenetic mechanism, namely a cellular defect in electrolyte transport.

Sweat electrolyte abnormality is present at birth and continuously throughout the patient's life. It has no relationship to the severity of disease or the extent of involvement of other organs. Chloride and sodium content of sweat are increased, sometimes being several times normal. As a diagnostic tool, the determination of sweat electrolytes has been most valuable. The clinical consequence of this abnormality has not been of significance, except for excessive and sometimes dangerous salt loss with prolonged exposure to heat and vigorous exercise (**heat exhaustion**).

The abnormality of mucus, its secretion and elimination, and the resultant obstruction cause most of the pathologic changes, which set the stage for its many serious and eventually fatal complications. Because of the presence of large numbers of mucus-secreting elements in the pancreas and tracheobronchial tree, these organs are particularly susceptible and are almost always involved in cystic fibrosis.

The term *cystic fibrosis* was originally intended to describe the pathologic changes in the pancreas, where dilated glands and ducts, fibrosis, and degeneration of parenchyma are characteristic features. Pancreatic insufficiency, causing inadequate digestion and absorption of food, may result in severe malnutrition in these patients, mostly when they are not properly treated.

The lungs are involved to varying degrees in virtually all patients with cystic fibrosis. Transepithelial electrolyte transport, which normally controls the amount and composition of the mucosal fluid, is markedly abnormal in this disease. The resultant thick and dehydrated mucus and impairment of mucosal cilia causes airway obstruction and a wide variety of pathologic changes of cystic fibrosis. Atelectasis, pneumonia, bronchiectasis, bronchiolectasis, bronchitis, peribronchitis, emphysema, abscess, and fibrosis are seen in various combinations. Obstruction and retained secretions pave the way for bacterial infection, which plays a major role in the development, perpetuation, and progression of most of these pulmonary complications. *Staphyloccus aureus* and *Pseudomonas aeruginosa* are the most common pathogens infecting the lungs in cystic fibrosis. The latter organism can be isolated from the sputum of almost all adult patients with this disease. Chronic sinusitis and nasal polyps are frequently present, especially in older patients.

Clinical Manifestations. Pancreatic insufficiency is the cause of most gastrointestinal manifestations of cystic fibrosis, which include abdominal distension, abnormal stools, and malnutrition despite good appetite. Sometimes obstructive complication of the gastrointestinal tract may occur. *Meconium ileus* is due to plugging of the distal end of the small intestine by putty-like meconium in the newborn. The intestinal obstruction in this condition is usually present at birth.

There are other extrapulmonary manifestations, including hepatobiliary disease and reproductive system malfunction, whose discussion is beyond the scope of this book.

Pulmonary involvement, which results in the most important and potentially fatal manifestations of cystic fibrosis, eventually occurs in all patients. The time of onset of clinical pulmonary manifestations is quite variable; they may be apparent within a few weeks of birth or may occur years later. Cough is the earliest and the most common symptom, which is initially nonproductive, but may shortly become productive of thick and tenacious sputum. Repeated bouts of respiratory-tract infection cause frequent exacerbation of these symptoms. With progressive and irreversible damage to the lungs, dyspnea is soon added to the clinical picture. Dyspnea may become quite severe with advancing disease. Some patients may present with episodic breathlessness and wheezing suggestive of asthma. Recurrent exacerbation of respiratory tract infection in the form of bronchitis and/or pneumonia is a typical feature of cystic fibrosis. Hemoptysis, which may be massive, is not uncommon in these patients. Spontaneous pneumothorax, a common occurence in cystic fibrosis, should be suspected when a sudden exacerbation of dyspnea occurs.

On *physical examination*, in addition to the evidence of malnutrition and poor body development, signs of pulmonary involvement are frequently present. The chest may be barrel-shaped and hyperresonant to percussion. Changes in breath sounds with varying adventitious sounds are often detected. In the advanced stage, the patient may be in respiratory distress, using the accessory respiratory muscles. Cyanosis and other signs of respiratory failure, including cor pulmonale, eventually occur. Clubbing of fingers and toes is a common finding in cystic fibrosis, which is almost always present in adult patients.

Radiographic Study. The radiographic examination of the chest in patients with pulmonary involvement usually shows evidence of diffuse hyperinflation, increased lung markings, and irregular densities (Fig. 11–2). Mucoid impaction and areas of atelectasis may be demonstrated. Frequent pulmonary infection usually manifests radiographically by new infiltration and occasionally by abscess formation. Pneumothorax and/or mediastinal emphysema may be manifest in some. Sinus x-ray films are almost always abnormal in adults with cystic fibrosis.

Diagnostic Studies and Other Laboratory Findings. Sweat test is the simplest

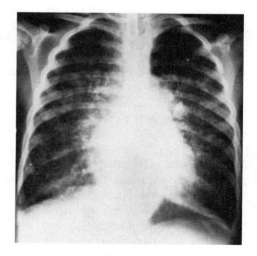

Figure 11–2. Chest radiograph of a child with severe cystic fibrosis. Bilateral irregular parenchymal infiltration and hyperinflation are demonstrated.

and reliable method for the diagnosis of cystic fibrosis. If performed properly, a positive test (i.e., a sweat chloride concentration of over 60 mEq/L) is diagnostic in an appropriate clinical setting. Because of a somewhat higher concentration of sweat electrolytes in normal adults and because of their increase in conditions other than cystic fibrosis, the diagnostic specificity of the test in adults is less than in children. Its results should, therefore, be interpreted with caution, especially when the clinical presentation is atypical. A small number of patients have been described who have incomplete expression of their disease, which may be limited to pulmonary manifestations with normal or borderline sweat electrolytes. With a wider availability of cystic fibrosis gene detection, it may become the diagnostic test of choice. Tests for cystic fibrosis gene detection is especially useful for identification of its carriers and for genetic counseling among the family members of a patient with known disease.

Pulmonary function tests in cystic fibrosis usually show evidence of obstructive ventilatory impairment and hyperinflation. Vital capacity is markedly diminished while residual volume is increased up to several times predicted normal. Blood gas abnormalities in cystic fibrosis occur in late stages of the disease.

Management. The greatest challenge in management of patients with cystic fibrosis is related to pulmonary complications. Gastrointestinal manifestations are usually controlled by proper diet, vitamins, and pancreatic enzymes. Despite significant advances in knowledge and understanding of pulmonary problems in cystic fibrosis and availability of effective therapeutic measures, patients with this dreadful disease still succumb to pulmonary complications.

The treatment of these patients should be started very early in the course of their disease before the development of irreversible pulmonary damage. As was indicated earlier, the common denominator of lung lesions is obstruction of airways due to bronchial secretions. Therefore, the principle of management will center around removal of these secretions and alleviation of obstruction. The role of antibiotics in treatment of these patients is evident from the importance of bacterial infection in causing many of the pulmonary complications.

In considering the measures for removal of mucopurulent secretions, it should be recalled that these secretions are thick and very tenacious; therefore, the importance of proper humidification and other methods for their loosening should be emphasized. Dry air and respiratory irritants should be avoided. Use of mist tents and other methods of humidity therapy has resulted in some success in helping to reduce sputum viscosity and in making coughing and postural drainage more effective. The argument for and against regular use of mist tents at night continues, although there is a steady decline in their use.

Expectorants such as potassium iodide or glycerol guaiacolate have no demonstrable beneficial effect. Mucolytic and enzymatic agents, such as acetylcysteine and pancreatic dornase, despite their in vitro effect, have not been clinically useful to any significant degree. Effective cough is most important for removing secretions; it should always be a part of the patient's daily routine. The effectiveness of time-honored postural drainage is proven by recent clinical studies. It should be carried out systematically, as discussed and illustrated in Chapter 10. Gentle chest tapping, cupping, or use of mechanical devices may help the effectiveness of postural drainage. Proper exercise is also known to improve the tracheobronchial clearance. IPPB has no therapeutic role in these patients; it may even be harmful.

Antibiotic therapy is one of the most important aspects of management of patients with cystic fibrosis. The antibiotic is usually given therapeutically and, occasionally, prophylactically. Staphylococcal infection, which is the most common bacterial infection earlier in the course of cystic fibrosis, should be treated with a proper antibiotic. *Pseudomonas aeruginosa* is isolated from the sputum of these patients with increasing frequency as the disease advances. Once established, this organism is rarely, if ever, totally eradicated despite the use of potent antibiotics. However, with infectious exacerbations or development of pseudomonas pneumonia, it should be vigorously treated with appropriate antimicrobial agents.

Lung lavage with normal saline solution has resulted in variable success in some patients with severe and life-threatening pulmonary involvement. Aerosolized antibiotic therapy has given various results. Surgery has been rarely considered for resection of localized lesions or control of massive hemoptysis. Nutritional support is an important part of comprehensive management of patients with cystic fibrosis.

Course and Prognosis. In most cases of cystic fibrosis, the severity of pulmonary complications determines the outcome. The degree of pancreatic insufficiency has no significant effect on the ultimate outlook if properly treated with adequate nutrition and replacement therapy. The increase in average life expectancy from less than 2 years to about 27 years in the past 40 years is the result of early diagnosis, availability and use of effective antibiotics, comprehensive management plan, and recognition of milder cases. Although some patients die in infancy or early childhood, an increasingly large number survive to ages of 30 to 40 years, occasionally even longer. Death from cystic fibrosis beyond the neonatal period is due to pulmonary complications such as overwhelming infection or respiratory failure. For some unknown reason(s), female patients with cystic fibrosis tend to have more rapid decline in their pulmonary function than do male patients. Recurrent pneumothorax denotes a poor prognosis.

Male patients with cystic fibrosis are almost always sterile, and the pregnancy rate in female patients is markedly diminished.

BIBLIOGRAPHY

Berger HA, Welsh MJ. Electrolyte transport in the lungs. *Hosp Pract*. 1991; 26(3):53–59.

Cerny FJ. Relative effects of bronchial drainage and exercise for in-hospital care of patients with cystic fibrosis. *Phys Ther*. 1989; 69:633–639.

Davis PB, di Sant'Agnese PA. Diagnosis and treatment of cystic fibrosis: an update. *Chest*. 1984; 85:802–809.

de Boeck C, Zinman R. Cough versus chest physiotherapy: A comparison of the acute effects on pulmonary function in patients with cystic fibrosis. *Am Rev Respir Dis*. 1984; 129:182–184.

Dubinsky WP. The physiology of epithelial chloride channels. *Hosp Pract.* 1989; 24(1): 69–82.

Elborn JS, Shale DJ. Lung injury in cystic fibrosis. *Thorax.* 1990; 45:970–973.

Fick RB Jr. Pathogenesis of pseudomonas lung lesion in cystic fibrosis. *Chest.* 1989; 96:158–164.

Krauss RD, Rado TA. Review: current approaches to the molecular and physiological basis of cystic fibrosis. *Am J Med Sci.* 1989; 298:334–341.

Lloyd-Still JD, Wessel HV. Advances and controversies in cystic fibrosis. *Semin Respir Med.* 1990; 11:197–210.

Mouton JW, Kerrebijn KF. Antibacterial therapy in cystic fibrosis. *Med Clin North Am.* 1990; 74:837–850.

Reisman JJ, Rivington-Law B, Corey M, et al. Role of conventional physiotherapy in cystic fibrosis. *J Pediatr.* 1988; 113:632–636.

Rommens JM, Iannuzzi MC, Kerem BS, et al. Identification of the cystic fibrosis gene. *Science.* 1989; 245:1059–1080.

Rossman CM, Waldes R, Sampson D, Newhouse MT. Effect of chest physiotherapy on removal of mucus in patients with cystic fibrosis. *Am Rev Respir Dis.* 1982; 126:131–135.

Shwachman H, Kowalski M, Khaw K-T. Cystic fibrosis: a new outlook. *Medicine.* 1977; 56:129–149.

Spector ML, Stern RL. Pneumothorax in cystic fibrosis. *Ann Thorac Surg.* 1989; 47:204–207.

Welsh MJ, Fick RB. Cystic fibrosis. *J Clin Invest.* 1987; 80:1523–1526.

SECTION *IV*

Restrictive Lung Diseases

CHAPTER 12

Chronic Diffuse Infiltrative Diseases: Idiopathic Pulmonary Fibrosis

Chronic diffuse infiltrative diseases of the lung include many heterogeneous pathologic conditions with common clinicoradiologic features that justify their discussion under one heading. In contradistinction to chronic obstructive pulmonary disease, they are characterized by reduced lung volumes with *normal* expiratory flow rates and are, therefore, also referred to as chronic *restrictive* lung diseases. They are radiographically recognized by diffuse, bilateral, and more or less persistent densities that are predominantly interstitial. Gas transport abnormality, reflected in reduced diffusing capacity and manifested by arterial hypoxemia, is one of their main features. Their course is chronic, and diffuse fibrosis is the ultimate pathologic process in most of these conditions.

This chapter will begin by discussing the idiopathic pulmonary fibrosis as the prototype of this group of pathologic conditions. It will be followed by a concise version of the differential diagnosis of chronic diffuse infiltrative diseases. In the next three chapters, some of the more common and better-defined entities in this category of diseases will be considered.

IDIOPATHIC PULMONARY FIBROSIS

Idiopathic pulmonary fibrosis is a chronic diffuse lung disease of unknown cause characterized clinically by chronic, slowly progressive dyspnea: radiographically, by widespread interstitial infiltrate; physiologically, by restrictive ventilatory impairment; and pathologically, by chronic inflammation and progressive fibrosis. It is also known by various other names of which *cryptogenic fibrosing alveolitis* is most descriptive. Idiopathic pulmonary fibrosis is differentiated from other conditions presenting with a similar picture by its lack of causative relation with known diseases or etiologic agents.

Pathogenesis and Pathology. Although the cause of idiopathic pulmonary fibrosis is unknown, the chronic inflammation at the alveolar level (alveolitis), which precedes fibrosis, suggests continuous or repeated insult to the lung tissue. It seems that the alveolar macrophages have a central role in maintaining the **alveolitis** by recruiting other inflammatory cells, especially the polymorphonuclear leukocytes. The damage to the alveolar cells is probably the result of enzymes and other chemical compounds released by these cells and macrophages. Toxic oxygen radicals, generated by granulocytes, are considered to play an important role in this process. By releasing certain mediators, macrophages also increase the number of **fibroblasts** that are essential for the development of fibrosis. The cause of the stimulation and the accumulation of macrophages to initiate and sustain the inflammatory process is not precisely determined, but there is some evidence that **immune complexes** produced locally may play an important role. The questions of how the immune complexes are formed and what their antigenic components are have yet to be elucidated, although certain autoantigens such as altered immunoglobulins and constituents of connective tissue have been implicated.

Pathologic examination in the early stage of idiopathic pulmonary fibrosis shows evidence of patchy alveolitis with cellular infiltration predominantly by neutrophils and macrophages, and also including small numbers of lymphocytes and eosinophils. The alveolar walls are somewhat distorted and thickened with edema. With progression of the disease, there is derangement and loss of thin, type I alveolar epithelial cells with proliferation of cuboidal type II cells. Proliferation of fibroblasts and deposition of fibrous tissue result in further thickening and distortion of the alveolar walls. Based on the preponderance of cell types, several pathologic forms of idiopathic interstitial pneumonitis have been described. Whether they are due to varied cellular responses to the same disease process or representative of different diseases is not determined.

Pathophysiology. Restrictive functional impairment, a characteristic feature of diffuse pulmonary fibrosis, is the result of the increased elastic recoil of the lungs (decrease in **compliance**) and their reduced volumes. Despite higher mechanical work against greater elastic recoil of the fibrotic lungs, there is increased minute ventilation from a faster respiratory rate. Higher respiratory frequency is primarily the result of an increase in afferent respiratory impulses from the receptors of the lungs and the thoracic wall. Although the diffusing capacity is almost always reduced, mismatching of ventilation and perfusion is mostly responsible for arterial hypoxemia commonly seen in patients with diffuse pulmonary fibrosis. Because of the maintenance of an increased alveolar ventilation, arterial PCO_2 is frequently low. Hypercapnia is unusual in patients with diffuse interstitial lung disease. Increased pulmonary vascular resistance and eventual cor pulmonale are secondary to longstanding hypoxemia and reduced pulmonary vascular bed from extensive fibrosis.

Clinical Manifestations. Idiopathic pulmonary fibrosis is mostly a disease of the middle-aged with a 2:1 male-to-female ratio. **Dyspnea,** a cardinal symptom in patients with advanced pulmonary fibrosis, may be absent or mild in the early stage. Its onset is insidious and initially related to physical activity. Once developed, dyspnea is relentlessly progressive. A nonproductive cough is often present. Common complaints of weakness and easy fatigability are difficult to distinguish from exertional dyspnea.

Findings on physical examination depend on the disease stage. In advanced disease there is limitation of chest expansion. Rapid and somewhat shallow breathing is the usual pattern of respiration in patients with restrictive pulmonary disease. Fine crackles are very common findings on auscultation of the lungs, especially over the lower lung fields. The breath sounds may appear louder as a result of their enhanced transmission. Digital clubbing is often present. Cyanosis is common in more severe disease.

Roentgenographic Findings. Interstitial reticular and nodular density is the typical x-ray picture, which may involve both lung fields diffusely (Fig. 12–1). However, frequently it may be more severe in certain areas, such as the lower lungs, perihilar regions, or some other parts. In the early stages, the chest x-ray film may be normal, but usually the lungs appear hazy, like ground glass; a reticulonodular pattern develops later. Coarse trabeculation, mimicking honeycomb, usually is indicative of long-standing fibrosis. Progressive reductions in lung volumes can be appreciated better by comparing serial x-ray films. The CT scan of the chest, especially when performed with a high-resolution technique, is more sensitive in detecting early changes and for defining the lesions in detail.

Pulmonary Function Tests. Pulmonary function abnormalities in idiopathic pulmonary fibrosis, as in most cases of

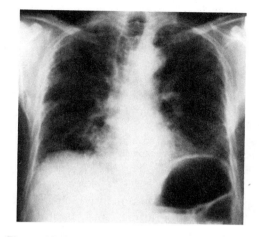

Figure 12–1. Advanced diffuse idiopathic pulmonary fibrosis. Lung volumes are reduced.

diffuse infiltrative lung diseases, have a restrictive pattern. The vital capacity, functional residual capacity, and total lung capacity are diminished. Unless there is concomitant airway obstruction, flow rates are normal. A schematic presentation of a typical spirographic tracing is seen in Figure 12–2. Reduction of diffusing capacity usually occurs earlier than changes in lung volumes. Arterial blood studies show a variable degree of hypoxemia and hypocapnia. Hypoxemia is usually made worse by exercise. Even in patients with a normal arterial PO_2, exercise may lower it significantly. Hypercapnia is observed only in the terminal stage of pulmonary fibrosis and when associated with obstructive changes.

Diagnosis. Although the clinical picture and radiographic findings are often suggestive, a lung biopsy is necessary for demonstration of characteristic histologic changes of fibrosis. Even then, the diagnosis of *idiopathic* pulmonary fibrosis cannot be made without proper

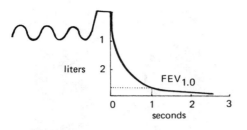

Figure 12–2. Forced spirogram in restrictive pulmonary disease. Vital capacity is reduced but flow rates are normal.

exclusion of conditions in which similar clinical, radiographic, and pathologic changes may occur. This necessitates a thorough history taking, careful physical examination, and performance of necessary laboratory tests. The biopsy may be obtained by the transbronchial method through a bronchoscope or percutaneously by a cutting needle. Thoracotomy and open lung biopsy are often required, however, for a better representative sampling and a more thorough pathologic study.

Bronchoalveolar lavage has been proposed as an alternative to biopsy. It is particularly useful for the detection of the early inflammatory stage of the disease when the treatment is more effective. Unfortunately, the study lacks diagnostic specificity. Among other tests that may help to determine the disease activity, radionuclide scanning with gallium 67 is commonly used.

Management. There is no known effective therapy for established pulmonary fibrosis. Patients with idiopathic diffuse pulmonary fibrosis usually have a relentlessly downhill course, and treatment with corticosteroids or other immunosuppressive drugs has little if any effect, unless the disease is treated in its early inflammatory stage. Therapeu-

tic benefit from these drugs, even with evidence of active disease, is variable and unpredictable.

In well-established pulmonary fibrosis, the treatment is mostly supportive and symptomatic. Prevention and prompt treatment of infection and avoidance of respiratory irritants and other noxious inhalants should be recommended, as for any patient with chronic pulmonary disease. In patients with severe hypoxemia, continuous oxygen therapy is indicated.

DIFFERENTIAL DIAGNOSIS OF CHRONIC DIFFUSE INFILTRATIVE DISEASES

An increasing number of patients who were thought to have idiopathic pulmonary fibrosis are being recognized in recent years as having additional pathologic changes of obliterating bronchiolitis with some areas of organizing pneumonia. Now generally known as *bronchiolitis obliterans organizing pneumonia* (BOOP), its cause as in idiopathic pulmonary fibrosis is undetermined. Its more patchy appearance on the x-ray film and its better response to corticosteroid therapy are some of its distinguishing clinical features.

In patients with clinical, radiographic, and pulmonary functional abnormalities suggestive of diffuse pulmonary fibrosis, other diagnostic possibilities should also be considered. Over 100 clinical entities have been described that have many of these characteristic features. They usually fall into the following categories of lung diseases:

1. Sarcoidosis
2. Immunologic

3. Environmental and occupational
4. Drug-induced
5. Circulatory
6. Neoplastic
7. Aspiration related
8. Related to physical agents
9. Infections
10. Miscellaneous

Sarcoidosis of the lung, which is discussed in the next chapter, is a granulomatous disease of unknown cause with a propensity for pulmonary fibrosis. Increasing evidence indicates that immunologic alteration is involved in its pathogenesis. The diagnosis is usually established by transbronchial lung biopsy.

Immunologic disorders as a cause of diffuse infiltrative lung disease include several heterogenous diseases, which are discussed in Chapter 14. **Extrinsic** *allergic alveolitis* and *connective tissue diseases* are the most common disorders in this category. They are usually suspected and may be diagnosed by history and characteristic clinical features. Certain laboratory studies, with or without tissue biopsy, are often necessary for their definitive diagnosis.

Drug-induced diffuse parenchymal disease is a well-known complication of some of the therapeutic agents. Anticancer drugs are by far its most common causes. Bleomycin, busulfan, methotrexate, and carmustine (BCNU) are the major offenders. Numerous other chemotherapeutic agents may occasionally result in lung injury. Nitrofurantoin (an antibacterial drug used for urinary tract infection) and amiodarone (an antiarrhythmic drug) are among other agents known for their significant pulmonary side effects. Pulmonary oxygen toxicity, discussed in Chapter 15, is another cause of diffuse lung injury and fibrosis.

Environmental lung diseases are discussed in Chapter 15. Diffuse infiltrative diseases among them include inorganic dust pneumoconioses and lung lesions from inhalation of noxious gases. An adequate occupational history, including information on the nature of dust or gas exposed to and severity and duration of exposure, is necessary for proper diagnosis.

Chronic pulmonary **congestion** from heart failure may appear as diffuse lung disease and is diagnosed by clinical presentation and its response to appropriate treatment. *Primary* or *metastatic lung* cancer may occasionally manifest as widespread pulmonary infiltration or interstitial density. Tissue biopsy is always diagnostic.

The *chronic aspiration* of gastric acid in patients with a predisposing condition, discussed in Chapter 17, has been implicated in causing pulmonary fibrosis. Among the physical agents, *x-radiation* is well known to cause lung injury in the form of pneumonitis and fibrosis. Radiation therapy for intrathoracic or extrathoracic malignancies is its cause. The areas of pulmonary reaction often coincide with the port of radiation, but occasionally other areas may also be affected. Use of certain anticancer drugs may potentiate the effect of radiation.

Diffuse infiltrative lung disease due to infection is often acute in its pulmonary and systemic manifestations; and, thus, it is usually diagnosed with little difficulty. Chronic lung infiltration from infection with mycobacteria and fungi is identified by proper bacteriologic and/or pathologic examination.

There are a number of other conditions in which diffuse lung infiltration and fibrosis may occur. These uncommon diseases include histiocytosis X (esosinophilic granuloma of the lung), alveolar proteinosis, pulmonary hemosiderosis, and certain rare heredofamilial diseases. For a more detailed and comprehensive discussion of the differential diagnosis of diffuse infiltrative lung diseases, the reader should consult the review articles listed in the Bibliography.

BIBLIOGRAPHY

Burkhardt A. Alveolitis and collapse in the pathogenesis of pulmonary fibrosis. *Am Rev Respir Dis.* 1989; 140:513–524.

Chrétien J. Interstitial lung disease—clinical presentation. *Postgrad Med J.* 1988; 64 (suppl 4):8–16.

Crystal RG, Bitterman BP, Rennard SI, et al. Interstitial lung diseases of unknown cause. *N Engl J Med.* 1984; 310:154–166, 235–244.

DePaso WJ, Winterbauer RH. Interstitial lung disease. *Dis Mon.* 1991; 37:67–133.

Drug-induced pulmonary disease. *Clin Chest Med.* 1990; 11:1–189.

Drugs that cause pulmonary toxicity. *Med Lett Drugs Ther.* 1990; 32:88–90.

Epler GR, Colby TV, McLoud TV, et al. Bronchiolitis obliterans organizing pneumonia. *N Engl J Med.* 1985; 312:152–158.

Hansell DM, Kerr IH. The role of high resolution computed tomography in the diagnosis of interstitial lung disease. *Thorax.* 1991; 46:77–84.

Müller NL, Miller RR. Computed tomography of chronic diffuse infiltrative lung disease. *Am Rev Respir Dis.* 1990; 142:1206–1215.

Panos RJ, Mortenson RL, Niccoli SR, King TE Jr. Clinical deterioration in patients with idiopathic pulmonary fibrosis: causes and assessment. *Am J Med.* 1990; 88:396–404.

Posiello RA. Radiation-induced lung injury. *Clin Chest Med.* 1990; 11:65–71.

Raghu G. Idiopathic pulmonary fibrosis: a rational clinical approach. *Chest.* 1987; 92:148–154.

Turner-Warwick M, Burrows B, Johnson A. Cryptogenic fibrosing alveolitis: clinical features and their influence on survival. *Thorax.* 1980; 35:171–180.

Wall CP, Gaensler EA, Carrington CB, Hayes JA. Comparison of transbronchial and open biopsies in chronic infiltrative lung diseases. *Am Rev Respir Dis.* 1981; 123:280–285.

CHAPTER 13

Sarcoidosis

Sarcoidosis is a systemic granulomatous disease of unknown etiology that may involve almost any body organ, particularly the lymph nodes, lungs, liver, spleen, skin, and eyes. The characteristic histologic appearance of epithelioid granulomas with little or no necrosis is not diagnostic by itself. The diagnosis is considered established when consistent clinical and radiographic features are supported by the histologic changes. Diseases of known causes with similar histologic features should be excluded.

Pulmonary involvement is perhaps the most important manifestation of sarcoidosis. Hilar and mediastinal lymphadenopathy, which is readily identifiable by the chest x-ray, is present in most patients.

Etiology and Pathogenesis. Although sarcoidosis is widespread throughout the world, its prevalence is very variable in different countries and even in different areas of the same country. It is much more common among blacks than whites in the United States. Sarcoidosis is rare in American Indians, Eskimos, and Chinese. Sarcoidosis is seen in all age groups, but the most common age at the time of diagnosis is in the 20 to 30 range. It occurs slightly more frequently in

females than in males, especially among blacks.

Although several theories on its etiology and pathogenesis have been proposed, and numerous attempts at identifying a causative agent have been made, the cause of sarcoidosis and the exact mechanism of its development have remained undetermined. Because there is a significant variation in its incidence among different groups according to their ethnic background as well as their geographic location, both genetic makeup and environmental factors seem to be involved in its etiology. Whatever the elusive cause may be, a special reactivity to the causative agent(s) is necessary for the expression of sarcoidosis in an individual. A unique and rather specific reaction of sarcoidosis patients to a product prepared from a sarcoid tissue is indicative of their special reactivity: an intradermal injection of such a product, known as Kveim antigen, to a patient with active sarcoidosis results in the development of granulomas at the site of injection; whereas a similar injection to an individual without sarcoidosis does not produce granulomas. This phenomenon suggests that sarcoidosis results from an interaction between this particular tissue reactivity and certain, as yet unknown, factor(s).

In recent years, studies of the cells obtained with the help of bronchoalveolar lavage have provided new information helpful in understanding certain aspects of the pathogenesis of sarcoidosis. These cells consist mainly of macrophages and lymphocytes. The latter are predominantly CD4-positive helper T cells. It has been shown that both macrophages and T lymphocytes are in an *activated* state capable of producing different chemical mediators.

Each of these cell lines, when activated, is able to stimulate the replication and the activation of the other with the help of the mediators. In addition to their mutual effects on the resident cells, they also recruit circulating lymphocytes and monocytes and direct their participation in granuloma formation. Macrophages seem to have a central role in initiating the cellular response and in setting the stage for granuloma formation of sarcoidosis. The inciting event in this process is unknown, although an antigenic stimulation is strongly suspected. It is the lack of modulation that, after the initial response, is responsible for perpetuating the reaction and producing more granulomas characteristic of sarcoidosis. It is, therefore, plausible that sarcoidosis is a state of enhanced immunologic reaction in which responses to antigenic stimuli are uncontrolled.

Pathologic Findings. Various organs may be the site of sarcoid reaction, but the lungs and the intrathoracic lymph nodes are among the most commonly involved. Sarcoid lesions in the lungs consist of disseminated nodules and variable fibrosis, although in the early stage, alveolitis with or without granulomas may be present. Marked scarring with fibrosis and hyalinization, cystic formation, honeycombing, and emphysematous changes are indicative of advanced disease. The histologic hallmark of sarcoidosis is the presence of numerous, closely similar granulomas composed mostly of epithelioid cells and occasional giant cells. In the lungs, the granulomas typically develop in peribronchial and subpleural interstitial tissues. Sometimes they are present in the bronchial mucosa. Fibrosis frequently accompanies the granulomas, some of which may be replaced by a relatively acellular mass of **hyaline** material. Significant necrosis is rare in sarcoid granulomas. It is interesting to note that histologic changes are frequently demonstrated in the lungs of patients with sarcoidosis who have no clinical or radiographic evidence of pulmonary involvement.

Clinical Manifestations. Symptomatology in sarcoidosis is quite variable because of differences in mode of onset, diversity of individual response, and involvement of various organs of the body. Different organs may be affected singly, in combination, or in sequence. Approximately half of the patients are asymptomatic or have minimal symptoms at the time of diagnosis. These are usually the patients with radiographic evidence of bilateral hilar lymphadenopathy (BHL). A more acute form of BHL is sometimes accompanied by fever, joint pains, and a purplish-red indurated rash on the extensor surface of legs and sometimes forearms (erythema nodosum). This type of onset occurs most often in young females.

In the chronic form of sarcoidosis,

symptoms, if present, can be divided into two categories: those related to the involvement of specific organs, and those due to constitutional manifestations. The latter symptoms include generalized weakness, fatigue, weight loss, malaise, and fever.

Although histologic involvement of the lungs can be demonstrated in the majority of patients, significant pulmonary symptoms develop in only about one-fourth of patients. These frequently include cough and dyspnea. Chest pain is not common and hemoptysis is rare. Dyspnea may be mild and only exertional, but it may progress to become extremely severe in advanced cases with marked fibrosis.

Full description of other symptoms due to the involvement of other organs is beyond the scope of this book. It should be mentioned, however, that sarcoidosis may involve almost any organ in the body. Most frequent complaints, besides the respiratory symptoms, are related to the eye and skin. Symptoms due to musculoskeletal, neurologic, cardiac, hepatic, and renal involvement may sometimes be present.

The physical examination may be entirely normal in many patients or it may reveal evidence of abnormality in various organs depending on their involvement. Enlargement of peripheral nodes, various skin lesions, enlargement of liver or spleen, signs of eye lesions, swelling of joints, and abnormal neurologic findings are among the extrapulmonary manifestations that sometimes can be detected in these patients. Physical examination of the chest usually is not rewarding even when there are gross changes in the radiographic films. In some patients, a few scattered rales and rhonchi may be heard. In more advanced cases when fibrosis has settled, physical findings of pulmonary fibrosis will be present.

Radiographic Findings. Radiographic changes in intrathoracic sarcoidosis may be due to lymph node enlargement, parenchymal pulmonary lesions, or combination of the two. Lymph node enlargement is characteristically localized in the hilar regions bilaterally in a more or less symmetrical fashion (Fig. 13–1). Enlargement of the right paratracheal nodes at the angle of the trachea and right main stem bronchus is also characteristic. Unilateral hilar node involvement is unusual. In most cases, lymph node enlargement subsides within 2 years. They may, however, persist and become calcified.

Radiographically demonstrable pulmonary lesions may occur without, accompany, or follow, but almost never precede, hilar lymphadenopathy. Pulmonary involvement is frequently diffuse and more or less evenly distributed throughout the lung fields. It usually has

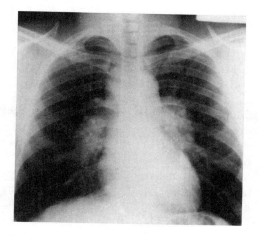

Figure 13–1. Bilateral hilar lymphadenopathy of sarcoidosis. Mediastinal nodes are also enlarged.

a reticulonodular pattern, but sometimes it may be predominantly alveolar. Some patients present with pulmonary infiltration as the first demonstrable evidence of sarcoidosis, and some may develop lung lesions later in the course of the disease. Most of the pulmonary infiltration slowly resolves, either completely or leaving only minor fibrotic residue. In some patients, however, fibrosis replaces the parenchymal infiltration, resulting in irregular and coarsely linear strands extending from the hili. Fibrosis is usually uneven in its distribution and may involve only certain portions of the lungs, particularly the upper lobes, distorting the normal hilar and vascular patterns. Retraction of fibrotic regions may accompany hyperinflation of the others. Sometimes, air-containing cysts or cavities are formed, which may harbor a fungus ball. Pleural effusion is an uncommon feature of sarcoidosis. Gallium-67 is usually taken up by active sarcoid lesions. Scanning with this radioisotope is helpful in defining the disease activity, as well as in following the response to therapy.

Pulmonary Function Tests.

Pulmonary function tests are frequently abnormal in sarcoidosis, even in patients with no radiographically demonstrable lung involvement. Ventilatory impairment usually has a *restrictive* pattern, although reduction in flow rates may occasionally be present. Lung compliance is commonly decreased. One of the most frequent abnormalities is low diffusing capacity. Arterial blood gas analysis may show variable degrees of hypoxemia, which become more evident with exercise. Arterial blood PCO_2 is frequently low.

Other Laboratory Findings.

Increased urinary calcium excretion and/or high blood calcium level may be demonstrated in some patients. Elevated serum gammaglobulin levels are common. An interesting finding in most patients with sarcoidosis is a high level of an enzyme that converts angiotensin I to angiotensin II (angiotensin-converting enzyme, or ACE). It is due to the increased production of this enzyme by the cells of sarcoid granulomas.

Diagnosis.

Diagnosis of sarcoidosis is considered established by consistent clinical and radiographic features together with histologic evidence from tissue biopsy. Sometimes the clinicoradiologic picture is so characteristic that the diagnosis of sarcoidosis can be made with reasonable accuracy without biopsy. The tissue for histologic examination may be obtained from a number of sites, but commonly mediastinal lymph nodes or lungs are preferred. With the advent of fiberoptic bronchoscopy, transbronchial biopsy has become the procedure of choice. Occasionally, an openlung biopsy may be necessary. Biopsy of peripheral nodes and liver may have a high yield, but has not been considered to be quite satisfactory for definitive diagnosis, particularly in atypical cases.

Other laboratory tests are available whose results may affect the diagnostic probability. Lacking specificity and sensitivity, however, these tests cannot be used for making or excluding the diagnosis of sarcoidosis. Measurement of serum ACE level, analysis of bronchoalveolar lavage fluid, and gallium-67 scanning are among such tests. They seem to be more useful for determination of disease activity and, sometimes, for assessment of therapeutic response.

Management.

Most patients with sarcoidosis require no treatment. Corticosteroids, and sometimes other immuno-suppressive drugs, are the only agents known to suppress the active process in sarcoidosis. Because of the significant side effects of these drugs, however, patients should be carefully selected for this type of therapy. The expected benefit of these agents should outweigh their potential harm to justify their use. Certain manifestations of sarcoidosis are definite indications for steroid therapy. These include progressive respiratory impairment, involvement of the eyes, cardiac sarcoidosis, central nervous system involvement, disfiguring skin lesions, and persistent elevation of serum calcium. The question of steroid therapy in less severe pulmonary involvement without significant respiratory symptoms has not been entirely settled. As most of these patients will have spontaneous remission, they may be observed closely and treated only when their disease shows progression.

Other antiinflammatory drugs and immunosuppressive agents are rarely used in treatment of sarcoidosis. Respiratory insufficiency and failure due to far-advanced disease with fibrosis are managed in the usual way discussed in other sections of this book.

Course and Prognosis. The frequency of limited forms of sarcoidosis and common spontaneous remissions make the prognosis favorable in the majority of patients. A fairly acute onset with bilateral hilar lymphadenopathy has excellent prognosis. More insidious disease involving the lungs may progress to pulmonary fibrosis. It is almost impossible, however, to predict accurately the longterm outcome. It has been estimated that about 65% of patients recover completely or have only minimal residual disease, and the remaining will have some degree of permanent disability due to pulmonary fibrosis or involvement of the eyes, kidneys, heart, or central nervous system. A small percentage of these patients may succumb to their disease early in life, mostly from respiratory failure.

Residual cystic or cavitary lesions from sarcoidosis, not uncommonly, may become the site for aspergillus infection, resulting in the development of a fungus ball (page 95). The cause of significant hemoptysis in sarcoidosis is usually from this complication.

BIBLIOGRAPHY

Abe S, Munakata M, Nishimura M, et al. Gallium-67 scintigraphy, bronchoalveolar lavage, and pathologic changes in patients with pulmonary sarcoidosis. *Chest.* 1984; 85:650–655.

Benatar SR. Pulmonary sarcoidosis—old problems and new insights. *Postgrad Med J.* 1988; 64 (suppl 4):56–63.

Crystal RG, Roberts WC, Hunninghake GW, et al. Pulmonary sarcoidosis: A disease characterized and perpetuated by activated T-lymphocytes. *Ann Intern Med.* 1981; 94:73–94.

Daniele RP. Sarcoidosis: diagnosis and management. *Hosp Pract.* 1983; 18(6):113–122.

Johns CJ, Scott PP, Schonfeld SA. Sarcoidosis. *Ann Rev Med.* 1989; 40:353–371.

Mitchell DN, Scadding JG. Sarcoidosis. *Am Rev Respir Dis.* 1974; 110:774–802.

Sharma OP. Sarcoidosis. *Dis Mon.* 1990; 36:474–535.

Thomas PD, Hunninghake GW. Current concepts of the pathogenesis of sarcoidosis. *Am Rev Respir Dis.* 1987; 135:747–760.

CHAPTER 14

Immunologic Diseases of the Lung

The importance of immunology in various diseases is well recognized. It seems that, in a broader sense, the immune system is involved in almost every pathologic condition of the lung regardless of its cause. As discussed in the previous two chapters, diffuse infiltrative lung diseases are mediated, at least partly, by immunologic reactions. In this chapter, following a brief discussion of immune responses and the basic immunologically mediated lung injuries, some of the infiltrative diseases in which immunology plays the major role are considered.

THE IMMUNE RESPONSE

Most biologic agents, as well as many foreign substances, when introduced into the lungs, or in any other organ of the body, elicit a set of highly regulated reactions that vary according to whether or not there was a prior exposure to such agents. These agents are called **antigens,** and the reaction to them is known as the *immune response.*

The immune response is mediated by a complex interaction of several groups of specialized cells, which together with various organs and tissues involved with their formation, differentiation, and localization make up the *immune system.* The principal cells in this system are different classes of lymphocytes, which with the help of their chemical products of immunoglobulins (**antibodies**) and **lymphokines** are primarily responsible for protecting the body against environmental pathogens. Other cells, however, such as monocytes, macrophages, and granulocytes (including mast cells) and certain enzymatic proteins known as *complements* play essential parts in immunologic reactions. They help and expand the function of immunologically active lymphocytes.

The initial introduction of an antigen into the body results in activation and proliferation of the lymphocytes that bear membrane **receptors** specific for that antigen, and in production of specific antibodies. Upon a repeat encounter of the sensitized lymphocytes with the same antigen, a faster and greater response occurs. The two major groups of lymphocytes in the immunologic system are T cells (thymus-dependent) and B cells (bone marrow-derived). T lymphocytes have both regulatory and **effector** functions, which are mediated by their separate subpopulations. With the help of their mediators and certain other cells, the effector cells are responsible for induction of inflammatory responses including delayed hypersensitivity reaction (cell-mediated immunity). Regulatory cells (memory cells) recognize specific antigens and regulate the functions of both effector T cells and B cells. Dependent on their membrane markers, T cells are also divided into two major groups of CD4-positive (T4) and CD8-positive (T8) cells. The CD4-positive cells include most of the regulatory cells that have helper function. On the other hand, CD8-positive cells, include most of the regulatory cells with suppressor function; they also include cytotoxic cells.

The B lymphocytes are the precursors of antibody-producing cells known as *plasma cells*. With their surface markers, B cells are capable of reacting to specific antigens, which stimulate them to manufacture specific antibodies. The regulatory T lymphocytes affect the extent of antibody production.

Macrophages, by presenting antigens to lymphocytes, play an important role in induction of the immune response. They are also important effector cells; they phagocytize microorganisms, attack the neoplastic cells, and remove foreign particles. Organisms coated by antibodies are phagocytized much easier by macrophages. With the mediation of some of the lymphokines, macrophages have an essential role in cell-mediated immunity and delayed hypersensitivity.

Immunologic response is therefore divided into two broad categories of humoral and cell-mediated immunities, depending on the mechanism involved. In humoral or antibody-mediated immunity, the B lymphocytes are the primary cells involved; whereas in cell-mediated immunity, the T cells and macrophages play the central role. However, these two types of immune response may occur together.

Although the immunologic response is one of the most important mechanisms of the body's defense against different pathogenic agents, this response can at times be detrimental and result in pathologic reactions. Allergic asthma is an example in which immunologic reaction to an inhaled antigen results in an asthmatic attack. One of the important characteristics of the immune response is its ability to distinguish between the body's own substances and foreign antigens. The lack of discrimination between self and nonself in certain disorders results in production of antibodies (**autoantibodies**) and sensitized lymphocytes against self-antigens. This pathologic response is the basis of conditions known as autoimmune disorders, such as systemic lupus erythematosus (see below).

IMMUNE MECHANISMS OF LUNG INJURY

Immunologic reactions involved in pathogenesis of different lung diseases are varied and often not precise enough for their satisfactory classification. However, four standard types of immunologically mediated tissue injury seem to be operative in the pathogenesis of most of the allergic and immunologic pulmonary disorders, including different infiltrative lung diseases.

Type I, or immediate hypersensitivity, is the basic immunologic reaction in common allergic diseases. This type of immune response is the result of interaction between an antigen and its specific antibody (IgE) on the surface of mast cells and basophilic leukocytes, which cause the release of several mediators such as histamine and leukotrienes from these cells. Allergic asthma is a good example of this type of reaction (Chapter 9).

In *Type II*, or cytotoxic reaction, the circulating antibody reacts with a component of the cell or tissue that acts as an antigen, resulting in cellular or tissue damage. Goodpasture's syndrome (pulmonary hemorrhage with nephritis) is considered to represent a hypersensitivity reaction of this type. In this disease, circulating antibodies are directed against the alveolar, as well as glomerular, basement membranes.

Type III, or **immune complex** reaction, is due to the presence of antigen-antibody complexes in tissues. These complexes, which result from a combination of antigens with their specific antibodies, are either deposited from the circulation or are formed locally. The tissue injury results from the activation of the complement system, which in turn attracts phagocytic cells. In the process, inflammation and necrosis of small blood vessels also develop. Pulmonary vasculitis may be part of the picture of certain systemic immunologic disorders of this type, such as systemic lupus erythematosus and allergic vasculitis. It is also suggested that part of the immunologic process in extrinsic allergic alveolitis is related to this type of hypersensitivity reaction.

Type IV, cell-mediated or delayed hypersensitivity, is mediated by sensitized lymphocytes to various agents, mostly infectious. The effect of antigen on the sensitized T lymphocytes is their proliferation and release of lympho-

kines that affect macrophages and other cells, resulting in characteristic inflammation in which both of these effector cells predominate. The basis of the tuberculin test and other similar tests is a delayed hypersensitivity reaction. This type of reaction plays a major role in immunity against many infections. It is also the cause of basic pathologic changes in certain infectious diseases such as tuberculosis and fungus disease. In extrinsic allergic alveolitis, type IV reaction seems to be an important feature. It plays a major part in organ transplantation and is responsible for graft rejection.

HYPERSENSITIVITY PNEUMONITIS (EXTRINSIC ALLERGIC ALVEOLITIS)

Hypersensitivity pneumonitis is an immunologically mediated, diffuse inflammatory lung disease resulting from the inhalation of antigenic and, mainly, organic dust. It may be acute, subacute, or chronic, depending on the severity and the duration of exposure.

Etiology and Pathogenesis. This disease was originally described in workers who stripped bark from maple logs; in the same year, similar illness was observed in farmers exposed to moldy hay. Since then, numerous other occupations have been implicated in causing acute or chronic lung disorders, which later have been shown to be due to inhalation of certain organic dusts of animal or vegetable (fungal) origin.

These conditions have usually been named according to the occupations associated with them. Table 14–1 includes some of the known types of hypersensitivity pneumonitis according to the sources of exposure and the causative agents. The complete list is longer and continues to grow. As shown in Table 14–1, the antigens causing these various conditions are mostly the spores of certain molds, particularly *thermophilic actinomycetes,* but sometimes they may be bacteria or animal proteins. The particle sizes are small enough to reach the alveoli where they evoke immunologic reaction.

Because of their common pathogenetic mechanism, indistinguishable pathologic and radiographic changes, and similar clinical manifestations, these various diseases should be considered as a syndrome due to multiple causes.

Immunologic features of hypersensitivity pneumonitis indicate the involvement of both type III (immune complex-mediated) and, more significantly, type IV (cell-mediated) mechanisms. The elevation of specific serum antibody titers, characteristic skin reaction to the antigen, time interval between exposure and symptoms, and demonstration of antibodies in the lung tissue are strongly suggestive of a type III reaction. Inflammatory changes of alveolitis are the result of the immunologic response, which includes granuloma formation. Sometimes a nonspecific reaction also plays a part in inflammation. Type I reaction may develop in atopic individuals resulting in allergic asthma.

Depending on the intensity, duration, and frequency of exposure to the antigen, two different forms of hypersensitivity pneumonitis may develop. The acute form is usually secondary to heavy exposure of short duration, whereas the chronic form is the result of light but prolonged or repeated exposures. A subacute form has also been described. It should be emphasized that there is a significant variation in individual susceptibility for the development of hypersensitivity pneumonitis, as is true with other immunologic diseases.

Pathologic Changes. Pathologic changes depend on the stage of the disease at the time of examination. In the acute stage, there is interstitial pneumonitis with infiltration of the alveolar walls by various cells, including lymphocytes and macrophages. Granuloma formation with epithelioid cells, lymphocytes, and multinucleated

TABLE 14–1. TYPES OF HYPERSENSITIVITY PNEUMONITIS

Type of Disease	Source of Exposure	Main Antigen
Farmer's lung	Moldy hay	*Micropolyspora foeni*
Humidifier lung	Humidifier	*Thermoactinomyces vulgaris,* amebas, *penicillium* spp
Bird breeder's lung	Pigeons, other birds	avian protein
Maple bark-stripper's lung	Moldy maple bark	*Cryptostroma corticale*
Bagassosis	Moldy sugar cane	*T vulgaris, T sacchari*
Mushroom worker's lung	Mushroom compost	*M foeni* or *T vulgaris*
Suberosis	Moldy cork dust	*Penicillum* spp
Sequoiosis	Redwood sawdust	*Pullularia* spp, *Graphium* spp
Wood pulp worker's lung	Wood pulp	*Alternaria* spp
Malt worker's disease	Moldy barley	*Aspergillus clavatus*
Cheese worker's lung	Moldy cheese	*Pennicillium caseii*
Detergent worker's lung	Detergents	*B subtilis*

giant cells, resembling sarcoid reaction, can be demonstrated in some sections. Bronchioles may show evidence of obstruction with organizing endobronchial exudate. Acute vasculitis of the alveolar capillaries has also been described. In the subacute stage, interstitial thickening with beginning fibrosis and changes of chronic bronchiolitis are demonstrated. In the chronic form, the basic pathologic feature is interstitial fibrosis, indistinguishable from diffuse pulmonary fibrosis of other causes or of unknown etiology.

Clinical Manifestations. The clinical picture depends on the degree and mode of exposure, as well as the responsiveness of the individual. In susceptible persons, several hours after usually heavy exposure to organic dusts, symptoms resembling those of a respiratory-tract infection will develop. Chills, fever, malaise, cough, dyspnea, and chest tightness are the usual presenting symptoms. Wheezing is not a feature of allergic alveolitis unless the patient also develops a type I hypersensitivity reaction and responds with concomitant asthma. In the acute form, the symptoms resolve spontaneously within a few days, only to recur following another exposure. Physical examination in this stage may reveal fever, tachypnea, cyanosis, and bibasilar pulmonary rales.

Some patients have a more insidious presentation, with slowly progressive cough, dyspnea, weakness, and weight loss. This form of onset is seen in patients with prolonged but light exposure. The patient is not usually aware of the relationship of his symptoms with his occupation. Repeated or prolonged continuous exposure to organic dusts is one cause of diffuse pulmonary fibrosis. At this stage the symptoms are related to respiratory insufficiency.

Radiographic Findings. In the acute stage, the chest roentgenogram may show diffuse nodular or patchy infiltration. These changes usually clear with discontinuation of exposure. In the chronic form, reticular pattern of pulmonary fibrosis is the predominant radiographic finding.

Pulmonary Function Tests. Pulmonary function studies will indicate restrictive impairment with reduction in vital capacity, diminished compliance, and low diffusing capacity. These abnormalities are reversible in acute form. In chronic stage, in addition to restrictive ventilatory impairment, a certain degree of obstructive defect may be demonstrated.

Diagnosis. The most important source of information for the diagnosis of hypersensitivity pneumonitis is from a thorough and accurate history. Because of the multiplicity of antigens that can result in this disease, the variation in the duration and the severity of exposure, and the time delay between the exposure and the occurrence of symptoms, a detailed occupational history, including the exact nature of work and hobby, should be obtained. The subacute and chronic forms are particularly difficult to diagnose.

Abnormality of serum proteins and presence of certain antibodies, particularly precipitating antibody against a suspected antigen, are common findings in hypersensitivity pneumonitis. A positive precipitin test, however, is not diagnostic, as it may also be positive in healthy individuals who have been exposed to antigens without developing the disease. The value of positive skin reaction to suspected antigen is also limited. The most specific test of inhalation challenge with a suspected antigenic material is used primarily for research purpose. The demonstration of a positive response with development of symptoms, radiographic changes, and pulmonary functional abnormalities will be diagnostic. Bronchoalveolar lavage has not proven to be a helpful diagnostic test in hypersensitivity pneumonitis.

Management. As is true with all preventable diseases, the most effective measure is the avoidance of exposure to pathogenic agents. The acute symptoms usually subside spontaneously and require no treatment in mild cases. In more severe forms, corticosteroids will hasten the resolution and give symptomatic relief. Avoidance of further exposure to the responsible organic dust should be emphasized. In more chronic forms, removal of patients from the contaminated environment will prevent further progress of the disease.

GOODPASTURE'S SYNDROME

Goodpasture's syndrome is a relatively rare condition, but is the only pulmonary disease known to be due to type II or cytotoxic hypersensitivity reactions. Circulating antibodies against renal glomerular basement membrane are directed also against the alveolar basement membrane, causing both glomerular and alveolar damage.

This syndrome is manifested by episodic pulmonary hemorrhage from diffuse injury to the alveolar capillary wall and renal impairment. Patients are usually young males. For an unexplained reason, pulmonary hemorrhage occurs more often in smokers than in nonsmokers. It seems that the underlying lung injury from other causes, such as viral infection, may also predispose to alveolar hemorrhage in Goodpasture's syndrome. Common manifestations are hemoptysis, dyspnea, anemia, diffuse pulmonary infiltrate, and signs of kidney disease.

Radiographic study during an acute episode shows a pattern of patchy airspace consolidation distributed unevenly throughout the lungs. In several days, a reticular pattern replaces the consolidation, which may clear further until the next episode of pulmonary hemorrhage. The radiographic changes are due to intraalveolar accumulation of blood and fibrotic reaction. Antibasement-membrane antibody can be demonstrated in the serum of most patients. The diagnosis is usually confirmed by the demonstration of immunopathologic changes in a kidney or lung biopsy. Spuriously increased CO diffusing capacity (DL_{co}) in Goodpasture's syndrome is due to uptake of carbon monoxide by the blood retained in the alveolar spaces.

The prognosis of Goodpasture's syndrome is generally poor, and death usually results from progressive kidney failure. Treatment with corticosteroids and **immunosuppressive** agents has been of some benefit in a few patients. The most promising therapy appears to be **plasmapheresis** (plasma exchange) through which the offending antibody in the blood is removed.

A closely related condition involving the lungs, but without kidney lesion or evidence of antigen-antibody reaction, is referred to as *idiopathic pulmonary hemosiderosis*, which is primarily a disease of young children.

PULMONARY MANIFESTATIONS OF CERTAIN SYSTEMIC IMMUNOLOGIC DISEASES

Under this heading we shall briefly discuss some of the systemic, probably immunologic, diseases in which pulmonary involvement is a common manifestation. Although the exact etiology of these diseases is unknown, there is ample evidence to believe that an immune mechanism is playing a major part in their pathogenesis. Because of the presence of certain antibodies against some of the body proteins or cell constituents in several of these conditions, they are sometimes referred to as *autoimmune disorders*. As connective tissue and blood vessels are involved, they are also recognized under the appellation of collagen vascular disease.

Systemic Lupus Erythematosus

Lupus erythematosus (LE) is a systemic autoimmune disease with varied clinical manifestations. Vascular and connective tissue lesions are the major pathologic changes, involving primarily the skin and serous membranes, but almost any organ in the body may be affected. This disease is more common in women of childbearing age. The clinical course is usually chronic with frequent remissions and exacerbations. The major immunologic reaction is type III or immune complex-mediated, and vasculitis is an important pathologic change in systemic lupus. Antibodies are formed against different cell constituents, particularly cell nuclei and their proteins. The diagnostic

studies are based on demonstration of these antibodies and LE cell phenomenon. The latter consists of demonstration of neutrophilic white blood cells that have engulfed a homogeneous material derived from nuclei of other cells.

Involvement of the lung and the pleura is a common feature of systemic lupus erythematosus; as many as 70% of patients have been reported to show such involvement. Pleural reaction with effusion is a characteristic manifestation of this disease. Pleural effusions are frequently bilateral and small. Pleuritis may be associated with chest pain. Pulmonary parenchymal disease may be present without symptoms or abnormal physical findings.

Common radiographic findings are bilateral elevation of the diaphragm and platelike atelectasis in the lung bases. Transient lung infiltrates may also be seen. Chronic changes with fibrosis are fairly common findings in late stages of the disease. An acute form with symptoms suggestive of pneumonia may progress rapidly, resulting in respiratory failure. Pulmonary hemorrhage with hemoptysis, similar to Goodpasture's syndrome, is occasionally seen. Its mechanism is unclear. As patients with systemic lupus erythematosus are predisposed to infection, respiratory-tract infection should always be suspected and differentiated from lesions related directly to lupus.

Pulmonary function tests may be abnormal despite lack of clinical or radiographic evidence of lung involvement. Most common findings include reduced vital capacity, diffusing capacity, and pulmonary compliance, indicating restrictive impairment. Arterial blood studies may show varying degrees of hypoxemia, usually with hypocapnia.

Rheumatoid Disease

Rheumatoid disease, commonly known as rheumatoid arthritis, is a systemic disorder with predominant involvement of the joints and related structures, which may result in crippling deformities. Although its cause remains unknown, there is enough evidence to implicate an immune mechanism. Demonstration of antibodies against gamma-globulins in serum and joint fluid supports the concept of **autoimmunity** in the pathogenesis of rheumatoid disease. The antibodies are generally known as rheumatoid factors.

In addition to the characteristic joint lesions, other tissues and organs may be affected. Subcutaneous nodules, vasculitis, eye lesions, and pleuropulmonary manifestations are fairly common in patients with rheumatoid arthritis.

Pulmonary and pleural lesions in rheumatoid arthritis are probably the result of immune complex-mediated reaction and are associated with high titers of circulating rheumatoid factor. The incidence of pleuropulmonary involvement in rheumatoid disease is quite variable in the reported series. In some, over 50% of patients have been reported to show radiographic changes in the lung or pleura consistent with rheumatoid involvement. Although rheumatoid arthritis is much more common in women than men, pleuropulmonary manifestations are more prevalent among men.

Pleural involvement is probably the most common intrathoracic lesion in rheumatoid disease. A variable amount of pleural effusion, which has the features of an exudate, may be demonstrated. Very low glucose content of this fluid is characteristic of rheumatoid effusion.

Pulmonary parenchymal lesions in rheumatoid disease are conveniently divided into two categories:

1. The nodular lesions of variable size and number are detected by chest radiograph. The patients usually have no symptoms.
2. Diffuse interstitial pneumonitis and fibrosis are indistinguishable from idiopathic pulmonary fibrosis and similar pulmonary lesions of other causes.

Dyspnea is the most common presenting symptom; it may be associated with cough and chest pain. Radiographic findings are the same as in other forms of interstitial pulmonary fibrosis discussed earlier. Pulmonary function tests show restrictive impairment.

Rheumatoid arthritis, on rare occasions, may be the cause of upper airway obstruction from the involvement of the larynx. Abnormality of the mandible from long-standing rheumatoid arthritis may be the cause of obstructive sleep apnea syndrome.

A closely related condition is **ankylosing spondylitis,** which characteristically involves the spine and causes fixation of the thoracic cage. The chest of these patients in advanced cases shows overinflation and marked restriction of its movement. Occasionally apical lesions with fibrosis suggestive of tuberculosis may be seen on chest x-ray film. Although only a few patients may have respiratory symptoms, pulmonary function studies usually show a pattern of restrictive impairment with hyperinflation.

Progressive Systemic Sclerosis (Scleroderma)

Progressive systemic **sclerosis** is a disease that primarily involves the blood vessels and connective tissue and results in vascular insufficiency and progressive fibrosis of various organs. Its incidence is three times higher in females than males. There is increasing evidence that autoimmunity plays a major role in its pathogenesis. The resultant regulatory defect in the activity of fibroblasts with an uncontrolled collagen fiber formation seems to be the basic pathologic abnormality. Skin, musculoskeletal system, gastrointestinal tract, lungs, heart, and kidneys are frequently involved. Characteristic skin changes, especially of the face, may be diagnostic in typical cases. Scleroderma is a progressive disease and generally has a poor prognosis. Death is usually due to pulmonary complications, heart failure, or renal insufficiency.

Pulmonary manifestations are very common in progressive systemic sclerosis. Morphologic changes have been reported in up to 90% of the cases. The usual pathologic findings are interstitial fibrosis, bronchiolar dilatation, pleural fibrosis with adhesions, and vascular changes. Clinical manifestations include progressive dyspnea, cough, basilar rales, and evidence of cor pulmonale. Some patients may have significant pulmonary hypertension and cor pulmonale with little or no clinical or radiographic evidence of lung disease. This is due to primary involvement of pulmonary vessels resulting in their narrowing and occlusion, which may occur without significant parenchymal disease.

Radiographic findings are similar to changes due to pulmonary fibrosis from other causes. The earlier fine reticular pattern may progress to marked honeycombing, mostly in the lower lung fields. Changes in pulmonary hypertension may be noted, with or without increased parenchymal density.

As in other forms of chronic interstitial lung disease, pulmonary function tests show a pattern of restrictive impairment, including reduced diffusing capacity. Sometimes functional defect may be present without radiographic abnormality. Hypoxemia, mostly with exercise, and hypocapnia are common blood gas abnormalities.

In addition to the primary involvement of the lung, patients with progressive systemic sclerosis are prone to develop other pulmonary complications, particularly pneumonia. Esophageal abnormalities, very common manifestations of scleroderma, may also predispose these patients to aspiration.

Polymyositis

Polymyositis (*poly,* many, + *myositis,* inflammation of muscle) is a chronic inflammatory disease of striated muscles of unknown etiology. When the skin is also involved, it is referred to as **dermatomyositis.** Other organs, such as heart, lung, and gastrointestinal tract, also may be occasionally affected. Based on pathologic evidence and the presence of autoantibodies in the serum of patients with polymyositis, cell-mediated autoimmunity is considered to be its underlying pathogenetic mechanism.

Clinical manifestations are mostly related to involvement of skeletal muscles, resulting in progressive weakness of proximal muscles of the extremities as well as cervical, pharyngeal, and trunk muscles. Although the lungs may be directly involved by the disease process, causing interstitial pneumonitis and fibrosis, pulmonary complications are usually the result of swallowing difficulty and respiratory muscle weakness.

Indeed, bronchopneumonia, with or without respiratory failure, is the most common cause of death in polymyositis. Frequent use of large doses of corticosteroids and immunosuppressive drugs in the treatment of this disease has increased the infectious complications. Difficulty in swallowing predisposes to frequent episodes of aspiration. Respiratory muscle weakness impairs the effectiveness of cough and other forced respiratory maneuvers, increasing the risk of pulmonary infection. Furthermore, severe inspiratory muscle weakness results in ventilatory failure, which is frequently precipitated by an intercurrent bronchopulmonary infection.

A condition in which the clinical features of more than one of the aforementioned entities coexist is known as *mixed connective tissue disease*. Pulmonary manifestations, which are mainly due to diffuse interstitial fibrosis, are very common in this disorder. There are many other, rather uncommon, systemic diseases due to immunologic disorders that may involve the lungs. These include *polyarteritis nodosa, Sjögren's syndrome, Wegener's granulomatosis*, and other related conditions. Due to the limitation of the scope of this book, they will not be discussed. Interested readers are referred to other texts on pulmonary diseases and articles mentioned in the Bibliography.

BIBLIOGRAPHY

Baydur A, Morgan ES. Thoracic manifestations in rheumatoid arthritis. *Semin Respir Med.* 1988; 9:305–317.

Bienenstock J. The lung as an immunologic organ. *Annu Rev Med.* 1984; 35:46–62.

Daniele RP, Henson PM, Fantone JC III, et al. Immune complex injury of the lung. *Am Rev Respir Dis.* 1981; 124:738–755.

Dickey BF, Myers AR. Pulmonary disease in polymyositis/dermatomyositis. *Semin Arthritis Rheum.* 1984; 14:60–76.

Eagen JW, Memoli VA, Roberts JL, et al. Pulmonary hemorrhage in systemic lupus erythematosus. *Medicine.* 1978; 57:545–560.

Fauci AS, Haynes BF, Katz P, Wolff SM. Wegener's granulomatosis. *Ann Intern Med.* 1983; 98:76–85.

Fink JN. Hypersensitivity pneumonitis. *J Allergy Clin Immunol.* 1984; 74:1–9.

Leavitt RY, Fauci AS. Pulmonary vasculitis. *Am Rev Respir Dis.* 1986; 134:149–166.

Martens J, Demedts M, Vanmeenen MT, Dequeker J. Respiratory muscle dysfunction in systemic lupus erythematosus. *Chest.* 1983; 84:170–175.

Morgan PGM, Turner-Warwick M. Pulmonary haemosiderosis and pulmonary hemorrhage. *Br J Dis Chest.* 1981; 75:225–242.

Owens GR, Follansbee WP. Cardiopulmonary manifestations of systemic sclerosis. *Chest.* 1987; 91:118–127.

Quismorio FF. Clinical and pathologic features of lung involvement in system lupus erythematosus. *Semin Respir Med.* 1988; 9:297–304.

Reynolds HY. Immunologic lung diseases. *Chest.* 1982; 81:626–631, 745–751.

Salvaggio JE. Hypersensitivity pneumonitis. *J Allergy Clin Immunol.* 1987; 79:558–571.

Sullivan WD, Hurst DJ, Harmon CE, et al. A prospective evaluation emphasizing pulmonary involvement in patients with mixed connective tissue disease. *Medicine.* 1984; 63:92–107.

Urbano-Márquez A, Casademont J, Grau JM. Polymyositis/dermatomyositis: the current position. *Ann Rhum Dis.* 1991; 50: 191–195.

Wiedemann HP, Matthay RA. Pulmonary manifestations of collagen vascular diseases. *Clin Chest Med.* 1989; 10:677–722.

Environmental and Inhalational Lung Diseases

CHAPTER 15

Environmental Lung Diseases

Environmental lung diseases are pathologic conditions of the respiratory tract that result directly from the inhalation of various gaseous or particulate matters in the air. Most, but not all, of these conditions are job-related and are also known as occupational lung diseases.

ENVIRONMENTAL EXPOSURE

The lungs are continuously exposed to a variety of external pathogenic agents in the form of fine particles and gas suspended in or mixed with atmospheric air. This atmospheric contamination is mainly manmade in populated areas of the world and, for the most part, is related to industrial development. These environmental pulmonary pathogens of various origin and composition enter the lungs as aerosol, in gaseous form, or as a mixture of the two. The deposition and the absorption of these substances on the airways or gas-exchanging membrane are related to their physical and chemical characteristics, the anatomical arrangement of air passages, and the rate of air flow.

Particle size is a major physical factor in determining the site where the aerosolized materials will deposit. The anatomical structures of the airways and changes in direction of air flow through the continuously dividing air passages result in *inertial impaction,* which is the principal mechanism of large particle deposition in the respiratory tract. Particles larger than 10 to 20 microns (μ) in diameter are almost totally removed in the upper airways by this mechanism. Some of the smaller particles are also deposited by inertial impaction. Settling by *gravity* or *sedimentation* is another important mechanism for particle deposition in the respiratory tract; this is the major way of deposition for particles ranging in diameter from 0.1 to over 50 μ. Very small particles are deposited mainly by diffusion or Brownian motion. The majority of particles reaching the terminal airways and alveoli are less than 4 μ in diameter and are deposited by gravitational forces and Brownian action. Much smaller particles, which will have no appreciable deposition, will be exhaled. Although large particles do not reach the distal airways, asbestos fibers can be demonstrated in the lung parenchyma despite their sizable length (up to 100 μ). The very small diameter of these fibers, despite their length, is probably the reason for their slowed sedimentation and their ability to penetrate deeper into the lung tissue.

Pulmonary Defense Mechanisms

Gaseous agents entering the lungs encounter little, if any, resistance. This is understandable considering the main function of the lung, which is to draw in environmental gases and distribute them throughout the alveolar surface area. The only defenses that the lung may exhibit are temporary cessation of breathing as a reflex upon exposure to irritant gases, partial absorption of soluble gases on the moist surfaces of the airways, and detoxification by chemical combination. These defenses, however, are inadequate; with significant exposure, noxious gases will have their damaging effects.

Inhaled particulate matters, once deposited on different areas of the respiratory tract, are taken care of by several defense mechanisms. Particles deposited on the mucous surface of the nasal passages and other parts of the upper airways are readily disposed of by ciliary movements toward the pharynx, from where they are swallowed or coughed out. Sneezing and blowing the nose also help in expelling these particles mixed with nasal secretions.

The mucous blanket over the ciliated epithelium of the tracheobronchial tree is the major vehicle for particles deposited on its surface. Cilia are normally bathed in more serous fluid, called the *sol layer*, or periciliary fluid,

which facilitates their rhythmic beating. The mucus, or *gel layer*, actually floats over the sol layer, and only its undersurface is contacted by the cilia, which propel it from beneath (Fig. 15–1). Particular viscoelastic behavior of the tracheobronchial mucus is very helpful in its movement. The speed of mucus movement and, therefore, the transport of particles deposited on it has been estimated to be between 10 and 20 mm per minute, so that 90% of the material settled on the airway mucosa is physically cleared in less than 1 hour.

The irritating effect of certain particles and gases increases airway secretions. With repeated and chronic exposure, the mucous glands will hypertrophy and will secrete more mucus in response to a variety of inhaled irritants. This is the basic pathologic change of chronic bronchitis, which was discussed earlier. *Cough* is an important mechanism by which secretions and foreign particles are expelled. Irritation of the nerve endings in the airway mucosa by these materials stimulates the cough reflex.

Distal airways (bronchioles) and alveoli have no ciliated epithelium, mucous glands, or goblet cells; therefore, particles deposited in their lumen are removed with more difficulty. Alveolar clearance involves more complex pathways of cellular and fluid transport. Phagocytic cells in the alveoli (macrophages) play the major role in disposing of the particles reaching this part of the

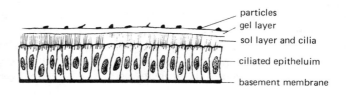

Figure 15–1. Mucous blanket on the ciliated epithelium.

particles
gel layer
sol layer and cilia
ciliated epitheluim
basement membrane

respiratory tract. In addition, alveolar surfactant, secreted by the type II alveolar cells, and fluid originating from capillary **transudation** help in transporting the particles toward the mucociliary escalator or in draining into the interstitial space and, thence, to the lymph channels. Disposal of particles from the alveoli is a very slow process, and the respiratory membrane remains exposed to their harmful effects until they are removed. Coating of the particles by secretory materials such as surfactant and certain chemical reactions, as well as enzymatic action, diminish their injurious effects.

Once phagocytized, particles are processed by the metabolic and enzymatic apparatus of the alveolar macrophages. The phagocytic effectiveness of these cells is influenced by a variety of **exogenous** as well as **endogenous** factors. Sometimes the offending agents impair the function of these cells. For example, silica causes death of macrophages, resulting in release of their enzymes as well as the silica particles.

When these primary disposing mechanisms fail to control the pathogenic factors from exerting their harmful effects, the secondary cellular and humoral defense mechanisms are brought into action. These mechanisms result in inflammation, which consists of dilatation and increased permeability of capillaries, exudation of fluid, and infiltration of white blood cells. The immunologic system plays a major part in this process. Macrophages are involved in presenting antigenic substances to the immunocompetent lymphocytes and, therefore, in helping them to initiate an immunologic response. It seems, therefore, that the pathologic changes are, at

least partly, the result of these secondary defense mechanisms.

Environmental pulmonary pathogens can be divided into four categories:

1. Infectious agents
2. Organic dusts
3. Inorganic dusts
4. Gases

Pulmonary diseases due to the agents in the first two categories have already been discussed in separate chapters. Some of the common diseases known to be due to inorganic dusts and certain gases will be reviewed in this chapter. Because of its importance in the pathogenesis of many pulmonary and extrapulmonary diseases, tobacco smoking will be discussed separately in Chapter 16.

ENVIRONMENTAL DISEASES DUE TO INORGANIC DUSTS

Diseases due to inhalation of inorganic dusts are generally referred to as **pneumoconioses** (*pneumo*, lung; *konia*, dust; *osis*, condition). Several factors will determine the outcome of exposure to such particles. These include chemical nature, particle size, severity and duration of exposure, and host factors. The latter are related to individual susceptibility, including the immunologic response and local handling of dust by bronchopulmonary defense mechanisms. Thus it is not uncommon for two individuals with the same degree of exposure to the same agent and under similar circumstances to have two quite different responses; one may remain unharmed, while the other may show evidence of significant lung disease.

Almost all cases of inorganic dust

pneumoconiosis are secondary to occupational exposure, particularly in the mining industry. There are other circumstances, however, where exposure to such mineral dusts is possible. Only with a thorough and detailed *occupational* and *environmental history* will the exact nature of these diseases become recognized. There are few or no clinical or radiographic features that can identify the cause of specific occupational lung disease.

The most important inorganic dusts causing pneumoconiosis are silicon dioxide (silica), silicates (asbestos, talc, kaolin, mica, etc.), and carbon (coal, graphite, etc.). Pneumoconioses due to less common causes, such as beryllium, iron, tin, aluminum, cobalt, and several others, will not be discussed.

Silicosis

Pneumoconiosis due to silica exposure is a fairly common chronic fibrosing disease of the lung that may occur in many occupations. Silica or silicon dioxide is a compound of the two most abundant elements of the earth's crust, oxygen and silicon. It is the main constituent of more than 95% of the earth's rocks. It occurs in a variety of forms, but the most common form is crystalline quartz. It becomes harmful when small respirable particles (less than 5μ in diameter) of crystalline silica are produced with its various industrial use. Sources of free silica dust include industries such as mining, quarrying, tunneling, stone masonry, road construction, sandblasting, stonecutting, abrasive industry, molding in foundries, pottery, and tile manufacturing. In many of these occupations, particularly in mining, the workers may be exposed to other particulate matters in addition to the silica dust, such as coal, asbestos, iron, and other minerals.

The development of silicosis depends on the particle size of the silica, its concentration in air, duration of exposure, and individual susceptibility. The particle size range that results in maximal alveolar deposition is 1 to 3 μ. The concentration of silica dust usually determines the rapidity of the onset of clinical manifestations of silicosis. Heavy exposure, sometimes seen in sandblasters, may result in a more acute form of silicosis after a relatively brief exposure. However, with a less heavy concentration, the disease requires many years of exposure to develop.

Pathogenesis and Pathology. Silica particles deposited in the alveoli are phagocytized by the macrophages. The interaction between these cells and silica seems to be pivotal in pathogenesis of silicosis. From in vitro studies, it is known that silica particles damage the macrophages and cause the release of intracellular enzymes as well as phagocytized silica. There is increasing in vivo evidence, however, that the release of inflammatory mediators from live macrophages is mainly responsible for pathologic changes of silicosis. Lymphocytes, neutrophils, and fibroblasts are all known to participate in the process. Immune mechanisms appear to have a significant role in silicosis. The impairment of function of macrophages is probably the cause of reduced defense of silicotic lungs against certain infections, especially tuberculosis.

The characteristic pathologic changes in silicosis are *silicotic nodules,* which are whorled and densely packed fibrotic lesions. They measure 2 to 3 mm in diameter and are unevenly scattered throughout the lungs, mostly in the upper lobes and the perihilar regions. These nodules are usually surrounded by distorted lung tissue, which may show emphysematous changes. Silica particles may be demonstrated in these lesions as well as in hilar and mediastinal lymph nodes.

The **coalescence** of nodular fibrosis, particularly in the upper lobes, results in the formation of irregular masses, which may become quite large and occasionally may show evidence of central cavitation. These changes are characteristic of *progressive massive fibrosis* (PMF), and are indicative of *complicated* silicosis. Such lesions have been frequently attributed to concomitant tuberculosis, atypical mycobacterial disease, or other infections. With progressive massive fibrosis, the upper lobes may become contracted, and the lower lobes may show evidence of emphysema, sometimes with large bullous changes.

Clinical Manifestations. Silicosis is a chronic disease, usually with an insidious onset after prolonged exposure to silica dust. It is not uncommon for the symptoms to develop many years after cessation of exposure. With heavy exposure, as seen in sandblasting, the symptoms may develop more rapidly. The pulmonary lesions of silicosis and associated disability are often progressive, despite removal of the patients from their dusty environment. Patients with simple silicosis are often asymptomatic. The main symptom with *complicated silicosis* is dyspnea, with or without cough. The severity of dyspnea is variable, but it is usually progressive. The history of cough and expectoration is often due to concomitant cigarette smoking. Other respiratory symptoms, such as hemoptysis or chest pain, are usually secondary to superimposed infection. Although tuberculosis and atypical mycobacterial infection are often implicated in the production of progressive massive fibrosis, clinical confirmation is difficult. Repeated bacteriologic studies are indicated, especially if the tuberculin test is positive. In more advanced complicated silicosis, respiratory failure may supervene.

Radiographic Findings. In the simple form of silicosis, multiple small nodular shadows can be demonstrated throughout the lung fields. For the development of radiographic changes, 10, 20, or more years of moderate exposure are necessary. However, with more heavy exposure, such as in sandblasting, roentgenographic changes may be demonstrated much earlier. In *complicated silicosis*, massive densities are seen in upper lung fields (Figs. 15–2, 15–3). Progressive change from a simple nodu-

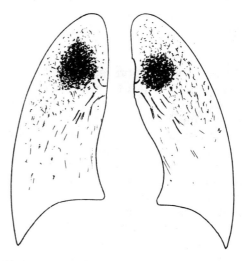

Figure 15–2. Progressive massive fibrosis of silicosis.

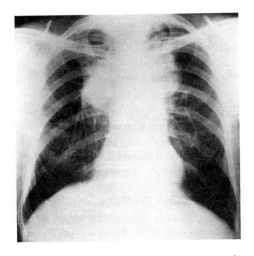

Figure 15–3. Chest radiograph of progressive massive fibrosis appearing as bilateral upper lobe masses. Both silicosis and coal workers' pneumoconiosis may cause this type of radiographic change.

lar form to massive fibrosis may take place within 5 years. With the development of massive fibrosis, the upper lobes show evidence of volume loss, with elevation of the hili and emphysematous changes of the lower lobes. In a small percentage of patients, characteristic eggshell calcification of hilar nodes may be present.

Pulmonary Function Tests. There is no characteristic pattern of pulmonary functional abnormality in patients with silicosis. In simple silicosis, the routine spirographic study is usually normal. In more severe disease, restrictive, obstructive, or mixed patterns of impairment may be demonstrated. Diffusing capacity and pulmonary compliance are frequently reduced. Serial pulmonary function studies are very important in evaluating the course and progression of the disease.

Management. There is no known effective treatment for any of the inorganic

dust pneumoconioses, including silicosis. However, preventive measures are most effective against acquiring these diseases. Awareness of health hazards associated with various industries is the first step, which should be followed by efforts in eliminating or reducing the exposure of the lungs to these offending agents. Proper ventilation of the work area; use of wet techniques; wearing of special masks, hoods, or respirators; and other methods of controlling the environment would markedly diminish the occupational hazards of silica exposure.

The principles of management of diffuse pulmonary fibrosis discussed earlier (Chapter 12) are equally applicable to well-established silicosis. Because of the increased risk of tuberculosis infection in patients with silicosis, necessary preventive and therapeutic measures should be taken against this complication. Patients with a positive tuberculin test without active tuberculosis are candidates for prophylaxis with isoniazid therapy.

Coal Workers' Pneumoconiosis

Coal workers' pneumoconiosis, commonly known as "black lung," is a chronic pathologic condition resulting from prolonged exposure to coal dust. The role of silica dust, often present with coal mining, is relatively small in coal miners' pneumoconiosis. There are occasional situations in coal mining, such as drilling operations in areas with significant rock strata, in which heavy silica exposure may result in silicosis. Although carbon is not a fibrogenic agent, with massive and prolonged exposure the clearance mechanisms of the lung are overwhelmed, and coal dust accumulates in terminal air spaces, resulting in pulmonary pathology.

As with other inorganic dust pneumoconioses, the severity and duration of exposure are among the major factors determining the pathologic changes due to coal dust inhalation. The area at which coal is cut, known as the coal face, is the dustiest part of the mine. Workers in this area are, therefore, exposed to a very high concentration of coal dust. The degree of exposure of workers in other areas of mining and transportation is variable. The incidence of pneumoconiosis in anthracite mining is much higher than in soft (**bituminous**) coal mining. It has been estimated that it takes at least 10 to 12 years of underground work for the development of coal workers' pneumoconiosis.

Pathogenesis and Pathology. The first reaction after the deposition of coal dust in the respiratory bronchioles and alveoli is phagocytosis of the particles by increasing numbers of macrophages. They move to the terminal bronchioles, from which they are removed by the mucociliary escalator. An excessive dust load results in overwhelming the pulmonary clearance mechanisms. Fibroblasts appear in this area, laying a thin network of reticulin fibers without significant collagen formation. The aggregations of macrophages and dust particles enmeshed in reticulin fibers is called *coal* **macules** (spots), as they appear as black dots on the lung sections. These spots are often associated with dilatation of respiratory bronchioles, called *focal* centrilobular emphysema. These changes are characteristic pathologic findings in *simple* coal workers' pneumoconiosis. The *complicated* form, as in silicosis, is characterized by massive fibrosis, involving mostly the upper lobes. However, in coal workers' pneumoconiosis, the lesions are black and, unlike silicosis in

which they consist of a conglomeration of silicotic nodules, they are amorphous and relatively homogeneous. They develop less commonly than in silicosis. Coal dust is also known to produce pathologic changes of chronic bronchitis. Cigarette smoking is, however, a much more important factor in causing bronchial mucosal changes than coal dust in coal miners who are smokers.

Clinical Manifestations. Simple pneumoconiosis produces no significant symptoms or signs. Coal workers with simple pneumoconiosis or clear chest x-rays who have significant symptoms, particularly dyspnea, usually have concomitant chronic bronchitis or emphysema probably unrelated to their exposure. In the complicated form, dyspnea, mostly with exercise, is often present. Expectoration of black material (**melanoptysis**) is common in coal workers, with or without pneumoconiosis. In the advanced and complicated form of disease, signs of respiratory failure, including pulmonary hypertension and cor pulmonale, may be present.

Radiographic Findings. Simple pneumoconiosis is characterized by reticular and nodular densities throughout the lung fields. The nodules are small and less defined that those of silicosis. Large shadows of 1 cm or more in diameter are indicative of complicated pneumoconiosis, known as progressive massive fibrosis (Fig. 15–3). These lesions are almost always restricted to the upper lung fields. They may sometimes cavitate.

Pulmonary Function Studies. The majority of nonsmoking patients with simple pneumoconiosis have no significant abnormality on routine pulmonary function studies. Some increase in residual volume, however, has been demonstrated in many coal workers with simple pneumoconiosis and sometimes without chest x-ray abnormalities. With special studies, evidence of small airway obstruction can be shown in most workers with significant coal dust exposure, even without radiographic abnormalities. Patients with complicated pneumoconiosis often have evidence of restrictive as well as obstructive impairment of pulmonary function. Diffusing capacity is often reduced. In most studies it has been demonstrated that in coal workers' pneumoconiosis smoking is by far the most important factor in producing respiratory symptoms and reducing ventilatory functions.

Management. The measures mentioned in management of silicosis are relevant in prevention of coal workers' pneumoconiosis as well. Early detection of radiographic changes in the latter condition and cessation of exposure, however, prevents further progression of disease, in contrast to silicosis in which the lesions may progress despite removal of patients from their environment. Patients with simple coal workers' pneumoconiosis who have no symptoms need no treatment. The principles of treatment of complicated disease are similar to those discussed in chronic obstructive pulmonary disease and pulmonary fibrosis.

Asbestos-Associated Diseases: Asbestosis

Asbestos Exposure. Asbestos is a generic name applied to a family of fibrous hydrated silicates, which have been widely used in industry because of their unique physical characteristics. Asbestos fiber is flexible, heat resistant, and extremely durable. Of the several forms of asbestos, chrysotile is most commonly used in North America. Until recently, this mineral was extensively used in the construction industry in the form of asbestos cement products, such as pipes, tiles, shingles, and other roofing products. The risks of exposure not only occur during their manufacture, but also when they are being cut, drilled, or demolished. In addition, there are numerous other uses, including manufacture of insulation materials, car brake and clutch linings, air filters, fire-resistant clothing, ship building and repairing, and undercoating of cars.

Recent legislation has resulted in a significant reduction in the widespread use of asbestos in the manufacturing industry in this country. Large amounts of asbestos, however, may still be released into the air during demolition and renovation of old buildings and ships, contributing to the atmospheric pollution. Moreover, many individuals are known who were exposed when asbestos use was uncontrolled. Asbestos carried in the clothing of workers has also been a source of exposure to other members of the household. Therefore, asbestos exposure occurs not only from work in mining, manufacturing, and use of its products, but also from neighborhood and other forms of contamination and general community asbestos air pollution. Although clinical **asbestosis** usually develops following more significant and prolonged exposure, the question of potential health hazards of low-concentrations of asbestos and short duration of exposure, such as its carcinogenic effect, has remained unanswered. A long interval, sometimes up to 30 or 40 years, between the time of exposure and development of neoplasia makes the evaluation of the cause-and-effect relationship even more difficult.

Pathology and Pathogenesis. Pleuropulmonary complications of asbestos exposure are pulmonary fibrosis, bronchogenic carcinoma, pleural effusion, pleural fibrosis, and mesothelioma. They may develop singly or, often, in various combinations. The term *asbestosis* is applied to pulmonary parenchymal reaction to asbestos and development of fibrosis. The mechanism of production of pleuropulmonary lesion by asbestos fibers is not entirely understood. It seems that initial injury to the terminal airways, alveolar walls, and interstitial tissue causes inflammatory reaction, which leads to fibrosis. The inflammation is primarily the result of activation of the alveolar macrophages. The participation of other inflammatory cells, notably neutrophilic leukocytes, and the release of inflammatory mediators and oxygen radicals seem to be important in progression of pathologic process. Shorter asbestos fibers are readily phagocytized and removed. However, longer asbestos fibers remain in distal airways and alveoli and continue to stimulate unsuccessful phagocytic activity, perpetuating inflammation and fibrous tissue formation. The fact that the pathologic process continues long after the exposure has ceased is strongly supportive of this pathogenetic concept.

Fibrosis in asbestosis, unlike silicosis, is nonnodular, involves mostly the lower lung fields, and is often accompanied by fibrous pleural thickening. The extent of fibrosis is variable; in the mild form there is thickened alveolar septa; in severe fibrosis the alveolar spaces are hardly visible. Advanced asbestosis is one of the causes of honeycomb lung. Asbestos fibers can be identified in these lesions, sometimes enveloped in an iron-containing protein film, giving them a characteristic feature. They are referred to as *asbestos bodies* or, more appropriately, *ferrugenous bodies.*

Pleural reaction involving the parietal pleura, with fibrous thickening and plaque formation, is a common manifestation of asbestos exposure. Pleural calcification is a frequent finding. Pleural effusion, sometimes bloody, is a fairly common form of pleural reaction to asbestos.

Bronchogenic carcinoma is a frequent complicating event in asbestosis. However, the relationship is mostly due to the combined effect of asbestos and cigarette smoking. Whereas the incidence of lung cancer in nonsmoking asbestos workers is somewhat higher than in the nonsmoking general population, heavy smokers who are also exposed to asbestos have an 80-fold to 90-fold greater predisposition to bronchogenic carcinoma. Therefore, the combined effects of cigarette smoke and asbestos are more multiplicative than additive.

Another malignant disease associated with asbestos exposure is malignant pleural (sometimes peritoneal) **mesothelioma.** This cancer appears to develop almost exclusively in individuals with asbestos exposure, and smoking has no effect on its incidence. The risk of developing malignant mesothelioma reaches its peak 30 to 35 years after initial exposure.

Clinical Manifestations. Clinical manifestations of asbestosis are similar to those presented by pulmonary fibrosis in general. There is a various gradation of symptoms from asymptomatic stage of early and mild cases to severe respiratory incapacity with advanced and severe fibrosis. The average period of exposure before developing symptoms is about 20 to 30 years. Symptoms rarely develop in patients with less than 10 years of exposure. Dyspnea, with or without cough, is the most common symptom. Physical examination often reveals basal pulmonary rales. Digital clubbing is a common finding.

The presence of pleural disease may manifest by deformity and restriction of the chest, dullness to percussion, and reduced breath sounds. Most patients with pleural plaques have no symptoms unless there is concomitant asbestosis. The most common symptom of malignant mesothelioma is chest pain, which may be followed by dyspnea and systemic symptoms of malignancy. Physical findings of pleural effusion are usually present.

Radiographic Findings. Parenchymal lung disease manifests by interstitial markings with reticular density, predominantly involving the lower lung fields. Cardiac and diaphagmatic outline may appear indistinct and "shaggy." Sometimes marked honeycomb pattern may be present. The lung volume is often diminished. Pleural changes are very common, including pleural thickening, plagues, calcification, and effusion. *Rounded atelectasis* is a characteristic radiographic finding that results from associated asbestosis with pleural effusion and fibrosis, in which a portion of the lung becomes trapped and atelectatic after the effusion is resorbed, and assumes a round shape. It may mimic a

neoplasm. Malignant mesothelioma frequently manifests with pleural thickening and effusion. Computed tomography (CT) scanning has proven to be very useful in studying patients with asbestos-associated pleural disease.

Pulmonary Function Tests. As in diffuse lung fibrosis in general, pulmonary function tests in asbestosis are indicative of restrictive ventilatory defect with reduced lung volumes and diffusing capacity. Flow rates are usually normal.

Management. Preventive measures and removal of patients from the contaminated environment at the first sign of disease are most important. Treatment of established asbestosis is the same as that of pulmonary fibrosis in general. In view of the marked increase in incidence of bronchogenic carcinoma among smokers exposed to asbestos, they should be strongly urged to quit smoking.

ENVIRONMENTAL PULMONARY DISEASES DUE TO NOXIOUS GASES

As a result of the combustion of fuel for locomotion, heating, and power production in various industries and photochemical reactions in the atmosphere, the inspired air may contain small concentrations of certain noxious gases, such as sulfur dioxide, nitrogen oxide, carbon monoxide, hydrocarbons, and ozone. Injurious effect of these gases on *healthy lung* at the concentration present in community air pollution has not been clearly demonstrated. However, many of these gases (as well as particulate matters), even in low concentrations, may play a contributing role in triggering and exacerbating symptoms from underlying bronchopulmonary disorders. On the other hand, exposure to higher concentrations of these gases that may occur accidently or, rarely, intentionally is known to be always harmful.

Acute Exposure to Irritant Gases

Irritant gases are known to cause inflammation of mucous membranes on contact. They are irritating both to the eyes and to the mucous membranes of the respiratory tract, resulting in a burning sensation, itching, and watering of the eyes; sneezing and runny nose; and coughing. These irritating effects are usually severe enough to force the exposed victim to escape whenever possible; therefore, exposure time will be brief, and the amount of inhaled gas will be small. The degree of irritation of the eyes and the upper airway mucosa is proportional to the water solubility of these gases. The more soluble the gas, the more irritating it is to these areas; and thus, the less likely it will produce a significant toxic effect on the distal airways and alveoli. It should, however, be noted that even the most soluble irritating gas can cause acute bronchiolar and alveolar damage if the victim is unable to escape and/or the inhaled dose is massive. The following is a list of some of the irritating gases that are known to cause respiratory tract injury:

- Ammonia (NH_3)
- Sulfur dioxide (SO_2)
- Chlorine (Cl)
- Nitrogen dioxide (NO_2)
- Ozone (O_3)
- Phosgene ($COCl_2$)

They are listed according to their water solubility, ammonia being the most soluble and phosgene the least soluble. Because of their high solubility, the first three gases on the list cause intense irritation of the eyes and the upper airway mucous membranes and, therefore, they cannot be tolerated to any extent that would cause a significant harmful effect to the lower respiratory tract. Only with massive accidental exposure in a situation from which the victims are unable to escape, will these gases result in serious bronchopulmonary injury. On the other hand, the last three gases on the list, which are much less water soluble and thus less irritating to the eyes and the upper airways, are better known for their injurious effect on the distal airways and alveoli.

The toxic effects of all of these gases to the respiratory tract are more or less similar. Hyperemia, edema, epithelial injury with mucosal sloughing, hypersecretion, and cellular reaction are usual tissue responses. Cough, increasing dyspnea, and cyanosis are common manifestations of heavy exposure to these agents. Radiographic changes of pulmonary edema become apparent within several hours. Hypoxemia may be severe and difficult to correct by oxygen administration.

A condition commonly known as *silo-fillers' disease* is caused by exposure to a high concentration of nitrogen dioxide, which is produced by fermentation of fodder in a silo. This gas and its polymer, being heavier than air, accumulate on top of silage as a reddish-brown "cloud." Upon exposure to this cloud, depending on the concentration of nitrogen dioxide and duration of exposure, various degrees of bronchopulmonary damage will ensue. Mild exposure may result in acute, self-limited bronchitis; heavy exposure may cause acute, sometimes fatal, pulmonary edema. There is a subacute form of clinical presentation in which the symptoms recur and persist after an apparent recovery.

Management of acute severe irritant gas injury is mostly supportive and symptomatic. As in hypoxemic respiratory failure from any cause, the first priority should be the correction of the hypoxemia. If oxygen administration by nasal cannula or mask does not correct the hypoxemia, or if there is progressive respiratory distress or inadequate spontaneous ventilation, mechanical ventilatory support will be needed as discussed in the management of respiratory failure (Chapter 25). The role of corticosteroids in the treatment of patients with irritant gas exposure is questionable. Complete recovery is the usual outcome in properly managed patients. However, sometimes residual functional impairment may be observed. Patients with pulmonary injury due to irritant gas exposure should have a close follow-up after their apparent recovery because of the possibility of recurrence.

CARBON MONOXIDE POISONING

Carbon monoxide has no *direct* injurious effect on the lungs. However, because of its ready absorption, its extreme affinity for hemoglobin and, therefore, its interference with oxygen transport and delivery, poisoning with CO gas causes significant mortality and morbidity as a result of the impairment of tissue oxygenation.

Sources of Carbon Monoxide
Carbon Monoxide (CO) is produced during incomplete burning of carbon or carbon-containing materials. Therefore,

it can occur from the burning of fuels such as coal, wood, gasoline, or natural gas in an atmosphere in which sufficient oxygen is not available for their complete combustion. Automobiles characteristically burn gasoline incompletely; as a result, CO may reach highly toxic concentrations inside the car from a defective exhaust or in a closed garage within a short period of time. This has become an increasingly common cause of suicidal or accidental poisoning.

A low concentration of CO with air pollution may become significant during heavy traffic, particularly in places like toll booths, tunnels, and congested expressways. Use of charcoal grills indoors for cooking or heating, faulty gas refrigerators, and heaters or burners supplied with various fuels may cause accidental poisoning in houses and trailer homes. The combination of incomplete combustion and insufficient ventilation is the usual setup for such an exposure. Natural gas, as used in the United States, does not contain CO and has replaced the older manufactured gas, which had a significant concentration of this gas. It is the incomplete combustion of presently used natural gas that produces CO. Many deaths not related to burns in fire and holocaust are due to CO poisoning, as will be discussed later.

Tobacco smoke contains a high concentration of carbon monoxide to which smokers are voluntarily exposed (see Chapter 16). Heavy cigarette smokers, as well as cigar smokers who inhale, have chronically high blood carboxyhemoglobin (COHb) levels. A small amount of carbon monoxide is endogenously produced by the normal breakdown of hemoglobin. Carbon monoxide is also the metabolic by-product of methylene chloride, the main ingredient of most paint removers. Inhalation of this product after its application in a poorly ventilated space may result in a significant increase in serum carboxyhemoglobin levels.

Toxic Effects of Carbon Monoxide

The most important effect of carbon monoxide is related to its extremely high affinity for hemoglobin and the production of carboxyhemoglobin, which impairs the ability of red blood cells to carry oxygen and deliver it to the tissues. Carbon monoxide and oxygen compete for the binding sites on hemoglobin molecules. The affinity for CO is about 240 times that for oxygen. Therefore, in competing for binding sites on hemoglobin molecules, CO is able to displace and readily replace O_2; to achieve an equal concentration of oxyhemoglobin and carboxyhemoglobin with a PO_2 of 100 torr at equilibrium, a CO tension of only 0.42 torr will be necessary. A CO concentration of less than 0.1% in inspired air with long enough exposure time will be sufficient to cause such a high COHb level.

Upon exposure to carbon monoxide, it is rapidly absorbed by diffusion via the alveoli until an equilibrium is reached, provided that an immediately fatal concentration is not inhaled. The COHb level at equilibrium is proportional to the CO concentration in inspired air (Fig. 15–4). The time required for equilibrium is inversely related to CO concentration. As in clinical situations the equilbrium is seldom reached, other factors in addition to inspired CO concentration and duration of exposure are important. They include metabolic rate, alveolar ventilation, and pulmonary blood flow.

In addition to reducing the oxygen-

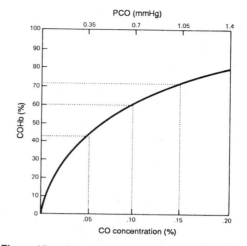

Figure 15–4. Relation of blood carboxyhemoglobin (COHb) levels and inspired carbon monoxide (CO) concentration at equilibrium. Note that at equilibrium CO concentrations as low as 0.1% result in very high and even fatal COHb levels in blood.

carrying capacity of hemoglobin, an equally important effect of CO on hemoglobin is the alteration in the position as well as in the shape of the oxyhemoglobin dissociation curve. The curve will be shifted to the left as the affinity of unoccupied binding sites of hemoglobin for oxygen is increased; and the curve will tend to change from its normal **sigmoid** shape to a hyperbolic curve. Both of these changes have profound effects on oxygen unloading at the tissue sites.

The question of the significance of CO binding to other hemoproteins, such as cytochrome oxidase in mitochondria and myoglobin in cardiac and skeletal muscle cells has not yet been satisfactorily answered. As these hemoproteins are important in oxygen metabolism, their putative involvement in CO intoxication would further impair cellular hypoxia. As pathophysiologic changes due to CO poisoning are all related to tissue hypoxia, the brain and the heart, which are highly sensitive to oxygen lack, are mostly affected.

Clinical Manifestations. The symptoms from carbon monoxide poisoning depends on the blood level of carboxyhemoglobin (measured as percent of total hemoglobin). A level of less than 10%, as seen in heavy smokers, causes no significant symptom in otherwise healthy individuals. In patients with coronary artery disease, however, there is lowering of the threshold for exercise-induced angina. Patients are usually symptomatic with carboxyhemoglobin concentrations of 20% and higher. Headaches, exertional dyspnea, dizziness, difficulty to concentrate, impaired judgment, incoordination, lethargy, and mental confusion are common manifestations. Nausea, vomiting, and other gastrointestinal symptoms may also be present. With higher concentrations of carboxyhemoglobin, loss of consciousness, convulsions, and deep coma will supervene. Fatal cases show carboxyhemoglobin levels of 60% to 80%. The symptoms develop more rapidly with exposure to higher concentrations of CO in air; sometimes CO is absorbed so fast that unconsciousness occurs suddenly and without warning symptoms.

Electrocardiographic changes indicative of myocardial hypoxia and various arrhythmias may be seen. Occasionally, there is evidence of acute myocardial infarction. Practically every organ may show functional impairment. Acute pulmonary edema, resulting from cardiac failure as well as from increased alveolar capillary leak, has been occasionally seen in severe CO poisoning. Various delayed neuropsychiatric manifestations are fairly common following severe CO intoxication. Chronic low-level CO poisoning, as commonly seen in heavy smokers, is a cause of increased red blood cells (**polycythemia**).

Diagnosis. Besides the history, there are very few clinical findings to help the diagnosis of CO poisoning. The cherry-red color of the skin and mucous membranes, frequently mentioned in most textbooks, is not a common finding in live victims. Once suspected, the diagnosis is readily made by measurement of the carboxyhemoglobin level in the blood by one of the available methods. As there is an excellent correlation between the blood COHb level and expired CO concentration, the measurement of the latter by one of the CO analyzers may be used as a rapid screening test.

Arterial blood PO_2, as expected, is normal; however, oxygen *content* will be reduced proportional to the carboxyhemoglobin level. If PO_2 and O_2 saturation studies are done independently, there will be a significant discrepancy between the calculated and measured O_2 saturation. Low PCO_2 is rather common. Metabolic acidosis may also be present due to lactic acid production of tissue hypoxia.

Management. Once the diagnosis of carbon monoxide poisoning is suspected, treatment should be initiated immediately and before the results of laboratory studies are reported. The most important step in the treatment of CO poisoning is the removal of the victim from the contaminated atmosphere. In mild cases without significant symptoms, a few hours of bed rest, with or without added inspired O_2, will usually suffice. The factors that facilitate CO elimination include alveolar ventilation and inspired oxygen tension. From the therapeutic point of view, increasing alveolar O_2 tension is the most important and practical measure. CO elimination is exponential, the average half-life being inversely proportional to the alveolar PO_2. A half-life of 5 hours breathing room air is reduced to 1 hour by the administration of 100% oxygen at atmospheric pressure. The half-life will be diminished further by the administration of oxygen in a hyperbaric chamber. The treatment goals in severe CO poisoning are to reverse tissue hypoxia and rapidly reduce the blood COHb level to below 10%. Both are achieved by the administration of 100% oxygen. Patients with severe CO poisoning are treated in the hospital. Oxygen therapy should be continued until the COHb level is below 10%. This usually takes several hours.

The role of hyperbaric oxygen in CO poisoning remains controversial. However, more rapid CO elimination and a better tissue oxygenation by hyperbaric oxygen therapy makes it an attractive method for the management of CO poisoning. If a hyperbaric chamber is readily available, it should preferably be used for treatment of patients with severe poisoning and significant cardiac or cerebral dysfunction. Otherwise, lack of response to 100% **normobaric** oxygen within 4 hours is considered by some to be an indication for transporting the patient to the nearest hyperbaric facility. The importance of close monitoring of the patients and their supportive care cannot be overemphasized. The persistence of coma or other neurologic sequelae is indicative of hypoxic brain injury, which requires a more prolonged supportive care.

SMOKE INHALATION

Smoke inhalation is the most important cause of morbidity and mortality among fire victims and fire fighters. The prognosis of most burns is often determined by the magnitude of concurrent smoke inhalation.

Pathogenesis and Pathology. Fire smoke is a complex mixture of gases, vapors, and particulate matter that result from combustion, evaporation, and **pyrolysis.** The latter is heat-induced decomposition of organic compounds in the absence of oxygen. The composition of smoke, therefore, varies not only because of the difference of the chemical makeup of substances that are burning, but also because of steady reduction in available oxygen that is being consumed by the fire. In addition to carbon monoxide, which is the major cause of poisoning from smoke, many irritant and caustic gases may be generated. They include aldehydes (especially **acrolein**), hydrogen chloride, oxides of sulfur and nitrogen, and ammonia. They cause direct injury to the respiratory tract by their irritating and corrosive effects. With the increasing use of synthetic materials containing isocyanate compounds in buildings and furnishings, hydrogen cyanide has become an important component of smoke from fires. This gaseous form of cyanide exerts its toxic effect by binding to cytochromes, thus interfering with the oxidative metabolism at the cellular level.

In addition to inhaling the noxious gases, fire victims in enclosed spaces breathe an air with a steadily diminishing concentration of oxygen and increasing concentration of carbon dioxide.

Although inhalation of hot air may cause thermal injury to the upper air passages, distal airways and alveoli are spared. The pathologic changes in the respiratory tract are mainly from irritant gases. These changes are complex and quite variable. Tracheobronchial mucosal edema, vascular congestion, and epithelial sloughing are often present. Alveolar edema is the result of leaky alveolar-capillary membrane. Bronchiolar damage may result in obliterative bronchiolitis. The pathologic changes begin to develop within several hours of exposure, but they may be delayed for a day or two, or even longer.

Clinical Manifestations. The clinical presentation varies considerably. The victim may be alert, drowsy, or unconscious, usually depending on the intensity of concomitant carbon monoxide poisoning. Lack of evidence of external burns does not exclude the possibility of significant smoke inhalation. Upper airways may look inflamed. Cough, with expectoration of black phlegm, is often present. Tachypnea, stridor, grunting respiration, and other signs of respiratory distress may not appear until several hours later. With the development of pulmonary edema, severe dyspnea and signs of marked hypoxemia, including shock, will be evident. However, because of frequent association with CO poisoning, cyanosis may not be manifest, despite profound hypoxemia. Therefore, the patient may suffer from an extreme degree of tissue hypoxia due to combined effect of carboxyhemoglobinemia and respiratory failure.

The concomitant effect of cyanide on cytochromes impairs oxygen utilization further. Cyanide poisoning should be suspected in comatose victims of fires in which plastic or other synthetic materials are involved, especially when the patients fail to recover after their blood carboxyhemoglobin levels are lowered.

Diagnosis. Radiographic changes of smoke inhalation may be minimal or totally absent initially. Bilateral pulmonary edema, however, may appear later. Early bronchoscopy is often recommended when, despite a high initial carboxyhemoglobin levels in patients with smoke inhalation, there is no clinical or radiographic evidence of pulmonary involvement at the time of presentation. The presence of mucosal changes distal to the larynx is a good predictor of subsequent development of respiratory difficulty. Alternatively, radionuclide ventilation scan may be used for this purpose, which has a high negative predictive value; that is, a normal distribution with a normal clearance of the radioactive tracer virtually excludes the diagnosis of significant distal airway damage from smoke inhalation.

Management. In smoke inhalation, in addition to treatment for CO poisoning, patients with pulmonary injury will require appropriate management. Because both clinical manifestations and radiographic changes may be delayed, all patients exposed to smoke should be carefully observed, especially when the carboxyhemoglobin levels are elevated. A patient with normal physical findings, a normal chest radiograph, and a safe level of carboxyhemoglobin level may be released after a short period of observation. If performed, a normal bronchoscopy or ventilation lung scan provides added assurance that late pulmonary complications will not develop.

In view of frequent association with CO exposure, oxygen should be administered immediately, while waiting for measurement of blood carboxyhemoglobin level. If cyanide poisoning is suspected and/or blood cyanide level is high, appropriate therapeutic measures should be undertaken without delay.

Patients with evidence of bronchospasm are treated with inhaled bronchodilators, and systemic corticosteroids if needed. Otherwise, there is no indication for corticosteroids in smoke inhalation. Prophylactic antibiotic therapy has not been proven to be effective in preventing pulmonary infections, which may develop in patients with severe lung injury. Such infections should be promptly and adequately treated once they occur.

With the development of progressive respiratory distress and persistent hypoxemia despite an adequate airway and oxygen therapy, mechanical ventilation will be necessary. Unless there is severe airway injury at the level of or proximal to the larynx, endotracheal intubation is preferred to tracheostomy. With severe pulmonary edema and intractable hypoxemia, positive end-expiratory pressure should be used, as discussed in management of acute respiratory distress syndrome (ARDS) (Chapter 25). Associated severe and extensive skin burn is known to increase the incidence and severity of ARDS with smoke inhalation.

AIR POLLUTION

In atmospheric air pollution, in addition to various gases, particulate matters in aerosolized form are also present. Chemical composition of these particulate pollutants varies, and usually includes carbon, metals, and other inorganic, as well as organic, compounds. Because of their very low concentrations, the lung defense mechanisms, discussed earlier, are normally quite adequate to prevent their harmful effects. However, in persons with underlying pulmonary disease and in individuals with hyperreactive airways or hypersensitivity states, the health hazard of air pollution with particulate matters may be significant. In mixed air pollution, particles are also important in their capacity for carrying noxious gases on their surface to distal air spaces, whereas such gases would have been removed by their solubility in the upper airways without carrying particles.

The effect of short-term exposure to noxious gases on healthy individuals at the concentration present in community air pollution has not been proved to be significant, and the respiratory consequences of long-term exposure in people without underlying chronic cardiopulmonary conditions, although suspected, have not been conclusively demonstrated. However, as with exposure to low concentrations of particulate matters, patients with chronic respiratory illness, such as asthmatics and persons with COPD, show evidence of significant deterioration of their symptoms and impairment of their respiratory function upon exposure to noxious gases of air pollution.

Air pollution is, therefore, considered to be a relatively weak respiratory pathogen but an important aggravating factor on preexisting pulmonary disease. However, because of the unavoidable, involuntary, and continuous nature of exposure and uncertainty regarding its long-term effect, air pollution has deservedly received much attention and caused worldwide public concern about its potential health hazards.

OXYGEN TOXICITY

The toxic effect of a high concentration of oxygen has been suspected since the discovery of this gas in the eighteenth century. Only in recent years, however, has its clinical importance been fully recognized, and its pathogenesis elucidated. Although the toxic effect of oxygen has been most extensively studied in relation to the respiratory system, it is also known that oxygen with high enough tension and sufficient duration of exposure may injure almost any organ system of the body through a complex biochemical reaction of cells. Its toxic effect on the retinal arteries of premature infants with development of a condition called **retrolental fibroplasia** is well known. With more judicious use of oxygen, monitoring arterial blood PO_2 and, thus, avoiding unnecessarily excessive PO_2, this **iatrogenic** eye disease and blindness are rarely seen nowadays.

Neurologic toxicity, such as convulsions, is observed with a very high oxygen tension, which can only be reached in environments such as hyperbaric chambers in which O_2 at pressure greater than 2 atm (atmosphere) is inspired.

The toxic effect of oxygen on any tissue is directly related to both its partial pressure and the duration of exposure. Without sufficient O_2 tension or sufficient time of exposure, injury will not result. Various effects of oxygen at high partial pressure are referred to as *hyperoxic syndromes.*

Pulmonary Oxygen Toxicity

As the lungs are exposed to higher partial pressures of oxygen than other organs in the body, the primary toxic effect of a high PO_2 in the normobaric range is on the lung tissue. This effect is entirely separate from the ventilatory effect of excessive oxygen administration in suppression of oxygen in hypoxic patients with hypercapnia. Another nontoxic, but nevertheless harmful, effect of oxygen is *absorption atelectasis,* which is due to the lack of nonabsorbable gas in the lungs and, therefore, is a function of FIO_2 rather than PO_2 of the inspired gas; whereas, pulmonary tissue damage of oxygen toxicity is related to the inspired oxygen tension rather than the FIO_2. A high concentration of oxygen is less damaging at a high altitude with low atmospheric pressures than it is at sea level. Moreover, astronauts who breathe 100% oxygen at a reduced ambient pressure show no evidence of toxicity.

The precise oxygen tensions and duration of exposure that result in toxic effects on the lungs have been difficult to establish. This is compounded by the fact that there is significant individual variation in susceptibility to oxygen toxicity. It is generally considered that clinically significant pulmonary toxicity occurs in individuals exposed to 100% oxygen at normobaric pressures when the exposure time is over 24 to 48 hours; however, mild and reversible effects may develop with shorter exposures. An entirely safe partial pressure of oxygen for humans has not been agreed upon by different investigators, but the likelihood of significant toxicity to the lungs at an inspired oxygen pressure below 0.6 atm is very small.

Pathogenesis and Pathology. Morphologic changes of oxygen toxicity with 100% oxygen and an exposure time of 6 to 24 hours occur in tracheobronchial mucosa, which can be demonstrated by bronchoscopy. However, studies by bronchoalveolar lavage indicate that early changes may be an alveolar-capillary leak from injury to the endothelial and type I epithelial cells. With more severe damage that occurs with longer exposure, interstitial and alveolar edema develops. When O_2 toxicity develops more insidiously, and following the acute exudative phase in surviving patients, the proliferative stage will occur. This stage is characterized by cellular infiltration, proliferation of type II alveolar epithelial cells, and beginning fibrosis.

Alveolar and capillary cell damage, therefore, appears to be the initial event in the pathogenesis of hyperoxic pulmonary toxicity. Cellular injury is not the direct effect of molecular oxygen, but is due to the toxic effect of highly reactive metabolites of molecular oxygen. These products, which are produced intracellularly, include free radicals, particularly superoxide anion, peroxides, and the hydroxyl radical. Normally, the cells are protected from the toxic effect of these products by antioxidant enzymes. One such enzyme, which is extremely efficient in detoxifying the superoxide radical, is **superoxide dismutase. Glutathione** is the primary intracellular antioxidant, which has to be constantly reduced by special enzymes to maintain this function. Vitamin E, also an antioxidant, is known to have protective effects against these toxic agents. During exposure to hyperoxia, the production of free radi-

cals and other oxidants overwhelms natural defenses against them, resulting in cell injury. Impairment of function of certain enzymes and inhibition of synthesis of DNA, protein, cellular lipid, and surfactant constitute the metabolic basis of tissue damage by these powerful oxidants.

Clinical Manifestations, Diagnosis, and Management. Persons exposed to 100% oxygen for less than 24 hours may develop tracheobronchitis manifested by a nonproductive cough and retrosternal pain that is aggravated by deep inspiration. In such patients, reduced vital capacity, low diffusing capacity, and changes in pulmonary compliance have been reported. Severe acute pulmonary oxygen toxicity manifests by symptoms and signs of respiratory distress syndrome.

In a practical setting, pulmonary oxygen toxicity should be suspected in patients receiving high concentrations of oxygen for several days and who develop unexplained diffuse pulmonary infiltration on radiographic examination, changes in pulmonary compliance, or increasing difficulty in oxygenating the arterial blood. These changes, however, are not specific for oxygen toxicity, and may well be due to other common disorders such as widespread pneumonia, heart failure, or other causes of alveolar-capillary leak. In most situations in which oxygen toxicity is suspected, there is significant hypoxemia requiring higher inspired O_2 tensions. In turn, the latter causes further lung damage and impairment of oxygen transport.

In view of the seriousness of hypoxemia in critically ill patients, withholding oxygen for fear of toxicity will be more disastrous in patients who are in need of prolonged oxygen support. However, the concentration of oxygen in these situations should not be more than what is needed for achieving an acceptable PO_2. Every effort should be made to improve oxygenation without increasing oxygen tension above the potentially toxic level. The correction of underlying pathophysiologic abnormalities, proper tracheobronchial toilet, control of heart failure, avoidance of excessive fluid administration, treatment of acid-base imbalance, optimal ventilation with adequate tidal volumes, and use of positive end-expiratory pressure will diminish the requirement for high inspired oxygen tension for adequate oxygenation.

The role of antioxidants, such as vitamin E and superoxide dismutase, in the management of pulmonary oxygen toxicity has not yet been established.

BIBLIOGRAPHY

Aberle DR, Balmes JR. Computed tomography of asbestos-related pulmonary parenchymal and pleural diseases. *Clin Chest Med.* 1991; 12:115–131.

Bateman ED, Benatar SR. Asbestos-induced diseases: clinical perspectives. *Q J Med.* 1987; 62:183–194.

Becklake MR. Asbestos-related diseases of the lung and pleura. *Am Rev Respir Dis.* 1982; 126:187–194.

Cahalane M, Demling RH. Early respiratory abnormalities from smoke inhalation. *JAMA.* 1984; 251:771–773.

Craighead JE, Mossman BT. The pathogenesis of asbestos-associated diseases. *N Engl J Med.* 1982; 306:1446–1453.

Davis GS. The pathogenesis of silicosis. *Chest.* 1986; 89 (suppl):166S–169S.

Davis WB, Rennard SI, Bitterman PB, Crystal RG. Pulmonary oxygen toxicity. *N Engl J Med.* 1983; 309:878–883.

Doll NJ, Stankus RP, Barkman HW. Immunopathogenesis of asbestosis, silicosis, and coal worker's pneumoconiosis. *Clin Chest Med.* 1983; 4(1):3–14.

Douglas WW, Hepper NG, Colley TV. Silo-filler's disease. *Mayo Clin Proc.* 1989; 64:291–304.

Garcia JGN, Griffith DE, Levin JL, Idell S. Tobacco smoke exposure in occupational lung disease. *Semin Respir Med.* 1989; 10:372–385.

Green GM, Jakab GJ, Low RB, Davis GS. Defense mechanisms of the respiratory membrane. *Am Rev Respir Dis.* 1977; 115:479–514.

Griffith DE, Levin JL. Respiratory effects of outdoor air pollution. *Postgrad Med.* 1989; 86(5):111–118.

Haponik EF, Crapo RO, Herndon DN, et al. Smoke inhalation. *Am Rev Respir Dis.* 1988; 138:1060–1063.

Hillerdal G. Rounded atelectasis. *Chest.* 1989; 95:836–841.

Ilano AL, Raffin TA. Management of carbon monoxide poisoning. *Chest.* 1990; 97: 165–169.

Jackson RM. Molecular, pharmacologic, and clinical aspects of oxygen-induced lung injury. *Clin Chest Med.* 1990; 11:73–86.

Morgan WKC, Lapp NL. Respiratory disease in coal miners. *Am Rev Respir Dis.* 1976; 113:531–559.

Peitzman AB, Shires GI III, Teixidor HS, et al. Smoke inhalation injury: evaluation of radiographic manifestations and pulmonary dysfunction. *J Trauma.* 1989; 29: 1232–1239.

Root WS. Carbon monoxide. In Fenn WO, Rahn H, eds. *Handbook of Physiology,* II. Washington, D.C.: American Physiology Society; 1965; 1087–1098.

Samet JM, Marbury MC, Spengler JD. Health effects and sources of indoor pollution. *Am Rev Respir Dis.* 1987; 136: 1486–1508, and 1988; 137:221–242.

Sleigh MA, Blake JR, Liron N. The propulsion of mucus by cilia. *Am Rev Respir Dis.* 1988; 137:726–741.

Thom SR. Smoke inhalation. *Emerg Med Clin North Am.* 1989; 7:371–387.

Waller RE. Atmospheric pollution. *Chest.* 1989; 96(suppl):363S–368S.

Weill H. Occupational lung diseases. *Hosp Pract.* 1981; 16(4):65–80.

Ziskind M, Jones RN, Weill H. Silicosis. *Am Rev Respir Dis.* 1976; 113:643–665.

CHAPTER 16

Tobacco Smoking

In several chapters of this book we have alluded to the role of smoking in causing or contributing to various respiratory disorders. This chapter focuses on the health consequences of tobacco smoking; it follows after a brief discussion of the physicochemical and biologic properties of cigarette smoke. As disease prevention is one of the primary responsibilities of health professionals, they should have a thorough knowledge and understanding of this manmade and entirely preventable health hazard. The unique position of providers of respiratory care affords them the opportunity and the obligation to inform their clients, as well as the general public, on the health effects of smoking and to help them stop their potentially dangerous smoking habits. Tobacco smoking is a very prevalent human behavior initiated by easily available psychosocial factors and continued by the addition of overpowering addictive forces. Although the avoidance of starting the habit is a relatively simple matter, smoking cessation after the establishment of psychological and physical dependency becomes a most difficult and complex task. As discussed later in this chapter, one of the most challenging responsibilities of health care providers is to equip their smoking clients with enough incentive and encouragement that their desire for giving up smoking overcomes their desire for smoking. Knowledge of health consequences of smoking alone is not enough for this purpose. It also necessitates the understanding of the dynamics of smoking, both as an acquired behavior and as an illness.

Since the first report of the U.S. Surgeon General on smoking and health in 1964, follow-up reports and numerous scientific studies have reaffirmed the conclusion of the original report and also have provided data on various health problems related to both voluntary and involuntary (passive) smoking. It seems that, at least in this country, most people are aware of many of the smoking-related diseases, yet the decline in cigarette consumption has been less than impressive; and teenagers and young adults continue taking up the habit in rather large numbers. However, development of new policies and legislation on restriction of smoking in certain public places and work areas, steady decline of social acceptability of smoking, and increasing public awareness of high-risk behaviors are some of the encouraging signs that the battle against smoking will eventually be won. Meanwhile, some 50 million Americans who are current smokers will need help for various health problems resulting from their smoking and for their struggle in giving it up.

HARMFUL CONSTITUENTS OF CIGARETTE SMOKE

A lighted cigarette produces about 4,000 known compounds and several thousand unidentified chemicals, some in gaseous form and most in aerosolized particulate form. Inhaled (mainstream) smoke is partly retained in, or absorbed from, the respiratory tract and partly exhaled. Sidestream smoke is the part that is released to the environment from the lighted end of the cigarette. The gaseous phase of the cigarette smoke includes carbon dioxide, carbon monoxide, oxides of nitrogen, hydrogen cyanide, aldehydes, ammonia, volatile nitrosamines, hydrocarbons, and free radicals. Carbon monoxide is the best-recognized harmful component of the gas phase. Its effects on hemoglobin and resultant impairment of oxygen delivery was discussed in the preceding chapter. Most other components are known to be respiratory irritants; some (especially hydrogen cyanide and aldehydes) are toxic to the respiratory cilia; and a few have **carcinogenic** potential. Gaseous components of smoke have been considered to play a major role in the pathogenesis of chronic obstructive lung disease. As respiratory irritants, they may provoke bronchospasm in individuals with hyperreactive airways.

"*Tar*" is the name given to the aggregate of the particulate matter in the cigarette smoke minus nicotine and moisture. In contradistinction to gases in the cigarette smoke, "tar" and nicotine are partly trapped in the filter tip. The amount of "tar" delivered in mainstream smoke in each cigarette constitutes its "tar" content. Therefore, it varies not only with the amount and brand of tobacco, but also the properties of the filter tip and the characteristics of the puffs. "Tar" contains numerous compounds known or suspected to be carcinogens, tumor promoters, or co-carcinogens. Among them, **polynuclear aromatic** hydrocarbons are the best-known carcinogens. The role of others such as **N. nitrosamine,** "tumorigenic" metals, and radionuclides in causing human lung cancer is less certain. "Tar" contents of American-made cigarettes have been steadily reduced during the past 35 to 40 years by processing and reconstituting of tobacco brands, changing the cigarette papers, and introducing more effective filter tips. These changes, however, have not yet favorably influenced the incidence of lung cancer among smokers.

Nicotine
Nicotine is by far the most important pharmacologically active substance in every form of tobacco and its smoke. It is the principal cause of physiologic addiction to smoking. People who smoke cigarettes or use other tobacco products chronically do so because of the nicotine content. The powerful addicting properties of nicotine are the cause of failure to quit smoking by most cigarette smokers who desire to quit and make numerous attempts to do so. Even the smokers who have tobacco-related illnesses and recognize the effect of smoking on their health have a very hard time giving it up. This type of behavior fits the definition of

drug dependence, and the drug in question is nicotine.

Once in the bloodstream, nicotine readily crosses the blood-brain barrier and is distributed in various parts of the central nervous system (CNS). It has a variety of complex CNS actions through its binding to the brain receptors. Among many of its pharmacologic effects, autonomic ganglia are better-known targets. In small doses nicotine stimulates both sympathetic and parasympathetic ganglia; in large doses, it has an opposite effect. **Catecolamines** (epinephrine and norepinephrine) released from the activation of the sympathetic nerves and adrenal gland are the cause of several of nicotine's biologic responses. They include the effect on the heart rate, myocardial contractility, vascular resistance, and mobilization of fatty acids. An increase in the blood level of other hormones associated with cigarette smoking is probably related to the effect of nicotine. Tolerance to some of the effects of nicotine is well recognized, which may develop quite rapidly. Unpleasant symptoms of dizziness, nausea, and vomiting in first-time smokers do not develop with repeat smoking, and other effects of nicotine are also attenuated. In habitual smokers, nicotine has a satisfying and pleasurable effect, which is at least partly the result of relief from unpleasant symptoms of abstinence. Arousal, relaxation, improved concentration and attention, and reduced anger and tension from stressful situations are some of the subjective beneficial effects. Withdrawal symptoms that occur in about 80% of smokers include restlessness, irritability, anxiety, impatience, impaired concentration, and strong desire or craving to smoke a cigarette. Most of the symptoms are accounted for by the withdrawal of nicotine, as they also occur with the cessation of smokeless tobacco and nicotine gum and are relieved by the administration of nicotine.

Nicotine is distilled from burning tobacco and carried on "tar" particles. The mainstream smoke of a filter-tipped cigarette on the average contains 15% of the nicotine in its tobacco, although it may vary depending on individual smoking characteristics. Most of the nicotine from cigarette smoke is absorbed through the wide surface of the alveoli after its inhalation. Its absorption from oral mucosa is negligible. However, nicotine in cigar and pipe smoke and in smokeless tobacco is absorbed from the oral mucous membrane. As drugs absorbed from sites other than the gastrointestinal tract bypass the liver, they are not detoxified and reach their target tissues or cells directly. Nicotine from the inhaled cigarette smoke reaches the brain within seconds of the first puff. The amount of nicotine that a smoker absorbs with each cigarette is determined not only by its nicotine content and the physical properties of its filter tip, but by the puff volume, depth of inhalation, rate of puffing, and duration of breath holding after each inhalation. These smoking patterns also affect the amount of gaseous material and "tar" to which the individual smoker is exposed.

Interposition of an effective filter tip and reduction of tar and nicotine content of most cigarettes made in the United States are ostensibly positive steps in reducing user exposure to these harmful agents. Lack of significant effect on the risk of some smoking-related diseases in users of low-yield cigarettes, however, indicates that the degree of exposure to the agents has not been appreciably reduced. As smoking behavior in habitual smokers is primarily a response to the levels of nicotine in their system, they adjust their smoking pattern accordingly. Therefore, smokers of low-tar and low-nicotine cigarettes tend to increase the number of cigarettes smoked and to use a pattern of smoking that yields the maximum amount of nicotine from each cigarette in order to maintain their accustomed nicotine level.

RELATIONSHIPS OF SMOKING AND DISEASE

The mortality and morbidity statistics clearly demonstrate that smoking is associated with increased rates of death and illness. Life expectancy at any given age is significantly shortened by cigarette smoking. It is estimated that for each cigarette smoked, an average of 5½ minutes of life is lost: a 30- to 35-year-old man who smokes two packs of cigarettes daily has a life expectancy 8 to 9 years shorter than a nonsmoker of the same age. The excess mortality in both smoking men and women is noted to be greatest for the 45- to 55-year-old age groups; therefore, smoking is associated with premature mortality. Judging from the prevalence of chronic illness and disability, the incidence of acute medical conditions, the number of days lost due to illness, and the frequency of hospitalization among smokers versus nonsmokers, there is a distinct and irrefutable correlation between smoking and morbidity. Smoking is also responsible for about 25% of all deaths and nonfatal injuries from fire. The following are some of the conditions known to be caused by or related to smoking.

Nonneoplastic Bronchopulmonary Diseases. The cause-and-effect relationship between smoking and chronic obstructive pulmonary disease (COPD) is well known. Over 80% of deaths from this disease are attributed to smoking. The etiologic role of smoking in chronic bronchitis and emphysema and its effect on precipitation and aggravation of asthmatic symptoms are discussed in related chapters. Cigarette smokers have a much higher frequency of respiratory symptoms. Both cough and expectoration are proportional to the amount and the duration of smoking. It has been demonstrated that even asymptomatic smokers have impaired ventilatory function when compared with nonsmokers of the same age. In addition to changes in ventilatory function, smokers show evidence of impairment of pulmonary clearance, including ciliary and alveolar macrophage functions. Respiratory infections are more prevalent and severe among cigarette smokers, particularly heavy smokers, than among nonsmokers. Smoking play a significant role in the severity of symptoms and disabililty in many patients with occupational lung disease, especially in coal miners. Postoperative pulmonary complications are seen more frequently in cigarette smokers than in nonsmokers.

Bronchogenic Carcinoma. Cigarette smoking is considered to be the most important causative factor in bronchogenic carcinoma. Its incidence is over 10 times higher in smokers than in nonsmokers. Certain histologic types are seen almost exclusively in smokers. The risk of developing lung cancer increases with the intensity and duration of smoking. Heavy and long-time smokers are the most likely victims, in whom the incidence may be as much as 70 times higher than in nonsmokers. Although cigarette smoking is associated with lung cancer in women, this relationship, for some unknown reasons, appears to be stronger in men. However, lung cancer mortality rates in women are increasing more rapidly than in men, and this apparent difference in susceptibility may not hold much longer. There are certain indications that the "tar" content of cigarettes is the major factor in the carcinogenesis of smoking. The higher the level of tar in the smoke reaching the lungs, the more is the risk of developing lung cancer. The incidence of lung cancer appears to be higher among cigarette smokers with chronic bronchitis than without. Certain occupational exposures, particularly to asbestos, act synergistically with smoking in causing lung cancer.

Laryngeal Cancer. Association between smoking and laryngeal cancer is as strong as in bronchogenic carcinoma. It has been estimated that about 84% of all the cases of laryngeal cancer are directly related to smoking. It seems that alcohol use has a synergistic effect with smoking. Higher incidence of cancer of the larynx in men as compared with women is at least partly due to higher alcohol consumption in men.

Other Malignant Neoplasms. Oral cancer is much more common in smokers of cigarettes, pipes, and cigars, especially among heavy smokers. Smokeless tobacco use (chewing and snuff dipping) has also been considered to be causally related. Carcinoma of the esophagus is also more prevalent among smokers. Alcohol use in smokers further increases the incidence of oral and esophageal cancers. Other malignancies associated with smoking include cancers of the pancreas, bladder, and kidney.

Coronary Artery Disease. The death rate from heart attack is much higher among smokers than among nonsmokers. It is estimated that about 25% of deaths from coronary artery disease are attributable to smoking. Cigarette smoking is considered to be one of the major risk factors for the development of coronary atherosclerosis. Smoking may also precipitate **angina pectoris** in patients with coronary artery disease. Both nicotine and carbon monoxide have been implicated in the development of these processes, as well as precipitation of coronary thrombosis. The incidence of myocardial infarction and sudden death in both men and women is much more prevalent among smokers. Smoking together with any other risk factors, such as hypertension, hypercholesterolemia, and diabetes increases the risk of heart attack to an alarmingly high level. It has been demonstrated that the efficacy of some of the antianginal medications is reduced by cigarette smoking. Smoking is a readily controllable risk factor. Smoking cessation not only rapidly reduces the risk of coronary artery occlusion, but also influences the outcome following myocardial infarction and coronary artery surgery.

Cerebrovascular and Peripheral Vascular Diseases. Cigarette smokers have higher death rates from stroke than do nonsmokers. Women on oral contraceptives who smoke have markedly increased risk for cerebrovascular accident. Heavy cigarette smoking is the most important recognizable risk factor for atherosclerotic peripheral vascular disease, which may result in progressive occlusion of arteries, especially of the lower extremities. Mortality from abdominal aortic aneurysm is two to three times higher in smokers than in nonsmokers.

Peptic Ulcer Disease and Other Gastrointestinal Disorders. Cigarette smokers have an increased prevalence of peptic ulcer and its complications as compared with nonsmokers. Smoking appears to reduce the effectiveness of standard ulcer treatment and to slow the rate of ulcer healing. "Heartburn," as a result of reflux of gastric juice to the esophagus, has been shown to increase with smoking.

Hematologic Disorder. Heavy smokers of cigarettes and cigars are known to develop secondary polycythemia, which is caused by chronically elevated blood carboxyhemoglobin (COHb) levels. Patients with chronic lung disease are particularly prone to develop this complication as a result of combined effects of chronic hypoxemia and high blood COHb levels on increased red-cell production.

Pregnancy. Smoking during pregnancy has a retarding effect on fetal growth as manifested by low infant birth weight and an increased incidence of prematurity. In addition, it seems that women who smoke during pregnancy have significantly greater risk of an unsuccessful pregnancy than those who do not smoke.

Smoking and Drug Metabolism. Cigarette smoking is known to alter the metabolism and pharmacologic effects of certain drugs. The best-known among drugs affected by smoking is theophylline. Smokers usually need a 50% increase in the maintenance dose of theophylline. It should also be noted that stopping smoking in chronic theophylline users, as during hospitalization, may result in theophylline toxicity if proper dosing adjustment is not made. Cigarette smoking and oral contraceptives may interact and increase the risk of thromboembolic events, such as stroke and coronary artery occlusion. Smoking reduces the effectiveness of H_2-blocking drugs and antacids in peptic ulcer disease.

Involuntary Smoking

Involuntary or *passive smoking* is defined as the inhalation by nonsmokers of the products of tobacco combustion generated by active smokers. Smoke from the burning end of cigarettes or other tobacco products (sidestream smoke) and the exhaled smoke not retained by the smoker are the source of this special form of indoor air pollution. It contains all the constituents of tobacco smoke, although in a lower concentration.

In recent years, the subject of involuntary smoking (also known as secondhand smoking) has received an increasing amount of public attention and has resulted in more controversy and dispute than any other aspect of smoking. It also is having a greater impact on smoking practices than ever before. As a result of increasing public awareness and concern about involuntary smoking, a growing number of private policies and public ordinances are being enacted and enforced.

Unlike the health effects of active smoking, which are on solid scientific grounds, information on involuntary smoking is sparce and often disputed. Acute exposure by normal subjects to the environmental tobacco smoke may result in many subjective symptoms, although objective changes are unusual. Eye irritation, nasal symptoms, headache, cough, and throat irritation are often reported. Persons with allergic disorders are especially prone to these symptoms, which are mostly due to the irritating effect of tobacco smoke rather than from allergic response. True allergy to tobacco smoke is a very rare occurrence. In asthmatic subjects, however, it may, as with other bronchial irritants, nonspecifically precipitate or aggrevate an asthma attack.

The effect of long-term exposure to environmental tobacco smoke on airways of normal adults is generally small or negligible. It is therefore doubtful that chronic exposure to secondhand smoke would increase the risk of chronic lung disease in nonsmoking adults. Several studies, however, have shown a significant association between parental smoking and prevalence of acute respiratory illnesses in infants and young children. These illnesses in turn have been implicated as a risk factor for developing COPD in older age. Childhood chronic exposure to household smoking may, therefore, play an indirect role in the pathogenesis of COPD. Although epidemiologic data point to an increased incidence of lung cancer among nonsmokers who are chronically exposed to secondhand tobacco smoke, the evidence is less than conclusive.

CESSATION OF SMOKING

One of the most challenging, as well as rewarding, tasks of the health care pro-

fessional is motivating a chronic smoker to stop smoking permanently. Although the majority of smokers would like to terminate their unhealthy habit, and have tried more than once, their success rate is disappointingly small. The reasons for establishing and maintaining the smoking habit are complex. Behavioral, psychosocial, and pharmacological factors are all important and should be considered in any smoking-cessation plan. Recently, increasing emphasis on personal responsibility for individual health maintenance and disease prevention seems to have a greater impact in giving up the smoking habit.

There are several stop-smoking programs and self-help groups which may be suitable for an individual smoker. In more difficult and recalcitrant cases, methods such as behavior modification, psychotherapy, with or without hypnosis, acupuncture, and drug therapy have been tried with encouraging results. The drug therapy method is based on the convincing evidence that the major factor in causing cigarette addiction, and therefore, in producing withdrawal symptoms, is nicotine. The use of nicotine and nicotine-like substances have been shown to ease the withdrawal from cigarettes. Chewing gums in which nicotine is incorporated and bound to an ion exchange resin provide controlled release of nicotine.

Several studies have shown that the early changes in the respiratory tract resulting from smoking are reversible and improve after smoking cessation. The progression of advanced and irreversible changes is usually halted when cigarette smoking is stopped. The risk of developing bronchogenic carcinoma and a host of other cancers in ex-smokers reaches the incidence in nonsmokers after about 15 years of abstinence. The benefit from smoking cessation on the cardiovascular system has also been dramatic.

In advising patients for smoking cessation, the health risks of their habit and the benefits from its cessation should be explained as they pertain to the individual health problem. Every effort should be made to facilitate the acceptability to give up smoking and to support the patient during the early abstinence period. Logically, smoking prevention should be primarily addressed to the persons most susceptible to the smoking habit, especially school-age children and adolescents. As the start of smoking is promoted by psychosocial forces from peer pressure and misleading advertisements, these should be carefully considered in any public health measures addressing the issues of smoking.

BIBLIOGRAPHY

Aronson MD, Weiss ST, Ben RL, Komaroff AL. Association between cigarette smoking and acute respiratory tract illness in young adults. *JAMA*. 1982; 248:181–183.

Beck GJ, Doyle CA, Schacter EN. Smoking and lung function. *Am Rev Respir Dis*. 1981; 123:149–155.

Belt WT Jr. Tobacco smoking, hypertension, stroke, and coronary heart disease: the importance of smoking cessation. *Semin Respir Med*. 1990; 11:36–49.

Benowitz NL. Pharmacologic aspects of cigarette smoking and addiction. *N Engl J Med*. 1988; 319:1318–1330.

Calverley PMA, Leggett RJ, McElderry L, Flenley DC. Cigarette smoking and secondary polycythemia in hypoxic cor pulmonale. *Am Rev Respir Dis*. 1982; 125:507–510.

CDC. *The health benefits of smoking cessation:* a report of the Surgeon General, 1990. Rockville, Maryland: US Department of Health and Human Services, Public Health Service, 1990; DHHS publication no. (CDC) 90-8416.

Crofton J, Masironi R. Chronic airway disease: the smoking component. *Chest*. 1989; 96(suppl):349S–355S.

Fiore MC, Pierce JP, Remington PL, Fiore BJ. Cigarette Smoking: the clinician's role in cessation, prevention, and public health. *Dis Mon*. 1990; 35:186–241.

Fisher EB Jr, Haire-Joshu D, Morgan GD, et al. Smoking and smoking cessation. *Am Rev Respir Dis*. 1990; 142:702–720.

Griffith DE, Garcia JGN. Tobacco cigarettes, smoking, smoking cessation, and chronic obstructive pulmonary disease. *Semin Respir Med*. 1989; 10:346–371.

Hale KA, Ewing SL, Gosnell BA, Niewoehner DE. Lung disease in long-term cigarette smokers with and without chronic air-flow obstruction. *Am Rev Respir Dis*. 1984; 130:716–721.

Health and Public Policy Committee, American College of Physicians. Methods for stopping cigarette smoking. *Ann Intern Med*. 1986; 105:281–291.

Henningfield JE, Nemeth-Coslett R. Nicotine dependence: interface between tobacco and tobacco-related disease. *Chest*. 1988; 93(suppl):37S–55S.

Huber GL. Physical, chemical, and biologic properties of tobacco, cigarette smoke, and other tobacco products. *Semin Respir Med*. 1989; 10:297–332.

Idell S, Garcia JGN. Mechanisms of smoking-induced lung injury. *Semin Respir Med*. 1989; 10:345–355.

Kikendall JW, Evaul J, Johnson LF. Effect of cigarette smoking on gastrointestinal physiology and non-neoplastic digestive disease. *J Clin Gastroenterol*. 1984; 6:65–78.

Knudson RJ, Knudson DE, Kaltenborn WT, Bloom JW. Subclinical effects of cigarette smoking. *Chest*. 1989; 95:512–518.

Koop CE. Smoking and cancer. *Hosp Pract*. 1984; 19(6):107–132.

Krzyzanowski M, Sherrill DL, Paoletti P, Lebowitz MD. Relationship of respiratory symptoms and pulmonary function to tar, nicotine, and carbon monoxide yield of cigarettes. *Am Rev Respir Dis.* 1991; 143: 306–311.

Mahajan VK, Huber GL. Health effects of involuntary smoking. *Semin Respir Med.* 1990; 11:87–114.

Nemery B, Moavero NE, Brasseur L, et al. Changes in lung function after smoking cessation. *Am Rev Respir Dis.* 1982; 125: 122–124.

Nicotine gum. *Med Lett Drugs Ther.* 1984; 26:47–48.

Tager IB, Weiss ST, Muñoz A, et al. Longitudinal study of the effects of maternal smoking on pulmonary function in children. *N Engl J Med.* 1983; 309:699–702.

Tashkin DP, Clark VA, Coulson AH, et al. Effects of smoking cessation on lung function. *Am Rev Respir Dis.* 1984; 130:707–715.

Tobin MJ, Suffredini AF, Grenvik A. Short-term effect of smoking cessation. *Resp Care.* 1984; 29:641–649.

US Department of Health and Human Services. Reducing the health consequences of smoking: 25 years of progress. A report of the Surgeon General, 1989. DHHS Publication no. (CDC) 89-8411.

Pulmonary Aspiration-Atelectasis

CHAPTER 17

Pulmonary Aspiration

Inhalation of endogenously produced secretions or exogenous substances into the airways beyond the vocal cords is referred to as *aspiration*. Aspiration, even in normal individuals, is a common event, which in most instances is mild, usually well tolerated, and often unrecognized. However, when clinically significant, it may have serious and sometimes fatal consequences. The development of respiratory complications depends on the amount and physicochemical characteristics of the aspirate, as well as the frequency and depth of aspiration.

MECHANISMS AND CAUSES OF PULMONARY ASPIRATION

Pulmonary defense mechanisms as related to respiratory tract infection and environmental lung diseases are briefly discussed in appropriate chapters (pp. 66 and 200). The defense against aspiration depends mainly on proper function of supraglottic and glottic structures, which through a complex yet coordinated interaction of muscles of deglutition and laryngeal reflexes are capable of protecting the more distal airways. Predisposing factors for pulmonary aspira-

tion are, therefore, the conditions that impair these important protective structures and their functions. Table 17–1 outlines the important and fairly common conditions in which pulmonary aspiration may occur. The dominant factor in most clinical situations associated with aspiration is impaired consciousness. Alcohol intoxication, seizure disorders, drug overdose, general anesthesia, cerebrovascular accident, head trauma, and other organic metabolic brain dysfunction are some of frequent causes. Both nasogastric intubation and tracheostomy are known to predispose to recurrent pulmonary aspiration. Swallowing difficulty from neurological disorders or structural lesions of the mouth, pharynx, larynx, and esophagus are other conditions associated with aspiration. Vomiting or regurgitation of gastric content together with most any of the above disorders makes pulmonary aspiration almost a certainty. It is not unusual for vomiting to occur with alcoholic intoxication, during cardiopulmonary resuscitation, with drug overdose, or following head injury. Impaired cough reflex is a common finding in patients with chronic recurrent aspiration.

Aspirated material may be oropharyngeal secretions, vomitus, regurgi-

TABLE 17–1. CONDITIONS PREDISPOSING TO ASPIRATION

Altered level of consciousness
  Alcoholic intoxication
  Drug overdose
  General anesthesia
  Seizure disorders
  Cerebrovascular accident
  Head trauma

Conditions affecting neuromuscular function
  Polymyositis
  Muscular dystrophy
  Myasthenia gravis
  Guillain-Barré syndrome
  Amyotrophic lateral sclerosis
  Multiple sclerosis
  Syringomyelia
  Parkinson's disease

Structural lesions of mouth, pharynx, larynx, and esophagus impairing swallowing

Other contributing factors
  Cardiopulmonary resuscitation
  Nasogastric tube
  Tracheostomy
  Gastric dilatation, gastroparesis
  Gastroesophageal reflux
  Frequent vomiting

tated gastric content, blood, food, drink, or other exogenous substances. These materials when aspirated may result in pathophysiologic changes related to three different mechanisms, each causing distinctive clinical syndromes of (1) infection, (2) toxic reaction, and (3) mechanical obstruction. These syndromes may develop alone or occur in various combinations. They may present as an acute single event or may manifest as a recurring and chronically debilitating condition. Infectious consequences of pulmonary aspiration are mentioned in Chapter 3 and, therefore, they will not be discussed further. In addition to bronchopulmonary diseases resulting from the aspiration of toxic fluids and me-

chanical effect of aspiration, a somewhat related subject of near-drowning will also be discussed in this chapter.

ASPIRATION PNEUMONITIS

There are several exogenous chemicals that under unusual circumstances may be aspirated, resulting in inflammatory reaction in the lungs; however, the most common and important problem of aspiration in clinical practice is related to gastric acid. For the purpose of this discussion, the term *aspiration pneumonitis*, which will be interchangeably used with the term *chemical pneumonitis*, will refer to pulmonary complication of aspiration of acid gastric content.

Pathogenesis and Pathologic Changes.
The main toxic effect of gastric juice stems from its high concentration of hydrochloric acid. The whole picture of aspiration pneumonitis can be produced by intratracheal injection of sterile hydrochloric acid in experimental animals. Its effect has been considered to be a chemical burn related to the very low pH of the aspirate. Data from animal studies indicate that a pH of less than 2.5 and a volume of at least 1 mL/kg of weight are necessary for an aspirate to cause a significant lung injury. However, in clinical situations other factors, such as distribution of the aspirated material and the presence of food particles, also affect the outcome of the aspiration of the gastric content. Chemical effect of gastric acid on respiratory tract is almost immediate and, with enough volume, quite extensive, owing to its rapid distribution. Although the acid is neutralized within a

few minutes, the damage has already occurred.

Pathologic changes usually consist of extensive acute inflammatory reaction, which together with alveolar and capillary injury results in exudation of fluid into and around the airspaces. The lungs are heavy and edematous with areas of hemorrhage. The early parenchymal changes are peribronchial, which become more diffuse in advanced stages. The mucosa of bronchi are often destroyed. The lesions following pulmonary aspiration are more severe in dependent portions of the lungs (ie, lower lobes and posterior segments of upper lobes). The right lung is usually involved more than the left because of its bronchus offering easier access to the aspirated material. In more severe cases the entire lung fields are involved.

Reduction of pulmonary compliance, ventilation-perfusion imbalance, intrapulmonary shunting, and severe hypoxemia are the usual pathophysiologic consequences of aspiration pneumonitis.

Clinical Manifestations.

Despite its frequent occurrence in various clinical situations, the diagnosis of aspiration pneumonitis without history or witness of vomiting and aspiration is almost impossible to make. Most often it is presumed or suspected in patients with the aforementioned predisposing factors and consistent clinical picture. Aspiration of small amounts of gastric content may cause no symptom or sign; however, if a sufficient volume of highly acid gastric secretion is aspirated, a distinct picture of acute respiratory distress develops. Usually within 2 to 5 hours following aspiration of liquid gastric content, there is abrupt onset of dyspnea, tachypnea, cyanosis, and tachycardia. Fever may or may not be present. Some patients become hypotensive and develop clinical shock. There is often evidence of bronchospasm with diffuse wheezing; frothy pink sputum and pulmonary rales are commonly present. The symptoms and signs become progressively worse unless appropriate treatment is instituted.

The most characteristic laboratory feature of aspiration pneumonitis is severe hypoxemia, which is often difficult to correct with increased FIO_2. Arterial blood PCO_2 is usually reduced unless there is significant ventilatory impairment. Blood gas abnormalities may be present right after aspiration, before development of a full clinical picture or radiographic changes. This may be an important clue in early diagnosis of aspiration pneumonitis.

Severe aspiration pneumonitis is one of the multiple causes of adult respiratory distress syndrome (see Chapter 25).

Radiographic Findings.

The chest x-ray may show bilateral diffuse mottling, more marked in dependent lung regions (Fig. 17–1). The changes may be limited to a few segments or lobes in less severe cases, the location of which will depend on the patient's body position at the time of aspiration.

Management.

Because of extreme seriousness of aspiration pneumonitis, which often has a fatal outcome, every effort should be made toward its prevention. Close observation of patients at risk of aspiration, such as patients with impaired consciousness; proper positioning of patients; appropriate preparation before general anesthesia;

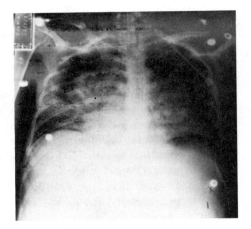

Figure 17–1. Chest radiograph of severe bilateral aspiration pneumonitis. There is diffuse interstitial and airspace infiltration in both lung fields (noncardiac pulmonary edema).

precautionary measures and immediate care of patients with seizure disorders; and close watch of patients with indwelling nasogastric tube, mostly if they are being fed through the tube, are some of the important measures that help in reducing the incidence of aspiration. The administration of a water-soluble antacid or an H_2 receptor antagonist, before general anesthesia, especially when there is a question about the gastric content, results in a significant reduction in the occurrence of serious aspiration penumonitis. Because commonly used particulate antacids are known to produce pulmonary injury when aspirated, they should not be used for this purpose.

Once aspiration is witnessed, immediate proper positioning of patient and suctioning of the airways should be undertaken. Tracheal lavage with saline solution or attempt to neutralize gastric acid with bicarbonate solution may be more harmful than beneficial.

The most important aspect of treatment of aspiration pneumonitis is correction of hypoxemia by administration of oxygen. Bronchodilators, such as aminophylline or beta-adrenergic stimulating agents, may be tried. If hypoxemia cannot be corrected by simple means, intubation and mechanical ventilation, usually with positive end-expiratory pressure, will be necessary. As is true with most cases of acute respiratory distress syndrome, the correction of hypoxemia is the most important part of management of aspiration pneumonitis.

The role of corticosteroids in the management of aspiration pneumonitis remains controversial. Once the full clinical picture has developed, their use has no demonstrable effect. Administration of steroids immediately following aspiration or within a few hours has been commonly practiced, despite lack of conclusive evidence for their benefit. Antibiotic therapy for prophylaxis against bacterial infection is another unsettled question in the management of aspiration pneumonitis. However, because of a high incidence of pulmonary infection following aspiration, periodic bacteriologic examination of sputum, as well as close clinical evaluation and follow-up radiographic studies, should be performed for the early detection of infection and its proper treatment.

Chronic Recurrent Aspiration
In contrast to the acute dramatic clinical picture, aspiration, if mild but chronic and recurrent, may produce more insidious and protracted symptoms. Transient recurrent fever, chronic cough and wheezing, subtle radiographic changes, and even progressive pulmonary fibrosis may be due to chronic aspiration of

gastric content in patients with esophageal disorder and/or impaired consciousness. The management of such patients is often difficult and usually unsuccessful because of the nature of the underlying predisposing conditions. Surgical interventions which are based on separating the airway from the alimentary tract, necessitate a tracheostomy with or without the closure of the larynx. Supraglottic or glottic closure, laryngotracheal separation, and tracheoesophageal diversion are some of the surgical techniques for this purpose. The tracheoesophageal diversion procedure, in which the proximal tracheal segment is connected to the esophagus, is potentially reversible and easier to perform. It would allow secretions and oral intake that may pass into the larynx to enter the esophagus. The decision for any of these interventions requires the considerations of many factors, which include lack of response to simpler measures, patient acceptability, prognosis of the underlying chronic disease, and patient's life expectancy.

Hydrocarbon Pneumonitis

Hydrocarbon pneumonitis usually results from the aspiration of accidentally ingested hydrocarbons such as kerosene, gasoline, or certain household compounds (furniture polishes) containing hydrocarbons. It is most commonly seen in young children after inadvertent ingestion of such substances. In adults it may occasionally occur with suicidal attempts, industrial accidents, or siphoning of gasoline. Because of their low viscosity and very low surface tension, hydrocarbons, once aspirated, spread throughout the lungs. Being lipid solvents, they are directly toxic to the lung tissues, causing widespread

injury and inflammation of the airways and alveoli. The clinical picture of hydrocarbon pneumonitis is one of rapidly progressive pulmonary edema with severe hypoxemia. The diagnosis is often suggested by the odor of the patient's breath.

The prevention of further aspiration is most important in the management of hydrocarbon pneumonitis. Measures that may cause vomiting should be avoided. Adequate oxygenation by supplemental oxygen, constant positive airway pressure (CPAP), or mechanical ventilation with positive end-expiratory pressure (PEEP), depending on the severity of the disease, will be necessary. The role of corticosteroids in its management has not been established.

MECHANICAL EFFECT OF ASPIRATION: FOREIGN-BODY ASPIRATION

Aspiration of solid or liquid material may cause ventilatory impairment and other pulmonary complications by mechanical airway obstruction. These materials may be inert or have limited toxic effect on the lungs.

Aspiration of foreign bodies can occur at any age, but it is most common in children between the ages of 1 and 3. The usual objects include nuts, seeds, pins, coins, and beads. Depending on the size and shape of solid material in relation to the airway, a variable degree of obstruction will result. Large objects will lodge in the larynx, causing upper airway obstruction. This was discussed in Chapter 7 along with other causes of upper airway obstruction. Smaller objects may lodge in one of the main-stem bronchi or more distally. The shape of the object will determine whether the obstruction will be complete from the beginning or will become complete secondary to tissue reaction to traumatic or toxic effect of the aspirated material. Because of the direction of the right main-stem bronchus, foreign bodies lodge in right lung bronchi twice as often as the left.

The initial symptoms of foreign-body aspiration are choking, cough, respiratory distress, and wheezing. A large body occluding the larynx results in suffocation; a smaller object in the larynx will cause hoarseness or complete loss of voice and croupy cough. As a result of laryngeal spasm and/or edema, obstruction may become complete if the object is not removed. Lodging of a foreign body in one of the bronchi will cause irritating cough and varying degrees of dyspnea, depending on the size of the obstructed bronchus and degree of obstruction. Localized wheezing or absent breath sounds may be detected.

Radiographic examination may show the aspirated object if it is radiopaque, or secondary changes may be demonstrated. Complete obstruction of a main stem or a lobar bronchus results in atelectasis; incomplete blockage may behave as a check valve and cause overinflation of the involved lung or lobe. This can be demonstrated better by comparing inspiratory with expiratory films.

Bronchoscopy is decisive in making the diagnosis and is essential for the removal of bronchial foreign bodies.

If untreated, the foreign body in a bronchus will result in late infectious complications, including pneumonia, lung abscess, empyema, and bronchiectasis. Frequently, the early symptoms of

foreign-body aspiration are transient and may be forgotten; therefore, late complications may be its only manifestations. The importance of bronchoscopic examination in these situations cannot be overemphasized.

Aspiration of any liquid material in large enough volume produces abrupt suffocation by total obstruction of air passages. Sometimes aspiration of a massive amount of vomitus may be the cause of respiratory arrest. This is not an uncommon terminal event in certain debilitated patients, particularly with impaired cerebral or other neurologic functions. Only immediate tracheal suctioning may be lifesaving. In massive hemoptysis, the cause of death is often due to mechanical obstruction of the airways from inundation of blood. It is often said that the patient with massive hemoptysis may "drown in his own blood."

DROWNING AND NEAR DROWNING

Drowning is death from asphyxiation as a result of submersion, but in *near drowning* the victim survives at least temporarily following such an accident. Near-drowning victims may suffer from *secondary drowning*, which is death from delayed complications following apparent recovery. Despite declining death rate from drowning in the United States in recent years, over 5,000 individuals, mostly young, still die from drowning each year. This number is only a small fraction of annual submersion accidents in this country.

Pathogenesis and Pathophysiology. In drowning the following sequence of events takes place. The initial period is characterized by panic at the time of submersion and violent struggle to reach the surface. Breath holding, which is a common reaction, will last until rapidly progressive hypoxemia and hypercapnia stimulate the respiratory center, forcing the victim to inhale. The entrance of water into the larynx causes intense laryngospasm. About 10% to 15% of drowning victims die from asphyxia due to glottic spasm without water entering into the lung; this is referred to as "dry drowning." The remaining victims aspirate the water into the tracheobronchial passages all the way to the terminal airways and alveoli. In either event the essential problem is related to respiratory arrest, which results in severe hypoxemia, acidosis, and death.

The distinction between freshwater and seawater drowning was unduly emphasized in the past. Although an occasional patient may have significant problems with water and electrolyte imbalance or other disturbances as a result of aspiration of hypotonic (fresh) or hypertonic (sea) water, the major clinical problems in all near-drowning victims, regardless of the composition of water, are related to hypoxia and acidosis.

Severe hypoxemia and respiratory acidosis may result in myocardial depression and reduced cardiac output. Marked impairment of tissue perfusion from peripheral vasoconstriction and low cardiac output, together with arterial hypoxemia, causes a profound tissue anoxia and lactic acidosis. Cerebral hypoxia is the cause of altered mental state and unconsciousness.

Near-drowning victims, after being rescued, may have diminished or no respiration. Hypoxemia and respiratory acidosis from lack of ventilation are sustained or even worsened with the development of pulmonary edema, which may occur during and/or after the rescue. Aspirated water, alveolar capillary leak, loss of surfactant, and myocardial depression may contribute to the development of pulmonary edema. The amount of aspirated water varies, but most near-drowning victims do not aspirate more than 4 mL/kg of body weight. This amount of fluid cannot by itself result in significant pulmonary edema. Increased alveolar capillary leak, which plays a more important role, may be due to injury from hypertonic salt solution of seawater, severe hypoxia, neurogenic effect, and the presence of other dissolved or particulate matters in aspirated water. Loss of surfactant, especially with freshwater aspiration, enhances pulmonary edema and also causes atelectasis. In severe near drowning, therefore, a clinicopathologic picture of ARDS develops. Ventilation-perfusion mismatch and intrapulmonary shunting may persist until the victim's full recovery. In some patients initial success in restoring adequate ventilation and oxygenation is followed by progressive respiratory distress and death (secondary drowning).

It has been demonstrated that hypothermia, which may occur in near-drowning victims from cold water, will have some protective effect against permanent central nervous system damage of anoxia (anoxic encephalopathy).

Clinical Manifestations. Upon rescue, a near-drowning victim is usually unconscious or agitated and confused, cold, and cyanotic. Respiration is often absent; otherwise tachypnea, cough, and frothy pink expectoration may be noted and rales and rhonchi may be heard. The pulse is often difficult to feel, and heart sounds are difficult to hear. Because of severe vasoconstriction, blood pressure is usually hard to measure. Neurologic examination shows varying degrees of cerebral dysfunction.

Chest radiograph in near drowning may be initially normal despite significant respiratory impairment. More often, patchy infiltrates or diffuse pulmonary edema are noted. These changes may develop later. Blood-gas abnormalities are always present; hypoxemia, hypercapnia, low serum bicabonate level, and very low blood pH are commonly seen. Varying patterns of electrocardiographic abnormalities can often be demonstrated. In seawater near drowning, serum sodium and chloride may be high.

Management. The primary objectives of treatment of near-drowning victims should be prompt restoration of ventilation, adequate oxygenation, and correction of acidosis. The initial stage of therapy should be on-the-scene emergency care with usual diligent resuscitative procedures (ie, establishment and maintenance of an adequate airway, mouth-to-mouth breathing or use of a hand respirator with supplemental oxygen if available, and application of cardiac massage if there is no heart beat). If near drowning is suspected to be the result of a diving accident, the possibility of head and neck injury should be considered and appropriate measures taken. Emergency care should be continued during the transportation of the victim to the hospital. At the hospital, in addition, the victim should be intubated if he or she remains unconscious, and mechanically ventilated with an adequate supply of oxygen. Positive expiratory pressure may be required for proper oxygenation. If the patient is conscious and breathes spontaneously, he or she should be kept in the hospital for observation and monitoring of clinical signs and blood gases, while receiving supplemental oxygen. It is not uncommon that the near-drowning victim, after apparent initial recovery, develops progressive respiratory distress. Other therapeutic measures should include restoration of fluid, electrolyte, and acid-base balance. Under certain circumstances, ionotropic drugs and diuretics may be used. Although infectious complications involving the respiratory tract are common, prophylactic antibiotic use is not recommended. Such infections should be watched for and treated promptly once recognized. Corticosteroids have not been proven to be beneficial for prevention or treatment of pulmonary complications in near drowning. Their use, however, is sometimes recommended for treatment of cerebral edema and increased intracranial pressure (ICP), which occurs commonly as a result of prolonged brain anoxia.

Neurologic status after initial resuscitation is the best indicator of outcome in most patients. Near-drowning victims who breathe spontaneously and are conscious have a very good prognosis. However, it should be emphasized that many patients who remain comatose, even for a prolonged period, are known to recover, often with restoration of most of their neurologic functions. Therefore these patients should be maintained with proper intensive care during their unresponsive state and, later, be subjected to vigorous rehabilitative measures. The usefulness of "cerebral salvage" techniques, such as induction of hypothermia, ICP monitoring, and barbiturate coma, is not well established.

BIBLIOGRAPHY

Brin MF, Younger D. Neurologic disorders and aspiration. *Otolaryngol Clin North Am.* 1988; 21:691–699.

DePaso WJ Aspiration pneumonia. *Clin Chest Med.* 1991; 12:269–284.

Eisele DW, Yarington CT Jr, Lindeman RC. Indications for the tracheoesophageal diversion procedure and the laryngotracheal separation procedure. *Ann Otol Rhinol Laryngol.* 1988; 97:471–475.

Gonzalez-Rothi RJ. Near drowning: concensus and controversies in pulmonary and cerebral resuscitation. *Heart Lung.* 1987; 16:474–482.

Holroyd HJ. Foreign body aspiration: potential cause of coughing and wheezing. *Pediatr Rev.* 1988; 10:59–63.

Huxley EJ, Viroslav J, Gray WR, Pierce AK. Pharyngeal aspiration in normal adults and patients with depressed consciousness. *Am J Med.* 1978; 64:564–568.

Joyce TH III. Prophylaxis for pulmonary acid aspiration. *Am J Med.* 1987; 83(suppl 6A):46–52.

Karlson KH Jr. Hydrocarbon poisoning in children. *South Med J.* 1982; 75:839–840.

LeFrock JL, Clark TS, Davies B, Klainer AS. Aspiration pneumonia: a ten-year review. *Am Surg.* 1979; 45:305–313.

Limper AH, Prakash UBS. Tracheobronchial foreign bodies in adults. *Ann Intern Med.* 1990; 112:604–609.

Modell JH, Graves SA, Ketover A. Clinical course of 91 consecutive near-drowning victims. *Chest.* 1976; 70:231–238.

Nelson HS. Gastroesophageal reflux and pulmonary disease. *J Allergy Clin Immunol.* 1984; 73:547–556.

Orlowski JP, Abulleil MM, Phillips JM. The hemodynamic and cardiovascular effects of near-drowning in hypotonic, isotonic, or hypertonic solution. *Ann Emerg Med.* 1989; 18:1044–1049.

Redding JS. Drowning and near drowning. *Postgrad Med.* 1983; 74(1):65–97.

US Department of Health and Human Services. Aquatic death and injuries—United States. *MMWR.* 1982; 31:417–419.

Wolkove N, Kreisman H, Cohen C, Frank H. Occult foreign-body aspiration in adults. *JAMA.* 1982; 248:1350–1352.

Young RSK, Zalneraitis EL, Dooling EC. Neurological outcome in cold water drowning. *JAMA.* 1980; 244:1233–1235.

CHAPTER 18

Pulmonary Atelectasis

Although atelectasis, in the strict sense of the word (*ateles,* imperfect; *ektasis,* expansion), refers to incomplete expansion of the lung at birth, it is generally used in broad terms to include partial or complete collapse of lung tissue that has previously been expanded. Atelectasis may involve an entire lung or be limited to any portion of it, from a lobe to the smallest lung unit. It is one of the most common changes in the lung that can occur under numerous conditions.

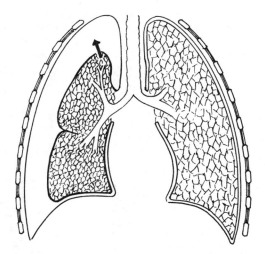

Figure 18–1. Collapse of the right lung as a result of elimination of negative intrathoracic pressure with pneumothorax.

Pathogenesis. To understand the development of atelectasis, it is important to consider the mechanisms that normally keep the lungs expanded. The natural tendency of the lungs to collapse is opposed by the tendency of the chest wall to expand. At the resting position (functional residual capacity, FRC), these two forces are oppositely equal; as a result, there is a negative (subatmospheric) pressure between the lung and thoracic wall (pleural pressure). Once this negative pressure is eliminated, as a result of conditions such as pneumothorax or pleural effusion, the underlying lung will collapse (Fig. 18–1).

The volume of individual alveoli is determined by an opposing negative intrathoracic pressure, which tends to expand them, and elastic recoil together with *surface tension* of the alveoli, which tend to collapse them (Fig. 18–2). The presence of **surfactant** reduces the surface tension of the alveoli. As the alveoli diminish in volume during expiration, reduction in surface area of alveolar wall results in increased thickness and change in configuration of lipid-protein structure of surfactant layer; thus alveolar surface tension is lowered (Fig. 18–3). This protective mechanism prevents col-

243

lapse of alveoli when they reach a certain volume at which they would have collapsed without the presence of such a surface-tension-lowering agent. Reduction or absence of surfactant, which occurs in numerous pulmonary pathologic conditions, is one of the most important contributory factors in production of atelectasis.

There is a significant difference in the volume of alveoli in various lung regions. At FRC, the alveoli in the upper lung zones are already expanded, while those in the lung bases have smallest volumes and, therefore, are capable of increasing their volumes much more during inspiration. The lower lung regions contribute much more to pulmonary ventilation than the upper ones, and they are, at the same time, more predisposed to atelectasis.

Continuous ventilation of the lung regions assures an adequate supply of air to the alveoli. The cessation of air replenishment, as may happen from the obstruction of the supplying bronchus, results in the resorption of air and, therefore, atelectasis (absorption atelec-

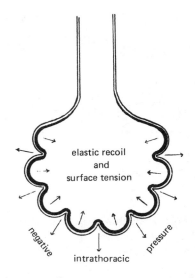

Figure 18–2. Forces determining the alveolar volume.

tasis, Fig. 18–4). Complete obstruction of the bronchus of a lobe will result in absorption of its air within 24 hours. If the lobe is filled with oxygen, atelectasis will occur much more rapidly. Sometimes the obstructing lesion will act as a one-way valve, allowing the air to escape from a lobe during various expira-

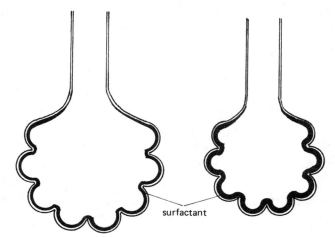

Figure 18–3. Reduction of alveolar surface tension during expiration, resulting from increased thickness of surfactant layer.

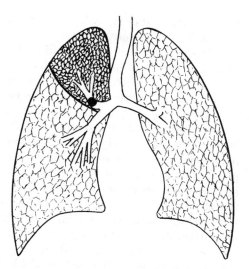

Figure 18–4. Atelectasis of the right upper lobe as a result of occlusion of its bronchus.

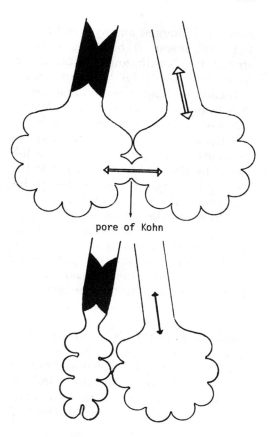

pore of Kohn

Figures 18–5 and 18–6. Collateral communication between the alveoli (pore of Kohn). Such a communication, when open, prevents alveolar atelectasis with distal airway obstruction (Fig. 18–5). Adequacy of collateral ventilation depends on the degree of alveolar inflation; with partial deflation, the communication may close (Fig. 18–6).

tory efforts but preventing its entrance during inspiration. This results in more rapid development of collapse. However, the reversal of function of such a one-way valve causes hyperinflation.

The obstruction of airways more distal to a lobar bronchus may or may not result in collapse of a corresponding portion of the lung. The effect of obstruction then will depend on the presence and the function of *collateral communication* between adjacent alveoli (Fig. 18–5 and 18–6). The most significant collateral ventilation occurs through the *pores of Kohn*, which are openings or discontinuities of alveolar walls. Adequacy of collateral ventilation depends on the degree of inflation of the lungs; with partial deflation the communications may close.

Normally the variation in depth of respiration with such acts as sighing, yawning, talking, laughing, crying, coughing, exertion, and excitement ensures periodic expansion of the areas of

the lungs that otherwise would collapse. In patients who are anesthetized, sedated, or obtunded from other causes, or when they are on a constant-volume ventilator, such periodic deep breathing does not occur. Although their ventilation may be adequate for gas exchange, they do not expand the lungs sufficiently for collateral ventilation between the alveoli, some of which may have plugged airways, and atelectasis will result. It has been demonstrated that continuous ventilation at fixed and low tidal volumes causes reduction of lung volume (atelectasis). Preexisting bronchopulmonary disease will hasten this complication.

Regional reduction or cessation of pulmonary blood flow is usually followed by diminished ventilation to the corresponding region. Atelectasis in this situation is always incomplete.

In many clinical situations there is usually a combination of two or more of the above-mentioned pathogenetic mechanisms. In addition, atelectasis may result from compression of the lung (eg, by large tumors or cysts) and scarring.

Etiology. From the discussion on pathogenesis, it is clear that a varying degree of atelectasis may be seen under numerous circumstances (Table 18–1). Indeed, atelectasis is one of the most common complications that occur in both medical and surgical patients, with or without preexisting pulmonary disease.

The presence of air or fluid in the pleural space will result in the collapse of underlying lung. Atelectasis is a common mode of presentation of patients with bronchogenic carcinoma due to airway obstruction. A foreign body in a bronchus or other endobronchial lesions may manifest by atelectasis. The compression of bronchi by lesions, such as enlarged lymph nodes or an abnormal blood vessel, may result in collapse of the corresponding part of the lung. Inadvertent intubation of the right main-stem or intermediate bronchus with an endotracheal tube causes atelectasis of the left lung, and sometimes the right upper lobe. In many instances, a mucous plug may be the culprit, such as with asthma, chronic bronchitis, prolonged mechanical ventilation, and debilitated individuals with suppressed cough. Some degree of atelectasis is very common in patients with drug overdose. Atelectasis is part of the pathologic changes in

TABLE 18–1. MECHANISMS AND CORRESPONDING COMMON CAUSES OF ATELECTASIS

Mechanisms	Causes
1. Elimination or reversal of negative pleural pressure	Pneumothorax, pleural effusion
2. Bronchial obstruction (absorption atelectasis)	Accumulated secretions, mucus plug, endobronchial neoplasm, foreign body, bronchial compression, intubation of right mainstem or intermediate bronchus
3. Lack or loss of surfactant	Respiratory distress syndrome, near drowning
4. Impaired diaphragmatic function	Phrenic nerve paralysis, high spinal cord injury, upper abdominal or thoracic surgery, abdominal distention, splinting from pain
5. Fixed and low tidal volume breathing	Improper ventilation setting, unconsciousness, immobility
6. Reduced pulmonary blood flow	Pulmonary embolism
7. Scarring	Rounded atelectasis (asbestosis)
8. Compression of lung	Large intrathoracic tumor or cyst, tension pneumothorax or hydrothorax

bronchiectasis and cystic fibrosis. Pneumonias may result in some volume loss of the involved lung. Partial atelectasis is common in pulmonary embolism. One of the characteristic features of respiratory distress syndrome in infants and adults is pulmonary volume loss.

Atelectasis is a well-recognized postoperative pulmonary complication. In addition to thoracic surgery, upper abdominal operation is frequently complicated by atelectasis. Various mechanisms are responsible for this common problem in postsurgical patients. Immobility, sedation, pain, reflex splinting of the diaphragm, dressings, and binders result in significant impairment of deep breathing and coughing. It has been demonstrated that there is a significant reduction in diaphragm activity in the postoperative period and also a shift from predominantly abdominal (diaphragmatic) to rib-cage breathing. Reduced ventilation, small airways obstruction due to secretion, and lack of collateral ventilation cause basilar atelectasis. Superimposed infection, pulmonary embolism, and fluid overload are among other contributory factors in the development of atelectasis in both postoperative and in critically ill patients.

As mentioned in Chapter 15, rounded atelectasis is caused by collapse of a portion of the lung as a result of pleural effusion and fibrous pleural adhesion in which the trapped segment, unable to expand, rolls into a rounded mass. Although it may rarely result from various pleuropulmonary conditions, atelectasis is a characteristic finding in asbestosis.

Pathophysiology. Atelectasis results in absent or reduced ventilation of the involved area of the lung and the proportional reduction of the lung volumes. Both FRC and vital capacity (VC) are diminished. Although as a result of pulmonary vasoconstriction, blood flow to the atelectatic region tends to diminish, ventilation-perfusion mismatching and intrapulmonary shunting are the usual pathophysiologic changes in atelectasis that cause hypoxemia.

Clinical Manifestations. Symptoms related to pulmonary atelectasis are frequently overshadowed by the presence of underlying pathologic conditions. Most patients with mild or small atelectasis have no symptoms referable to it. When present in more significant atelectasis, the symptoms are nonspecific. Dyspnea, cough, fever, and chest discomfort may suggest atelectasis under certain circumstances, such as following major surgery. Changes in lung mechanics in patients on a mechanical ventilator or increasing oxygen requirement for adequate oxygenation may indicate atelectasis. Physical findings are usually present in patients with collapse of a lung or lobe. Flattening of the chest wall with reduction of its expansion, deviation of trachea to one side, elevation of diaphragm, dullness to percussion, and diminished or absent breath sounds are some of the signs of pulmonary atelectasis. With less extensive involvement, physical findings are less impressive and less suggestive. The presence of basal rales and diminished breath sounds are the most common findings in postoperative atelectasis.

Pulmonary atelectasis is an important cause of ventilation-perfusion abnormality and hypoxemia. The latter may be the only manifestation of atelectasis.

Radiographic Changes. Although the radiographic examination is the most important in diagnosing atelectasis, it may be normal or unrevealing when smaller lung units are involved (micro-atelectasis). Radiographic signs, when present, may be both direct and indirect. Direct radiographic signs include increased density and reduction of the volume of a whole lung or part of it. Increased density, however, does not appear until a significant volume of air is absorbed or expressed from the involved lung, except when there is other associated parenchymal disease. Displacement of interlobar fissures, elevation of diaphragm, mediastinal shift, hilar displacement, alteration of bronchial and carinal angles, and changes in chest wall are among the indirect signs of atelectasis (Figs. 18–7 and 18–8). Frequently, underlying pulmonary disease may be identified. There are known patterns of radiographic changes with various lobar and segmental atelectasis. Their description is beyond the scope of this book.

Platelike atelectasis is a radiographic term applied to linear shadows of increased density, mostly situated in the lung bases in a roughly horizontal position. They are due to atelectasis of the alveoli in lower lung fields not related to specific bronchial distribution. Platelike atelectasis is frequently due to diminished diaphragmatic movement as a result of intraabdominal disease or surgery. As mentioned earlier, the combination of reduced ventilation, small airways obstruction due to secretion, lack of collateral ventilation due to inadequate inflation of the alveoli, and presence of fluid in alveoli will result in this type of atelectasis.

In many instances the diagnosis of the underlying cause of atelectasis, par-

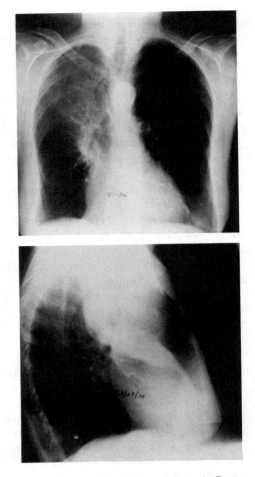

Figures 18–7 and 18–8. Lobar atelectasis. Posteroanterior and lateral chest radiographs showing atelectasis of the right upper lobe.

ticularly when it involves a lung, a lobe, or a segment, will require bronchoscopic examination.

Management. The prevention and the treatment of underlying conditions are the most important and effective measures against pulmonary atelectasis. In view of the multiplicity of the causes of atelectasis, we shall only outline certain principles of management, rather than discuss specific therapeutic measures.

In some instances atelectasis is a corollary to a more important basic disease, the treatment of which will solve the problem. Withdrawal of air or fluid from pleural cavity, removal of foreign body from the bronchus, and resectional surgery for neoplasms are a few examples. However, in the majority of cases, as discussed earlier, there is a combination of several factors that should be considered for proper management.

Inadequate lung inflation from pain, sedation, mental **obtundation,** and many other causes should be prevented by encouragement of periodic deep-breathing and other lung-expansion maneuvers. Such maneuvers have proven useful for both prophylactic and therapeutic purposes. Incentive spirometry is the most commonly used technique. Chest physiotherapy and the use of dead-space rebreathing tubes, blow bottles, and intermittent CPAP by facial or nasal masks are other methods that can be effective in preventing and treating atelectasis. The use of IPPB has declined significantly in recent years, mainly because of availability of simpler and more effective techniques. The choice of any of these methods depends on the circumstances in which atelectasis commonly occurs and on the patient's ability and willingness to cooperate. Nasal CPAP has proven particularly useful in poorly responsive patients. In cooperative and fully alert patients, simple deep-breathing exercises or incentive spirometry will suffice. Cough not only helps in clearing the airways but also increases ventilation and lung expansion. Because bronchial secretion is a major factor in producing atelectasis, every effort should be made in its removal by cough, postural drainage, and suctioning. Adequate humidification with proper hydration and inhalation therapy will prevent drying of secretions and facilitate their removal. The presence of underlying chronic bronchopulmonary conditions increases the need for these measures.

Both critically ill patients and patients with tracheal intubation, on or off ventilator, should be given special attention in treating or, better, in preventing atelectasis. Such patients are greatly handicapped by their inability to cough and clear their tracheobronchial tree. With their serious underlying problems with lungs and other organs, the development of atelectasis, even in mild form, is poorly tolerated and will markedly impede their recovery. Adequate bronchial hygiene and close monitoring of their ventilatory status, lung mechanics, blood gases, and chest radiographs are essential for prevention and early detection of atelectasis. The use of fiberoptic bronchoscopy in management of atelectasis in these patients has been rewarding. Kinetic therapy making use of rotating beds has shown to be beneficial in preventing pulmonary complications, including atelectasis, in critically ill patients, especially in those with head and neck injuries. The importance of the role of allied health professionals, particularly respiratory therapists, nurses, and physiotherapists, in the prevention and treatment of atelectasis in both surgical and medical patients cannot be overstressed.

BIBLIOGRAPHY

Bartlett RH. Respiratory therapy to prevent complications of surgery. *Respir Care.* 1984:29:667–677.

Bateman JRM, Newman SP, Daunt KM, et al. Is cough as effective as chest physiotherapy in the removal of excessive tracheobronchial secretions? *Thorax*. 1981; 36:683–687.

Celli BR, Rodriguez KS, Snider GL. A controlled trial of intermittent positive pressure breathing, incentive spirometry, and deep breathing exercises in preventing pulmonary complications after abdominal surgery. *Am Rev Respir Dis*. 1984; 130:12–15.

Duncan SR, Negrin RS, Mihm FG, et al. Nasal continuous positive airway pressure in atelectasis. *Chest*. 1987; 92:621–624.

Ford GT, Whitelaw WA, Rosenal TW, et al. Diaphragmatic function after upper abdominal surgery in humans. *Am Rev Respir Dis*. 1983: 127:431–436.

Gentilello L, Thompson DA, Tonnesen AS, et al. Effects of a rotating bed on the incidence of pulmonary complications in critically ill patients. *Crit Care Med*. 1988; 16:783–786.

Hammon WE, Martin RJ. Chest physiotherapy for acute atelectasis. *Phys Ther*. 1981; 61:217–220.

Marini JJ. Postoperative atelectasis: pathophysiology, clinical importance, and principles of management. *Respir Care*. 1984; 29:516–528.

Mintzer RA, Sakowicz BA, Blonder JA. Lobar collapse: usual and unusual forms. *Chest*. 1988; 94:615–620.

Paul WL, Downs JB. Postoperative atelectasis. *Arch Surg*. 1981; 116:861–863.

Reines HD, Harris RC. Pulmonary complications of acute spinal cord injuries. *Neurosurgery*. 1987; 21:193–196.

Roukema JA, Carol EJ, Prins JG. The prevention of pulmonary complications after upper abdominal surgery in patients with noncompromised pulmonary status. *Arch Surg*. 1988; 123:30–34.

Scuderi J, Olsen GN. Respiratory therapy in the management of postoperative complications. *Respir Care*. 1989; 34:281–291.

Stiller K, Geake T, Taylor J, et al. Acute lobar atelectasis: a comparison of two chest physiotherapy regimens. *Chest*. 1990; 98: 1336–1340.

Neoplastic Diseases of the Lung

CHAPTER 19

Lung Cancer

Malignant tumors of the lung may be primary, originating in the lung, or metastatic, having their site of origin in other areas of the body. Lung cancer refers to malignant neoplasms that start in the lung tissue. Although any tissue of the lung may undergo malignant change, by far the most common malignant neoplasm in the lung originates from the bronchial mucosa and is called bronchogenic carcinoma. *Lung cancer* and **bronchogenic carcinoma** are used interchangeably in this chapter.

Incidence. Primary lung cancer at present is the most common malignancy in the United States, and is one of the leading causes of death. A steady rise in its incidence in the past half-century among males is recently becoming more evident among females. The alarming yearly increase in its incidence shows no signs of slowing or leveling off, and it is feared that it will continue. Presently, one-fourth of Americans dying from cancer die from bronchogenic carcinoma. Although its incidence is lower among females, it is rising much faster than in males. Since 1986, lung cancer has become the leading cause of death from cancer in women as it has been the case for men for a long time.

Etiology. The exact cause and pathogenesis of cancer in general remains unknown. Certain factors, however, have been incriminated in its causation. In lung cancer, there is an indubitable relationship of prolonged inhalation of air pollutants to its occurrence. Among the pollutants, cigarette smoke has been the most important. Ninety percent of patients with lung cancer are cigarette smokers. As discussed in Chapter 16, a strong correlation exists between intensity and duration of cigarette smoking and development of lung cancer. Longtime heavy smokers are particularly at high risk. A smoker of two packs per day for 20 years has almost 70 times higher risk for developing lung cancer than nonsmokers. Certain histologic types of cancer (ie, small-cell and squamous-cell carcinomas) are almost exclusively observed among smokers. The risk of developing lung cancer diminishes with cessation of smoking; after 15 or more years of abstention from cigarette smoking, the risk of lung cancer approaches that of people who have never smoked.

There seem to be other factors that, when combined with smoking, enhance the carcinogenic effect of the latter. Exposure to asbestos dust and radioactive substances is known to have such an effect. The combined effects of cigarette smoking and asbestos exposure are more multiplicative than additive. This is probably also true in regard to heavy smoking and exposure to naturally occurring radon gas found in certain homes. Moreover, the fact that the incidence of lung cancer is higher in urban populations than in rural dwellers with the same degree of smoking exposure suggests that other pollutants in the atmosphere may play a role in lung cancer. Industrial exposure to certain inorganic and synthetic substances has been implicated in the etiology of lung cancer in some instances. However, cigarette smoking remains the major offender. The presence of scars and other chronic lung lesions appears to predispose to lung cancer. Cigarette smokers with COPD have a higher incidence of lung cancer than those without COPD.

Bronchogenic carcinoma is seen predominantly between the ages of 45 and 75 with a peak incidence at age 70. It is a rare occurrence below the age of 35.

Pathology. Pathologic changes are quite variable and depend on the histologic type, location, duration of disease, tumor size, metastasis, and secondary effects on the surrounding tissues and organs. Except for a small percentage of cases, lung cancer is bronchogenic (ie, it arises from bronchial mucosa). About half of the cases are centrally located; that is, their site of origin is in the large airways. The other half are peripheral, arising from smaller airways. However, this distinction is often difficult in advanced stages. The upper lobes, particularly the anterior segments, are more commonly involved than the lower lobes, and the right more than the left.

Although there are several different histologic forms of primary lung cancer, four major types of bronchogenic carcinoma have been recognized, which, in addition to their distinctive pathologic characteristics, show different epidemiologic, clinical, radiographic, and prognostic features. They account for 95% of primary lung cancers.

- The *squamous-cell* or epithelial type comprises about one-third of lung cancers and is the most common cell type in men. It is pathologically characterized by keratin formation, bridging between the cells, and the development of large well-outlined islands of cancer cells. Most of these carcinomas are centrally located, arising from the major bronchi. Because of their exposure to the bronchial lumen, exfoliated tumor cells are often detected in bronchial secretions. Their metastasis is mainly local, involving surrounding structures and regional lymph nodes.
- *Adenocarcinoma* has the same incidence as the squamous-cell type, but is the most common lung cancer in women. It is frequently a peripheral lesion, has a glandular architecture, and may produce mucin. Distant metastasis is common.
- The *large cell undifferentiated* carcinoma is made of large cancer cells that have no resemblance to squamous-cell type or adenocarcinoma. It usually presents as a large peripheral tumor. About

10% to 15% of lung cancers are of this type.

- The above-described cell types are collectively referred to as non-small-cell lung cancer (NSCLC) to differentiate them from the *small-cell lung cancer* (SCLC), which has distinctive biologic, histologic, and clinical features. The tumors in this group are rapidly growing carcinomas that metastasize to thoracic and extrathoracic sites early, and have a very poor prognosis. Most of them originate from central airways, grow submucosally, and involve the mediastinal nodes. Between 15% and 25% of bronchogenic carcinomas are small cell in type. Many of these tumors, by secreting different hormones, have various endocrine functions. Oat-cell carcinoma is the most common and the best-known category of this highly malignant disease.

Secondary pathologic changes resulting from lung cancer are due to obstruction or compression of structures such as bronchi, blood vessels, and nerves producing various complications. The most common ones, atelectasis, pneumonia, and lung abcess, are due to bronchial obstruction. Metastasis is very common with lung cancer; almost every case ending in autopsy shows metastasis, and over half of the cases at the time of diagnosis have evidence of metastasis. Locally, it usually spreads to the pleura, chest wall, and mediastinal structures. The lymph nodes, liver, bone, brain, and adrenal glands are among common sites for distant metastasis.

Clinical Manifestations. Practically every patient with lung cancer goes through an asymptomatic phase, which comprises the major part of its course. Many patients may even remain symptom-free despite radiographic or bronchoscopic evidence of tumor. Symptoms, when present, are nonspecific and varied depending on location of cancer, its size, rapidity of its growth, cell type, and presence of underlying bronchopulmonary disease (Table 19–1). The most common symptom is cough, which unfortunately does not concern most patients because of the frequent concomitance of chronic bronchitis. In these situations, usually change of characteristics of cough and expectoration may warn the patients. Bloody sputum, which occurs in about half of the patients during their illness, may be the initial symptom making the patient seek medical advice. Severe hemoptysis is much less common. Chest pain of variable intensity and other characteristics is fairly common in lung cancer. It may be mild and felt as heaviness or ache, or it may be very severe and unremitting. The presence of pain does not necessarily indicate pleural or chest-wall involvement, although significant steady pain is highly suggestive of this complication. Dyspnea may be due to tumor causing obstruction of major airways or large pleural effusion, but often it is due to presence of significant underlying bronchopulmonary disease. Hoarseness of recent onset usually indicates involvement of the laryngeal nerve, especially the left. Compression of the superior vena cava manifests by vascular congestion and edema of the face, neck, and upper extremities (Superior vena cava syndrome).

TABLE 19–1. PRESENTING SYMPTOMS OF LUNG CANCER

Thoracic symptoms
  Cough
  Dyspnea
  Hemoptysis
  Chest pain
  Wheezing
  Dysphagia

Systemic and extrathoracic symptoms
  Weight loss
  Anorexia
  Weakness, fatigue
  Bone and joint pain
  Swelling of face and arms
  Hoarseness
  Various neurologic symptoms

It is not unusual for bronchogenic carcinoma to manifest as a pulmonary infection such as pneumonia or lung abscess. Systemic symptoms of weight loss, weakness, fatigue, and anorexia, which are common to most advanced malignant diseases, are frequently observed in patients with lung cancer. Other symptoms may be due to distant metastasis to different organs, such as bone, brain, and liver.

Physical examination may be entirely normal in the early stage of lung cancer. In advanced cases, the physical findings frequently are due to bronchial obstruction and other complications or metastasis. Localized wheezing, alteration of breath sounds, or other signs of atelectasis, pneumonia, or pleural effusion may be present. Signs of metastasis to extrathoracic structures may be detected on first presentation or may develop later in the course of the disease. In addition to evidence of weight loss and muscle wasting, there are numerous other manifestations of lung cancer that are not related directly to its local or metastatic effects and are known as

paraneoplastic syndromes. Various endocrine syndromes are due to the secretion by the tumor of certain hormones or hormone-like substances. However, the mechanism in many others such as hematologic, musculoskeletal, neurologic, and cutaneous syndromes are not clearly known. Digital clubbing, a fairly common finding in patients with bronchogenic carcinoma, is another example of paraneoplastic syndromes.

Radiographic Findings. The diagnosis of lung cancer in the majority of patients is strongly suspected by routine chest radiography. Unfortunately, by the time a lung cancer becomes radiographically evident it is already in the invasive stage and is often unresectable. Radiography, therefore, is not an ideal method for diagnosing lung cancer in its early and curable stage. X-ray screening at regular intervals, as carried out in certain centers, has not been demonstrated to add significantly to the overall survival rate from lung cancer. It has been estimated that by the time a lung cancer becomes radiographically detectable it has completed two-thirds to three-quarters of its natural course.

Radiographic changes are quite variable and nonspecific; however, certain manifestations are characteristic. X-ray findings are due to the shadow cast by the tumor itself and secondary pulmonary changes due to bronchial obstruction, infection, or other complications (Fig. 19–1). A peripheral lung lesion may manifest as a small, more or less circumscribed density due to the tumor itself, usually referred to as solitary pulmonary nodule or coin lesion. The most common secondary changes are due to bronchial obstruction with development of atelectasis, obstructive pneu-

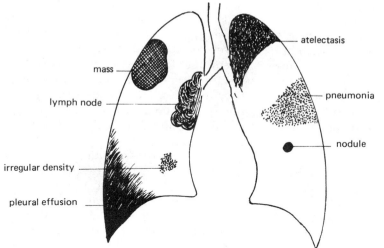

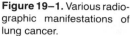

Figure 19–1. Various radiographic manifestations of lung cancer.

monia, and rarely hyperinflation. Hilar or mediastinal mass due to direct invasion by tumor or metastasis to the lymph nodes may be observed. Pleural effusion, which may be massive, is sometimes the only radiographic manifestation of lung cancer. The chest x-ray may show evidence of other complications, such as a paralyzed diaphragm or rib lesions.

Different histologic types of lung cancer often have characteristic radiographic features. Most adenocarcinomas manifest as peripheral lesions. Oat-cell carcinoma may present as a large hilar or mediastinal mass (Fig. 19–2). Squamous-cell carcinoma frequently causes bronchial obstruction. Cavitation is common in a peripheral mass due to squamous-cell cancer. The most common radiographic manifestation of large-cell undifferentiated carcinoma is a large peripheral mass.

Special radiologic techniques may be used for further investigation of a suspicious lung lesion. These include fluoroscopy, tomography, bronchogra-

phy, and pulmonary angiography. Thoracic CT scan has proven to be very useful for better delineation of the original lesion and for detection of nodal metastasis. CT scanning of the chest, abdomen, and head is an important part of the staging for lung cancer.

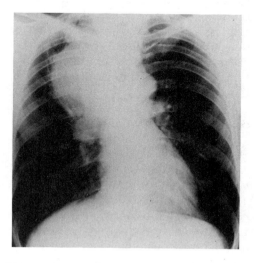

Figure 19–2. Bronchogenic carcinoma. Rapidly growing oat-cell carcinoma involving the right upper lobe and mediastinum.

Other Diagnostic Procedures

Patients who have a suspicious radiographic lesion or present with unexplained symptoms or signs, such as hemoptysis, unremitting cough, or localized wheezing, are subjected to diagnostic procedures that will help in identification, localization, histologic examination, evaluation of extent of the lesion, and detection of metastasis.

Sputum Cytology. One important diagnostic study is the cytologic examination of the sputum. The value of sputum examination in various bronchopulmonary diseases and methods of its proper collection have been discussed elsewhere (Chapter 2). Early morning, deep-cough technique is most satisfactory if sputum can be produced spontaneously. Otherwise, methods such as heated aerosol therapy or, preferably, ultrasonic nebulization may be used for sputum induction. Cytologic examination in expert hands has been successful for diagnosis in up to 90% of the cases of bronchogenic carcinoma of squamous-cell type. It is much less useful for detection of small-cell carcinoma because of its frequent submucosal location. Cytologic examination of pleural fluid, if present, may be helpful for the diagnosis of lung cancer, as well as for confirmation of pleural metastasis.

Bronchoscopy. This procedure is now routinely done on almost every patient suspected to have bronchogenic cancer. The advent of the fiberoptic bronchoscope has significantly increased the usefulness of bronchoscopy in detecting and locating lesions, even when they are situated in the airways as small as subsegmental bronchi. In addition, biopsy, bronchial secretion, and washing can be obtained for histologic and cytologic studies. Transbronchial biopsy in more peripheral lesions and brushing have become much easier with the fiberscope. The transbronchoscopic needle for aspiration of peripheral pulmonary nodules and mediastinal lymph nodes is a new and useful addition for diagnosing and staging lung cancer.

Mediastinoscopy has been frequently used for evaluation of patients with lung cancer for resectability and sometimes for diagnostic purpose. Other biopsy methods include biopsy of peripheral lymph nodes, various forms of percutaneous needle biopsy or aspiration of the lung lesion, and biopsy of pleura and other metastatic sites. Radioisotope scanning of liver, brain, and bones is very useful in detecting metastases to these sites. All of these studies, as well as radiologic examination of the chest, are useful not only for diagnosing but also for staging lung cancer. By staging, an accurate assessment of the primary tumor regarding its exact location, size, invasion of neighboring structures as well as involvement of regional lymph nodes, and other metastases is made. Staging is very useful in deciding the most appropriate therapy and in determining the prognosis.

Management. Surgical resection is the most preferred therapeutic approach in management of patients with non-small-cell lung cancer. Unfortunately, the majority of patients at the time of diagnosis of lung carcinoma are not operable because of advanced disease with evidence of metastasis, location of lesion, or poor general or respiratory state. Of 100 cases of lung cancer, about 25 are usually considered to be operable at the time of diagnosis. Some of them may turn out to be unresectable at the time of thoracotomy. About 25% of resectable cases live 5 years or longer after surgery. Despite significant improvement in diagnostic methods and surgical techniques, 5-year survival of lung cancer patients remains and 10%.

Radiotherapy, alone or combined with surgery, has not significantly improved the survival rate in non-small-cell carcinoma; however, it is a valuable therapy for palliation such as relieving bronchial obstruction, compression of intrathoracic structures, or pain due to skeletal metastasis. Various modalities of chemotherapeutic trials for cure still in progress. Although in some cases small-cell lung cancers are cured by surgery, chemotherapy with or without radiotherapy is the treatment of choice. These tumors are highly responsive to appropriate chemotherapeutic agents, which, in many cases, result in an appreciable increase in survival time.

Lung cancer remains an important health problem and continues to kill more and more people each year. Prevention by avoidance of known causative factors, particularly cigarette smoking, seems to be the best-known approach to this dreadful health problem at this time.

BIBLIOGRAPHY

Bone RC, Balk R. Staging of bronchogenic carcinoma. *Chest*. 1982; 82:473–480.

Carr DT. Malignant lung disease. *Hosp Pract*. 1981; 16(1):97–115.

Eddy DM. Screening for lung cancer. *Ann Intern Med*. 1989; 111:232–237.

Gadzar AF, Linnoila RI. The pathology of lung cancer: changing concepts and newer diagnostic techniques. *Semin Oncol*. 1988; 15:215–225.

Goodman GE, Livingston RB. Small cell lung cancer. *Dis Mon*. 1989; 35:779–825.

Haskell CM, Holmes EC. Non-small-cell lung cancer. *Dis Mon*. 1988; 34:61–108.

Hyde L, Hyde CI. Clinical manifestations of lung cancer. *Chest*. 1974; 65:299–306.

Jett JR, Cortese DA, Fontana RC. Lung cancer: current concepts and prospects. *Ca*. 1983; 33:74–86.

Johnson MR. Selecting patients with lung cancer for surgical therapy. *Semin Oncol*. 1988; 15:246–254.

Lillington GA. Management of solitary pulmonary nodules. *Dis Mon*. 1991; 37:271–318.

Little AG, Stitik FP. Clinical staging of patients with non-small-cell lung cancer. *Chest*. 1990; 97:1431–1438.

Sider L. Radiographic manifestations of primary bronchogenic carcinoma. *Radiol Clin North Am*. 1990; 28:583–597.

Symposium on Recent Advances on Lung Cancer. *Clin Chest Med*. 1982; 3(2):217–454.

US Department of Health and Human Services. Office of Smoking and Health. *The Health Consequences of Smoking: Cancer*. A report of the Surgeon General, 1982.

Webb WR, Golden JA. Imaging strategies in the staging of lung cancer. *Clin Chest Med*. 1991; 12:133–150.

Lungs in
Circulatory Disorders

CHAPTER 20

Disorders of Pulmonary Circulation

The major components of pulmonary circulation are:

1. the right heart chambers which act as reservoirs and pump mixed venous blood to
2. a system of pulmonary arteries and arterioles, which distributes the blood to

3. the capillary bed, which is the gas-exchanging site, and
4. a system of venules and veins, which collects the arterialized blood and returns it to the left side of the heart for distribution to the body (Fig. 20–1).

The functional part of pulmonary circulation is the capillary bed, which has a surface area of about 70 m², or 40 times the body surface area, where gas exchange with alveoli takes place.

The pulmonary vascular bed is a low-resistance system; therefore, the pressure required to circulate blood through it is low. These pulmonary vessels are also very distensible and can adapt to increased blood flow, as occurs with exercise, without corresponding increase in pressure. The vessels are under control of the autonomic nervous system, and influenced by factors such as vasoactive substances, hypoxemia, changes of alveolar oxygen tension, and acidosis. Regional changes in pulmonary blood flow occur as a result of gravity and variation in ventilation. The lowermost parts of the lungs (ie, the bases in upright position) have the highest perfusion per unit lung volume. Poorly ventilated or nonventilated lung

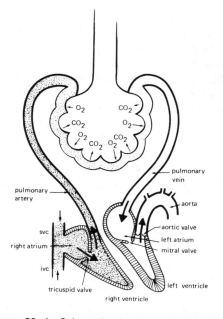

Figure 20–1. Schematic drawing of pulmonary circulation.

regions have reduced blood flow. On the other hand, reduction in regional perfusion, such as with occlusion of a branch of the pulmonary artery with an embolus, results in diminished ventilation of that area.

In addition to pulmonary circulation, the lungs receive arterial blood through bronchial arteries, which are branches of the thoracic aorta. They supply arterial blood to the walls of the tracheobronchial tree down to and including the terminal bronchioles. The venous return partly enters the pulmonary veins, causing a small amount of shunting.

Disorders of pulmonary circulation may be the result of various abnormalities in the lungs, its blood vessels, or the heart. Vascular changes are an integral part of pulmonary pathology from various causes. These changes may be the result of direct injury by the disease process or indirect effect through the abnormality of blood gases, particularly hypoxemia. Pulmonary blood vessels may be occluded by a local thrombus or, more commonly, by an embolus. They may be obstructed by primary vascular disorders. The close anatomic and physiologic relationship between the heart and the lung is the cause of their mutual effect in pathologic conditions. The function of the right heart chambers is often affected by lung disorders in which pulmonary vessels are involved. In addition, hypoxemia and disturbance in acid-base balance, which are common in severe lung disease, will have an adverse effect on the function of the myocardium. On the other hand, a malfunctioning left side of the heart results in circulatory disturbances in the lung, which may progress to overt heart failure and pulmonary edema.

In this chapter, the major disorders of pulmonary circulation, that is, the effect of heart failure on the lung, pulmonary embolism, pulmonary hypertension, and cor pulmonale are discussed.

CARDIAC PULMONARY EDEMA

Cardiac pulmonary edema is defined as abnormal accumulation of fluid in the lung tissue and/or alveolar spaces due to an increase in pulmonary microvascular pressure, which in turn results from abnormal heart function.

Etiology and Pathogenesis. Despite the fact that blood in the pulmonary capillary is separated from the alveolar space by only a very thin membrane, measuring no more than 0.5μ in thickness, the alveoli are normally kept free of excess fluid. This is accomplished by the integrity of permeability characteristics of this membrane and the balance of forces across this membrane, particularly between capillary hydrostatic pressure and plasma oncotic pressure. Although normally the plasma colloid osmotic (oncotic) pressure far exceeds the capillary hydrostatic pressure, the presence of other forces favors the movement of fluid out of the intravascular compartment. These forces are the negative hydrostatic and oncotic pressures of the pericapillary or interstitial space (Fig. 20–2). As demonstrated in the equation in Figure 20–2, the rate of fluid filtered from the capillary lumen to the interstitial space is determined by these forces, as well as the characteristics of the membrane separating the capillary blood from the interstitial space. Permeability of this membrane to colloids (proteins) affects the plasma-interstitial fluid oncotic gradient.

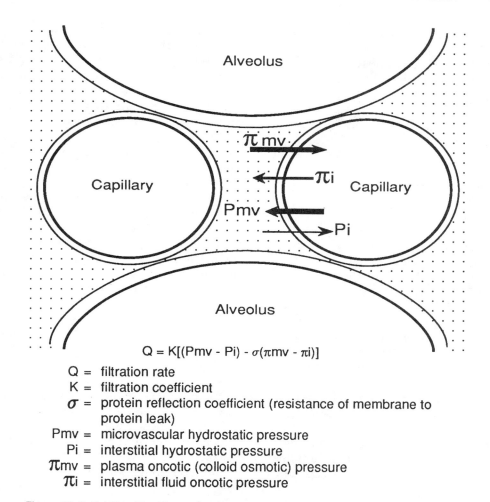

$$Q = K[(Pmv - Pi) - \sigma(\pi mv - \pi i)]$$

Q = filtration rate
K = filtration coefficient
σ = protein reflection coefficient (resistance of membrane to protein leak)
Pmv = microvascular hydrostatic pressure
Pi = interstitial hydrostatic pressure
πmv = plasma oncotic (colloid osmotic) pressure
πi = interstitial fluid oncotic pressure

Figure 20–2. Relationship of forces that determine the rate of fluid filtration from the capillaries to the interstitial spaces of the lungs. Normally these forces result in filtration of a small amount of fluid, which is readily absorbed by the lymphatics.

Variable amounts of fluid that are normally filtered into the interstitial space are readily reabsorbed by the lymphatic channels at this space. However, under pathologic conditions, when the rate of fluid filtration exceeds the absorptive capacity of the lymphatics, pulmonary edema develops. The excess fluid initially accumulates in the interstitial tissue (interstitial edema), and later also floods the alveolar spaces (alveolar edema).

In cardiac failure, pulmonary edema results from an increase in the microvascular hydrostatic pressure that, by increasing the transcapillary pressure, forces the fluid out of the capillary into the interstitial space.

Normally, the outputs of the two sides of the heart are so well adjusted that, despite tremendous changes in circulation with various activities, neither side will be overloaded and, thus, the lungs will not be flooded with blood. This is due to close similarity of the behavior of the two ventricles, which beat at the same rate under various influences and obey *Starling's law of the heart*. This law states that the stretching of the heart muscle, as occurs when more blood returns to the heart, increases the force of its contraction, therefore expelling more blood. Starling's law of the heart is the major mechanism by which the right and left ventricles maintain equal output. A disturbance in balance between the output of the two sides of the heart will result in overloading of one side of the circulation. In the event of failure of the left ventricle to handle its blood load, the pulmonary capillaries will be congested, and their hydrostatic pressure will rise.

In noncardiac pulmonary edema, which is the result of increased membrane permeability, proteins readily enter the interstitial space causing a reduction of colloid osmotic gradient between the plasma in the capillaries and interstitial fluid. As a result, the forces that oppose the microvascular hydrostatic pressure diminish, thus facilitating fluid accumulation in the interstitial space and from there, inside the alveoli. Also known as permeability pulmonary edema, this condition is a characteristic feature of the adult respiratory distress syndrome (Chapter 25).

Pulmonary edema is also known to result from increased negative intrathoracic and transpulmonary pressures. This may occur when a collapsed lung from a large pneumothorax or pleural effusion is rapidly reexpanded by removing the air or fluid from the pleural cavity too fast (re-expansion pulmonary edema). Pulmonary edema may also develop in upper airway obstruction as a result of forceful inspiratory efforts against the occluded airway. A sudden reduction of the interstitial hydrostatic pressure *and* an increased alveolar-capillary permeability have been implicated in the pathogenesis of pulmonary edema in these two, otherwise disparate, clinical circumstances.

By far the most common cause of pulmonary edema is increased pulmonary capillary pressure due to left-side heart failure from long-standing systemic hypertension, aortic or mitral valve lesion, arteriosclerotic heart disease, and different types of cardiac muscle disorder.

Pathophysiology. As a result of the accumulation of fluid in the interstitial and alveolar spaces, lung compliance diminishes markedly. Lung volumes and capacities are also decreased. The presence of fluid in the airways and edema of their walls cause increased airway resistance. The changes in compliance and airway resistance are not uniform throughout the lungs; as a result, the distribution of ventilation is altered. Marked mismatching of ventilation and perfusion and intrapulmonary shunting cause widening of the alveolar-arterial PO_2 difference and arterial hypoxemia. Reduced peripheral tissue perfusion from heart failure, as well as arterial hypoxemia, may result in significant tissue hypoxia and lactic acidosis.

Clinical Manifestations. Although pulmonary edema may develop without previous warning or antecedent symptoms of heart disease, most patients have a history of chronic and/or recurrent symptoms of heart failure. Dyspnea is the most common complaint. The mode of onset and characteristics of dyspnea are quite variable, depending on acuteness or chronicity and severity of disease. In mild forms of heart failure, shortness of breath is usually noticed during activity. As heart failure advances, dyspnea occurs with less and less effort until it is present even at rest. **Orthopnea** is a special type of dyspnea that occurs on recumbent position and is relieved by sitting. To avoid this symptom, the patient usually elevates the head of his bed or sleeps in a more or less sitting position. Orthopnea is a common manifestation of heart failure, but it also can be associated with severe lung disease.

Paroxysmal nocturnal dyspnea refers to an attack of severe dyspnea that occurs during the night and awakens the patient from sleep. After sitting upright for awhile, dyspnea improves and the patient returns to bed. The attack is due to an episode of acute but transient pulmonary edema, which can be demonstrated by physical examination and radiographic study.

In fully developed acute pulmonary edema, the patient experiences the sudden onset of dyspnea, which is very severe from the start and reaches the extreme degree within a short time. Cough productive of frothy and blood-tinged sputum is common.

Physical findings in mild heart failure are not striking; a few rales in the lung bases and, depending on duration of failure, a variable amount of peripheral edema may be present. In patients with acute severe pulmonary edema, the clinical picture is almost diagnostic. The patient is extremely dyspneic, tachypneic, apprehensive, and unable to lie down. The extremities are cool, clammy, and cyanotic. Rales and wheezes are heard throughout the lung fields. There

may be evidence of increased peripheral venous pressure manifested by engorged neck veins. The heart rate is rapid and may be irregular. Enlargement of the liver and peripheral edema may or may not be present. There is usually evidence of cardiac enlargement. Auscultation of the heart, although difficult because of a noisy chest, may reveal extra heart sounds and murmurs.

Radiographic Findings. Radiographic examination shows changes of pulmonary venous congestion with interstitial and air-space edema. In full-blown pulmonary edema, there is bilateral, more or less symmetrical, combined interstitial and air-space density involving mostly the lower lung fields and perihilar regions (Fig. 20–3). The vascular markings are prominent in upper lung fields. A variable amount of pleural effusion, usually bilateral, is commonly observed. The heart shadow is usually enlarged with prominence of the left ventricle. In less severe heart failure, radiographic findings are limited to changes of vascular markings and increased interstitial density.

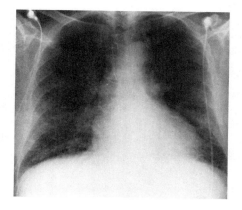

Figure 20–3. Radiograph of cardiac pulmonary edema. Note enlarged heart and predominantly interstitial edema.

Diagnosis. The diagnosis of pulmonary edema in a setting of known heart disease, characteristic clinical picture, and radiographic findings is usually easy. However, when pulmonary edema develops in critically ill patients, with or without the history of heart disease, in circumstances in which the clinical features are less clear, and there are other complicating disorders, the differentiation of cardiac from noncardiac pulmonary edema becomes a difficult diagnostic challenge. The measurement of pulmonary capillary pressure by a flow-directed, balloon-tipped catheter (Swan-Ganz) is most helpful in determining whether pulmonary edema is cardiac or noncardiac in origin. It is also a useful aid in choosing and guiding an appropriate treatment. As expected, pulmonary artery wedge pressure will be high in cardiac pulmonary edema and normal or low in noncardiac cases.

An uncommonly performed test for determination of the protein concentration of edema fluid, obtained by tracheobronchial suctioning, can also differentiate between the two forms of pulmonary edema. In cardiac pulmonary edema, the protein concentration is low, usually less than half that of the plasma; in noncardiac pulmonary edema, it is higher and closer to the plasma protein concentration.

Management. Acute pulmonary edema is a medical emergency requiring prompt and aggressive treatment. Respiratory specialists are frequently involved in the management of patients with this condition. In cardiac pulmonary edema, although therapeutic efforts are mostly directed toward improving the cardiac function and elimination of excess fluid, acuteness and severity of respiratory problems with marked derangement of arterial blood gases necessitate immediate treatment with oxygen administration, maintenance of adequate airways, and sometimes mechanical ventilatory support. The outcome of treatment of these desperately ill patients depends mainly on the coordinated efforts of both the cardiac and respiratory teams. In severely hypoxemic patients, especially when hypercapnia is also present, proper respiratory care is crucial for the efficacy of cardiac measures, because medications intended to improve cardiac function are usually ineffective in the presence of severe hypoxia and acidosis. As morphine is one of the mainstays of management of acute pulmonary edema, its respiratory depressant effect should be closely watched. Mechanical ventilatory support is indicated whenever there is evidence of hypoventilation or severe intractable hypoxemia. Positive end-expiratory pressure has been proved to be of benefit in cardiac pulmonary edema. Medical treatment usually includes the administration of rapid-acting diuretics, vasodilators, and inotropic drugs. Aminophylline is also commonly used.

Prognosis of cardiac pulmonary edema mainly depends on the underlying cause and other associated medical problems. Progressive pump failure and intractable arrhythmia are common causes of death. However, many patients also die from respiratory failure. Aggressive respiratory care and judicious use of mechanical ventilation, together with an appropriate cardiac regimen, have saved the lives of many such patients.

PULMONARY EMBOLISM

Pulmonary embolism is defined as the occlusion of the pulmonary artery or one or more of its branches by matter carried in the blood current. This matter is called **embolus,** which is most commonly a blood clot; however, it may be a fat particle, air, amniotic fluid, tumor or other tissue fragment, parasite, or foreign body. In the practical sense, pulmonary embolism refers to pulmonary arterial occlusion by a blood clot (**thromboembolism**) unless it is qualified by other causes such as fat embolism, air embolism, and so on.

A blood clot attached to its site of origin in a blood vessel or a heart chamber is called a **thrombus.** A thrombus becomes an embolus once it is detached from its origin and carried by the bloodstream.

Pulmonary embolism is one of the most common causes of morbidity and mortality among the adult population. Its true incidence is difficult to ascertain, but autopsy findings indicate that it is much more common than clinical estimates. Pulmonary embolism is a most common pulmonary pathologic finding at autopsy in large general hospitals.

Etiology and Pathogenesis. Nearly 90% of clinically significant pulmonary emboli result from deep-vein **thrombosis** (DVT) of the lower extremities. Any systemic vein and the right heart chambers, however, may be the site of thrombus formation and a source for pulmonary embolism. Risk of pulmonary embolism from the DVT confined to the calf and from superficial venous thrombosis is much less than when DVT extends to, or occurs at, the thigh.

Three important factors facilitate clot formation in a vessel: abnormal vessel wall, stagnation of blood, and increased coagulability. Although thrombosis may occur in the absence of any detectable predisposing factor, in most cases one or more of such factors are present.

Damage to the vessel wall, particularly to its inner layer, causes adherence of blood platelets and activation of clotting factors. **Phlebitis,** trauma to the vein, and inflammation about the veins, are examples in which local clotting takes place.

Venous stasis seems to be the most important factor in production of a thrombus. Many clinical conditions in which venous thrombosis and pulmonary embolism are observed cause venous stasis. Prolonged bed rest, immobility due to pain of trauma or surgery, presence of orthopedic cast, general debility, paralysis, pregnancy, varicose veins, heart failure, and many other medical or surgical conditions predispose to stagnation of blood, particularly in the lower extremities.

An increased clotting tendency of blood is known to occur following significant trauma, major surgery, pregnancy and childbirth, and malignant diseases. The role of birth-control pills in predisposing to thromboembolic disease is probably due to their effect on blood clotting. Hereditary or acquired quantitative or qualitative abnormalities of certain factors that control or inhibit clotting of circulating blood are uncommon but important causes of recurrent DVT and pulmonary embolism.

Once detached from its source, the blood clot is carried with the blood flow. From the vein, it travels to the right side of the heart and from there to the pulmonary arteries. Depending on its size, it lodges in various parts of the pulmonary artery. A very large embolus may occlude the main pulmonary artery; smaller ones will pass more distally. Because of the large blood flow to the dependent lung regions, they are most commonly involved with pulmonary embolism.

As a result of bronchial arterial blood supply, the occlusion of a pulmonary artery usually does not result in significant pathologic change in the lung parenchyma. A pathologic lesion, known as pulmonary **infarction,** occurs in about 10% of patients with pulmonary embolism, particularly when there is underlying cardiac disease.

Pathophysiology. Mechanical occlusion of a pulmonary artery results in nonperfusion of the part of the lung supplied by that artery. Continuation of ventilation of the nonperfused area will be wasted and, therefore, will add to dead-space ventilation.

Acute occlusion of a regional pulmonary artery results in changes of ventilation and perfusion of other lung regions causing additional $\dot{V}/\dot{Q}$ (ventilation-perfusion ratio) mismatching. Diversion of blood to nonoccluded branches of the pulmonary artery causes perfusion to exceed ventilation of the corresponding regions of the lungs, thus resulting in reduction of $\dot{V}/\dot{Q}$ ratio. Blood may even be forced to flow through nonventilated regions, causing intrapulmonary shunting. Lung volumes and compliance are usually reduced following pulmonary embolism. $\dot{V}/\dot{Q}$ mismatching and intrapulmonary shunting are the causes of an increased alveolar-arterial PO_2 gradient and hypoxemia. Hyperventilation, an almost uniform finding in pulmonary embolism, is secondary to the stimulation of lung mechanoreceptors. It occurs with or without hypoxemia.

Elevation of pulmonary artery pressure as a result of pulmonary embolism depends on the size of emboli and the presence or absence of underlying cardiopulmonary disease. As the right ventricle, because of its thin myocardium, is unable to generate high enough pressure, it may fail to maintain an adequate cardiac output if the pulmonary embolism is massive. Reduced cardiac output aggravates hypoxemia, which in turn increases the pulmonary vascular resistance further. Resultant systemic hypotension and circulatory failure are the usual cause of death in severe acute pulmonary embolism. Recurrent unresolved emboli may be the cause of chronic pulmonary hypertension (see below).

Clinical Manifestations. Clinical manifestations of pulmonary embolism vary greatly. The presence of significant underlying conditions often obscures or modifies the clinical picture. Many emboli, mostly when small, produce little or no symptoms and are hardly suspected. A large embolus may cause sudden death. In most cases, the symptoms are nonspecific and, unless the index of suspicion is high for pulmonary embolism, often ascribed to other conditions. The symptoms frequently experienced by patients with pulmonary embolism are dyspnea and chest pain. Dyspnea is by far the most common presenting symptom and has certain characteristics, such as its sudden onset, its severity out of proportion to clinical findings, and associated apprehension. Chest pain may be anginal type at the onset, but later becomes pleuritic in nature. Hemoptysis, although a very important symptom, is less common. Other symptoms include cough, faintness, and anxiety.

Physical examination may reveal evidence of **thrombophlebitis,** usually of lower extremities, manifested by pain, tenderness, and swelling. These findings, although very helpful for diagnosis, are lacking in over half of the patients with proven pulmonary embolism. In severe and massive pulmonary embolism, tachypnea, tachycardia, and cyanosis are the usual findings. Local decrease in breath sounds, wheezing, rales, pleural rub, and signs of pleural effusion may be present. Other findings, such as fever, changes in heart sounds, cardiac arrhythmia, and signs of cardiac failure or shock, are sometimes detected. Acute cor pulmonale refers to cardiac changes due to acute obstruction of pulmonary vasculature with embolism.

Radiographic Findings. The chest radiograph may be normal or show only minimal changes. Common findings include loss of lung volume, linear densities of atelectasis, elevation of one side of the diaphragm, evidence of pleural effusion, and parenchymal density of pulmonary infarction. More characteristic changes of local reduction in vascular markings and enlargement of a pulmonary artery in hilar region are observed uncommonly.

Laboratory Findings and Diagnosis. Arterial blood studies in patients with pulmonary embolism typically show low PO_2 and PCO_2. Although arterial hypoxemia is present in most patients, normal arterial PO_2 does not exclude the diagnosis. Widening of the alveolar-arterial PO_2 gradient, however, is almost always present; a normal gradient makes the diagnosis of pulmonary embolism unlikely.

The *electrocardiogram* may show certain abnormalities during pulmonary embolism, suggesting myocardial hypoxia or right ventricular strain.

Radioisotopic lung scanning is one of the most valuable clinical tools for the diagnosis of pulmonary embolism. A normal perfusion lung scan, for all practical purposes, excludes the diagnosis of pulmonary embolism. A defect in a perfusion lung scan, however, does not necessarily indicate the presence of pulmonary embolism, since there are many other causes for regional reduction in pulmonary blood flow. Any interpretation of the scan should be made in light of the patient's clinical and laboratory findings, and must never be made without concomitant review of plain chest x-ray films. Combination of ventilation and perfusion lung scanning is very helpful in differentiating pulmonary embolisms from other pulmonary conditions in which the abnmormality of perfusion is secondary to a ventilation defect.

Occasionally, *pulmonary* **angiography** will be necessary for definitive diagnosis of pulmonary embolism when the result of the above studies is not conclusive, and the patient has to undergo certain potentially risky therapeutic procedures.

Lower-extremity venography is another useful diagnostic study. The presence of a thrombus in a deep vein will support the diagnosis of pulmonary embolism in a proper clinical setting and an abnormal lung scan; a normal venography makes this diagnosis much less likely. Impedance plethysmography (IPG) is a noninvasive test that can detect up to 95% of acute thrombosis involving the deep veins of the lower extremities at the knee level of above. It is less accurate, however, for the diagnosis of DVT limited to the calf.

Management. As pulmonary embolism results from DVT, every effort should be made to prevent the formation of a clot in the deep veins. The patients at risk of developing DVT should be identified and the conditions that predispose them to venous stasis should be corrected. Proper positioning, active and passive exercises of lower extremities, early mobilization and ambulation, use of specially designed elastic stockings, and treatment of underlying diseases are some of the measures that can reduce the incidence of venous thrombosis and pulmonary embolism. The use of intermittent pneumatic compression devices are both simple and effective. They should be applied as early as possible *before* the development of venous thrombosis. Therefore, DVT should be excluded before their application. Prophylactic anticoagulation in high-risk patients and early anticoagulant therapy of DVT are effective in preventing pulmonary embolism.

Anticoagulation therapy with heparin remains the therapeutic method of choice for pulmonary embolism. Alleviation of hypoxemia with supplemental oxygen theapy is often indicated. Thrombolytic agents, such as streptokinase, are known to hasten the **lysis** of clots in peripheral veins and pulmonary arteries. They are not a substitute, but an addition, to anticoagulants. Their therapeutic benefit has been demonstrated in extensive DVT and massive pulmonary embolism associated with significant hemodynamic impairment. Bleeding, especially following recent surgery or from venous or arterial puncture site, is the main disadvantage of these agents.

Surgical therapy, such as ligation of the inferior vena cava or transvenous insertion of a filtering device, may be necessary in patients who for some reason or other cannot be anticoagulated or have recurrent embolism despite adequate anticoagulation. Currently, the Greenfield filter is the preferred device used as an effective mechanical means for preventing embolization of large-size and medium-size clots to the lungs. Made of stainless steel, this cone-shaped device is usually inserted via the internal jugular vein and placed inside the inferior vena cava below the renal veins. The filter is able to trap emboli larger than 3 mm in diameter without interrupting the blood flow.

PULMONARY FAT EMBOLISM

Inconsequential embolization of a small amount of fat particles to the lung and, possibly, to other organs is a common occurrence in trauma patients and during bone surgery. However, fat embolism syndrome, characterized by acute onset of respiratory distress often associated with fever, changes in sensorium, and the appearance of **petechiae,** is a relatively infrequent but serious complication of severe musculoskeletal trauma.

Etiology and Pathogenesis. Although fat embolism has been rarely demonstrated in association with soft-tissue injury, burns, and certain medical conditions, the vast majority of clinically recognizable cases of fat embolism follow multiple fractures, especially of long bones of the lower extremities and the pelvic bones. Despite continuation of disagreement regarding the mechanism of fat embolism, available data strongly suggest that fat particles from the injured sites, especially bone marrow, enter the blood via disrupted vessels (intravasation). This process is enhanced by movement of the fractured area from manipulation and lack of prompt splinting and immobilization. Embolized fat droplets become mostly lodged in the pulmonary microvasculature, while only a small fraction of them enter the systemic circulation and are carried to other organs.

The initial mechanical effects are soon followed by a chemical reaction from fatty acids, which are generated by the hydrolysis of the embolized fat. Although mechanical microvascular obstruction contributes to the clinical picture of fact embolism syndrome, it is mainly the local chemical effect of fatty acids that causes diffuse pulmonary injury and disruption of the integrity of the alveolar capillary membrane. Other factors, such as intravascular coagulation and platelet aggregation, also partake in this process. Exudation of fluid into and around the airspaces and reduction of alveolar surfactant complete a pathologic picture of adult respiratory distress syndrome (ARDS).

Pathophysiology. As with the other causes of adult respiratory distress syndrome, the characteristic pathophysiologic changes are reduced lung volumes and compliance with severe gas transport abnormality. Intractable hypoxemia, which is the most significant clinical problem with fat embolism, results from severe ventilation-perfusion mismatching and intrapulmonary shunting. Some of the neurologic manifestations of fat embolism are probably due to severe cerebral hypoxia, which aggravates the effect of cerebral fat embolism.

Clinical Manifestations. The clinical picture is composed of pulmonary and systemic manifestations. Usually 24 to 48 hours after serious injury, the patient presents with progressive respiratory distress with dyspnea, tachypnea, and cyanosis. Pulmonary rales and rhonchi may be heard. Fever and tachycardia are often present. Neurologic manifestations due to fat embolism to the brain include mental confusion, stupor, delirium, and coma. A characteristic sign, which is very helpful for diagnosis of fat embolism, is the occasional appearance of petechiae (small purplish-red spots caused by bleeding into the skin) over the neck, trunk, and conjunctivae.

Radiographic Findings. Radiographic examination usually reveals diffuse patchy densities due to alveolar edema. Similar changes, however, may be observed following severe trauma and shock without fat embolism.

Management. The principles of management of ARDS are applicable to the treatment of pulmonary fat embolism. Prompt correction of hypoxemia is the key to a successful outcome. Not uncommonly, this may require intubation, mechanical ventilation, and continuous positive pressure breathing. Among several therapeutic modalities used in management of fat embolism, corticosteroids have the most advocates. Large doses of corticosteroids have been shown to protect against fat embolism syndrome when used early in high-risk patients. Fat embolism, being a self-limited condition, usually has a better prognosis than ARDS from most other causes.

PULMONARY HYPERTENSION

The pulmonary vascular circuit is a low-pressure system due to the low resistance of pulmonary blood vessels. Moreover, because of the adaptability of this vascular bed, increased blood flow, as with exercise, normally does not cause significant elevation of its pressure. Systolic blood pressure in the pulmonary artery in the resting healthy adult averages about 24 mm Hg and diastolic about 10 mm Hg. The term *pulmonary hypertension* implies an increase in the pulmonary arterial pressure above the accepted upper limit of normal (ie, 30/16 mm Hg).

The mechanism of production of pulmonary hypertension is variable, as several factors, singly or in combination, affect pulmonary artery pressure. Increased pressure in the pulmonary circuit distal to capillaries (ie, left ventricle, left atrium, and pulmonary veins) results in elevated pulmonary artery pressure. Left ventricular failure, mitral valve disease, and occlusion of the pulmonary venous system are among the important causes of "postcapillary" pulmonary hypertension. However, the most common mechanism of elevation of pulmonary artery pressure is reduction in the total cross-sectional area of the pulmonary arterial bed ("precapillary" pulmonary hypertension). Three main processes result in increased pulmonary artery resistance: its (1) destruction; (2) obstruction; and (3) constriction. Because of remarkable distensibility of pulmonary blood vessels, the total area of this vascular bed must be decreased by more than 50% before any elevation of pulmonary arterial pressure develops.

Primary involvement of the pulmonary artery by conditions such as pulmonary vasculitis or its occlusion by pulmonary embolism results in pulmonary hypertension. Chronically increased blood flow to the lungs as seen in patients with congenital heart disease with left-to-right shunt (eg, atrial or ventricular septal defect) causes increased pulmonary arterial resistance and, hence, pulmonary hypertension.

By far the most common causes of pulmonary hypertension are chronic pulmonary disease and other conditions in which there is sustained hypoxemia. The mechanism involved may be due to significant reduction in pulmonary vasculature as a result of destructive changes in the lung or, more importantly, to the effect of hypoxemia on the pulmonary arteries. Low alveolar and arterial PO_2, when acute, causes constriction of pulmonary arteries; whereas when long-standing, it causes obstructive changes. Hypercapnia and acidosis enhance the effect of hypoxia. High-altitude residence is known to result in pulmonary hypertension through prolonged hypoxemia. In ventilatory insufficiency due to thoracic deformity, neuromuscular disease, sleep apnea syndrome, and primary hypoventilation, pulmonary hypertension may develop as a result of chronic hypoxemia. In chronic lung disease, both reduced vascular bed and increased pulmonary artery resistance due to hypoxemia, as well as hypercapnia and acidosis, contribute to pulmonary hypertension.

When there is no identifiable cause for increased pulmonary artery pressure, the diagnosis of primary, or idiopathic, pulmonary hypertension is made. This uncommon but clinically important disorder occurs mostly in young women. Exertional dyspnea, syncope, and chest pain are its common manifestations.

The diagnosis of pulmonary hypertension is usually suspected on clinical grounds. Radiographic finding of prominent pulmonary artery and its main branches is highly suggestive. Noninvasively, pulmonary artery pressure can be estimated with a reasonable degree of accuracy by Doppler ultrasonography. Cardiac catheterization for measurement of pulmonary artery and its wedge pressures is considered when postcapillary pulmonary hypertension is suspected. Pulmonary angiography is done when chronic thromboembolism involving large pulmonary arteries is suggested by radionuclide lung scan, and when surgery is seriously considered for its treatment.

CHRONIC COR PULMONALE

Clinical manifestation of pulmonary hypertension is through its effect on the heart, particularly the right ventricle. Chronic pulmonary hypertension leads to hypertrophy and eventual dilatation and failure of the right ventricle, as prolonged systemic arterial hypertension results in left ventricular hypertrophy and failure.

Chronic cor pulmonale is defined as changes in the right ventricle and its function due to elevation of pulmonary artery pressure resulting from diseases affecting the function or the structure of the lung or its vasculature.

Etiology. From the above definition, it is evident that the causes of cor pulmonale are many. The most common one is chronic obstructive lung disease. Chronic diffuse interstitial disease, severe destructive lung diseases following advanced tuberculosis or other chronic inflammatory conditions, cystic fibrosis, extensive resectional surgery, significant chest deformity, and **fibrothorax** are also common causes of chronic pulmonary hypertension and cor pulmonale.

Recurrent and unresolved pulmonary emboli, primary pulmonary hypertension, and other diseases involving the pulmonary vasculature may manifest by right ventricular hypertrophy and failure. Chronic upper airway obstruction, particularly in infants and children, due to enlarged tonsils and adenoids has been recently added to the list of disorders leading to chronic cor pulmonale. In chronic hypoventilation syndrome due to obesity, sleep apnea syndrome, neuromuscular disorders, or central nervous system malfunction, prolonged hypoxemia and perhaps hypercapnia result in pulmonary hypertension and right ventricular failure.

Clinical Manifestations. Because of the presence of significant underlying disease, clinical diagnosis of cor pulmonale is apt to be overlooked. Right ventricular hypertrophy is an early manifestation that is often difficult to prove clinically. Underlying pulmonary disease frequently prevents detection of changes in cardiac impulse or heart sounds. Most often the diagnosis of cor pulmonale is clinically made when there is evidence of right ventricular failure (ie, increased venous distention, peripheral edema, and enlarged liver).

Radiographic changes of cor pulmonale are usually present in more advanced cases. Signs of underlying pulmonary disease, enlarged pulmonary artery trunk and its main branches with attenuation of distal branches, and right ventricular hypertrophy are characteristic x-ray findings.

Electrocardiographic changes, especially the findings of right ventricular hypertrophy, if present, will be helpful. Cardiac arrhythmias are fairly common with cor pulmonale. By echocardiography and radionuclide ventriculography, the size and contractility of both ventricles can be determined. Cardiac

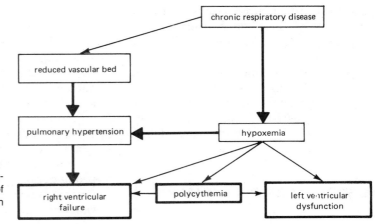

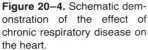
Figure 20–4. Schematic demonstration of the effect of chronic respiratory disease on the heart.

catheterization is rarely indicated in cor pulmonale.

Management. Effective management of cor pulmonale depends on understanding of the underlying cause and mechanism of its production. The treatment should be primarily addressed to correction of its cause. The importance of adequate ventilation and oxygenation cannot be overemphasized. If, despite optimal management, the patient remains chronically hypoxemic, continuous oxygen therapy is indicated. The use of a proper cardiac regimen, including rest, digitalis, and diuretics, is usually recommended when heart failure supervenes. It should be emphasized that the successful treatment of cor pulmonale depends much more on improving the underlying respiratory disorder, and that right-side heart failure is one of the complications of chronic pulmonary disease that can be prevented or at least delayed by its proper management.

As schematically demonstrated in Figure 20–4, chronic respiratory disease not only results in right ventricular failure, but also may affect the left ventricular function. Hypoxemia and acidosis are known to result in myocardial depression. Moreover, frequent presence of polycythemia, another complication of chronic hypoxemia, may also impair the cardiac performance.

BIBLIOGRAPHY

Allen SJ, Drake RE, Williams JP, et al. Recent advances in pulmonary edema. *Crit Care Med.* 1987; 15:963–970.

Boyd KD, Thomas SJ, Gold J, Boyd AD. A prospective study of complications of pulmonary artery catheterization in 500 consecutive patients. *Chest.* 1983; 84:245–249.

Crandall ED, Staub NC, Goldberg HS, Effros RM. Recent developments in pulmonary edema. *Ann Intern Med.* 1983; 99:808–822.

Cutaia M, Rounds S. Hypoxic pulmonary vasocontriction: physiologic significance, mechanism, and clinical relevance. *Chest.* 1990; 97:706–718.

Dinh Xuan AT, Higenbottam TW, Scott JP, Wallwork J. Primary pulmonary hypertension: diagnosis, medical and surgical treatment. *Respir Med.* 1990; 84:189–197.

Fabian TC, Hoots AV, Sanford DS, et al. Fat

embolism syndrome. *Crit Care Med*. 1990; 18:42–46.

Fedullo AJ, Swinburne AJ, Wahl GW, Bixby. Acute cardiogenic pulmonary edema treated with mechanical ventilation. *Chest*. 1991; 99:1220–1226.

Greenfield LJ, Wakefield TW. Prevention of venous thrombosis and pulmonary embolism. *Adv Surg*. 1989; 22:301–324.

Himelman RB, Struve SN, Brown JK, et al. Improved recognition for cor pulmonale in patients with severe COPD. *Am J Med*. 1988; 84:491–498.

Hull RD, Hirsh J, Carter CJ, et al. Pulmonary angiography, ventilation lung scanning, and venography for clinically suspected pulmonary embolism with abnormal lung scan. *Ann Intern Med*. 1983; 98:891–899.

Hull RD, Raskob GE, Coates G, Panju AA. Clinical validity of a normal perfusion lung scan in patients with suspected pulmonary embolism. *Chest*. 1990; 97:23–26.

Kelley MA, Carson JL, Palevsky HI, Schwartz JS. Diagnosing pulmonary embolism: new facts and strategies. *Ann Intern Med*. 1991; 114:300–306.

Klinger JR. Right ventricular dysfunction in chronic obstructive pulmonary disease: evaluation and management. *Chest*. 1991; 99:715–723.

Kollef MH, Pluss J. Noncardiogenic pulmonary edema following upper airway obstruction. *Medicine*. 1991; 70:91–98.

Moser KM. When unexplained dyspnea signals chronic obstructive thrombi. *J Respir Dis*. 1991; 12:295–307.

Moser KM. Venous thromboembolism. *Am Rev Respir Dis*. 1990; 141:235–249.

Peltier LF. Fat embolism: a perspective. *Clin Orthop*. 1988; 232:263–270.

Raskob GE, Hull RD. Diagnosis and management of pulmonary thromboembolism. *Q J Med*. 1990; 76:787–797.

Rich S, Levitsky, Brundage BH. Pulmonary hypertension from chronic thromboembolism. *Arch Intern Med*. 1988; 108:425–434.

Rich S. Primary pulmonary hypertension. *Prog Cardiovasc Dis*. 1988; 31:205–238.

Rounds S, Hill NS. Pulmonary hypertensive diseases. *Chest*. 1984; 85:397–405.

Sherry, S. Thrombolytic therapy for noncoronary diseases. *Ann Emerg Med*. 1991; 20:396–404.

Sibbald WJ, Cunningham DR, Chin DN. Non-cardiac or cardiac pulmonary edema? A practical approach to clinical differentiation in critically ill patients. *Chest*. 1983; 84:452–461.

Staub NC. The pathogenesis of pulmonary edema. *Prog Cardiovasc Dis*. 1980; 26:293–315.

Wiedemann HP, Matthay RA. Cor pulmonale in chronic obstructive pulmonary disease: circulatory pathophysiology and management. *Clin Chest Med*. 1990; 11:523–545.

Diseases of Pleura and Thoracic Wall: Trauma and Surgery of the Chest

CHAPTER *21*

Diseases of Pleura

ANATOMIC AND PATHOLOGIC CONSIDERATIONS

The pleura is a serous membrane that lines the inner surface of each side of the thorax, the upper surface of the hemidiaphragm, and the side of the mediastinum where, at the lung root, it deflects to envelop the lung. It invaginates into the interlobar fissures separating the lobes. Thus a closed space (or potential space) is developed around each lung with recesses between the lobes (Fig. 21–1). The part of the pleura that envelops the lung is called *visceral* pleura; the part that covers the interior of the thorax, the diaphragm, and the mediastinum is known as *parietal* pleura. Normally, the parietal and visceral pleurae are separated by a thin layer of fluid, which keeps their surfaces moist and smooth, allowing them to slide one against the other during the respiratory movement with minimum friction.

Because of close anatomic and physiologic relationship between the lung and pleura, the pathologic condition of one often affects the other. Most diseases of the pleura are secondary to pulmonary lesions that may or may not be apparent. On the other hand, significant disease of the pleura impairs the function of the underlying lung. In addition, as a result of proximity of many other organs, such as mediastinal structures and subdiaphragmatic viscera, the pleura may be involved in many other disease processes. As part of their manifestations or complications, several systemic diseases are known to affect the pleura. Among them, systemic lupus erythematosus

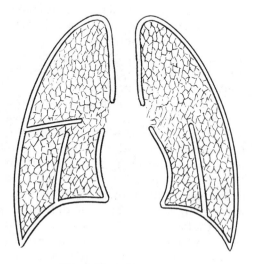

Figure 21–1. Pleural space.

and rheumatoid disease are the better known. Primary pleural disease is relatively uncommon.

Being a large interstitial space and because of its anatomic structure as a potential cavity with a subatmospheric pressure, the pleura usually manifests its disorders by the accumulation of fluids in its space. Heart failure, not infrequently, is associated with pleural effusion. Because of the immediate relation of the pleura with the lung and negative intrapleural pressure, the entry and accumulation of air in the pleural cavity (pneumothorax) occur fairly commonly.

Pleurisy, which is synonymous with pleuritis, refers to inflammation of the pleura with or without pleural effusion. It may be mild and transient due to common conditions, such as viral infection, or it may be more severe and indicative of serious illness.

The pleura, like most other tissues, responds to chronic inflammation by proliferation of fibrous tissue. Pleural fibrosis is a common reaction to many prolonged pathological states, and may result in adhesion of pleural surfaces. Calcium deposition may occur in old pleural fibrosis. Significant fibrous pleural thickening, with or without calcification, results in restriction of respiratory movement.

In view of the importance and the frequency of their occurrence, pleural effusion, empyema, and pneumothorax will be discussed in this chapter.

PLEURAL EFFUSION

Normally, a very small amount of fluid, which may be occasionally detected only by special radiographic study, is present in the pleural space, serving as a lubricant for pleural surfaces. Pleural effusion refers to the accumulation of an easily detectable *abnormal quantity* of fluid in the pleural cavity.

Pathogenesis. Fluid accumulation in the pleural space, as in any part of the body, is the result of imbalance between its formation and absorption. Continuous exchange of fluid in and out of the pleural cavity in normal state is so effectively balanced that only a very small amount of fluid is maintained. The difference between the hydrostatic pressure of blood capillaries in the parietal pleura (supplied by systemic circulation) and that of the capillaries of the visceral pleura (supplied mainly by pulmonary circulation) suggests that fluid is formed at the parietal pleura and absorbed by the visceral pleura. Recent studies in experimental animals indicate, however, that normally fluid is formed in the interstitial space of the parietal pleura, enters the pleural cavity, and then is absorbed via the lymphatics in the parietal pleura. The pleural lymphatics have a large reserve capacity, allowing them to absorb varying amounts of fluid, thus maintaining a constant small volume of fluid in the pleural space. Therefore, the pleural cavity normally behaves as an extention of the interstitial space of the parietal pleura.

In disease states, the balance of fluid formation and its absorption is upset, resulting in its accumulation in the pleural space. This occurs because of increased fluid formation, its reduced absorption, or a combination of the two. In pathologic conditions, the source of fluid and mechanism of its absorption may be different from those in a normal state. They also may vary depending on the nature of pathologic processes. For example, pleural effusion in cardiac pulmonary edema results from fluid leak across the visceral pleura from the lung.

When fluid accumulates as the result of a disturbance of the balance between transcapillary pressure and plasma oncotic pressure, it is a **transudate.** Increased capillary pressure in heart failure and reduced plasma oncotic pressure in certain kidney or liver diseases are the known causes of transudative fluid. This kind of fluid has a low specific gravity, a low protein content, and usually a low cell count. On the other hand, when increased fluid formation is due to increased capillary permeability, as in inflammation, it is an **exudate.** The exudative fluid has a higher specific gravity, higher protein content, and often an increased cell count. It may have a significant number of white blood cells, to the point of a gross purulent appearance.

The accumulation of pleural fluid in association with pneumonia is called *parapneumonic effusion. Pleural empyema* refers to the presence of pus in the pleural cavity; however, in practice, pleural fluid with a large number of polymorphonuclear leukocytes or the presence of **pyogenic** organisms has been considered to constitute an **empyema.** The accumulation of blood in the pleural cavity is called **hemothorax;** the presence of chyle (milky intestinal lymph fluid) is known as **chylothorax.** Concomitant presence of air with fluid results in **hydropneumothorax;** if the fluid is pus or blood, the terms **pyopneumothorax** or **hemopneumothorax** are applied, respectively.

Causes of Pleural Effusion. Pleural effusion may be associated with many different diseases, the majority of which involve the lung. Sometimes pleural effusion may be the most predominant manifestation of the lung disease. The following list gives the important causes of pleural effusion; the list is not complete and many other conditions may occasionally or rarely result in pleural effusion:

A. Transudate
1. Congestive heart failure.
2. Cirrhosis of the liver.
3. Kidney disease.
B. Exudate
1. Infections (bacterial, fungal, viral).
2. Neoplasms (primary, metastatic).
3. Pulmonary embolism.
4. Trauma and surgery.
5. Systemic diseases (lupus erythematosus, rheumatoid arthritis).
6. Intraabdominal diseases (subdiaphragmatic abscess, pancreatitis).
7. Idiopathic (cause cannot be determined).

The most common cause of pleural fluid in clinical practice is congestive heart failure, but various infections, neoplasms, pulmonary embolism, trauma and surgery, and certain systemic diseases are important in causing pleural effusion. Postoperative pleural effusion is a very common occurrence following upper abdominal surgery. The most common cause of massive pleural effusion, which may occupy the entire hemithorax, is metastatic cancer of the pleura. In adult males, it is more often from bronchogenic carcinoma and in adult females, from metastatic breast cancer. Tuberculosis, heart failure, and liver cirrhosis, however, may occasionally result in massive effusion. Sometimes empyema or hemothorax is massive.

Clinical Manifestations. The symptoms of pleural effusion may be absent or overshadowed by the symptoms of the underlying disease. Chest pain of the pleuritic type may be present at the onset when there is pleuritis, but it subsides once the fluid is formed and pleural surfaces are separated. The presence of a significant amount of fluid gives rise to dyspnea, which may be quite severe with massive effusion. The physical findings depend on the quantity of fluid. The typical signs are dullness to percussion, decreased vocal fremitus, and absent breath sounds over the fluid. Small effusions are not usually detectable on physical examination. Sometimes the sound of friction between the pleural surfaces may be heard on auscultation.

When a pleural effusion is large enough to cause significant displacement of the mediastinum to the opposite side, it is referred to as **tension hydrothorax.** In addition to severe dyspnea, patients with tension hydrothorax may be hypotensive from reduced cardiac output and have jugular venous distention.

Radiographic Findings. Radiographic study is the key for diagnosis of pleural effusion. Except for blunting of the **costophrenic** angle, small effusions may not be easy to identify in routine x-ray films, but they can be demonstrated by the lateral decubitus technique. In more typical cases with moderate amount of pleural fluid, characteristic homogeneous density in the dependent part of the **hemithorax** will be seen, which

obscures the diaphragm and fills the costophrenic angle. This density spreads upward, merging imperceptibly with the rest of the lung field (Fig. 21–2). In massive pleural effusion the entire hemithorax may be obscured by the fluid. Sometimes when the fluid is under significant pressure (tension hydrothorax), the mediastinum is pushed to the opposite side.

There are various atypical presentations of pleural fluid on chest radiographs, such as loculated fluid in a part of the pleural cavity, particularly in an interlobar fissure, or subpulmonic accumulation of fluid between the lung and diaphragm. In situations in which the diagnosis of plural effusion remains uncertain after appropriate standard radiographic studies, thoracic ultrasound, and/or CT scan would be very helpful both for the diagnosis and for the localization of plural fluid, especially when thoracentesis is being considered.

Examination of Fluid. Although the diagnosis of pleural effusion is often

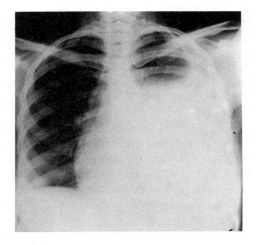

Figure 21–2. Radiograph of pleural effusion.

made prior to **thoracentesis,** sometimes it is necessary to ascertain its presence by diagnostic pleural tap. Frequently, this is done to obtain fluid for examination and occasionally for therapeutic reason. Etiologic diagnosis may be suspected from the clinical picture; however, examination of fluid is essential for definitive diagnosis in the majority of cases.

The gross appearance of fluid may give a significant clue; grossly bloody fluid following chest trauma or surgery, pus in empyema, or milky appearance in chylothorax are a few examples. Bloody effusion without history of chest trauma suggests malignancy or pulmonary embolism.

Fluid is usually examined for its cell count and differential. Presence of predominantly polymorphonuclear leukocytes is suggestive of pyogenic infection; predominance of lymphocytes may suggest tuberculosis or malignancy. In over 50% of pleural fluids due to malignancy, cytologic examination will be diagnostic. Determination of biochemical content of the fluid (eg, protein, sugar, and certain enzymes) will help in differentiating certain causes of pleural effusion. Determination of pleural fluid pH is also valuable in differential diagnosis. Bacteriologic examination of the fluid is of special importance in many instances, and probably should be done on all fluids obtained for diagnostic purpose.

Pleural Biopsy. In some cases the etiologic diagnosis of pleural effusion cannot be made despite careful examination of the fluid and other clinical and laboratory studies. Pleural biopsy then becomes necessary; with one of the biopsy needles presently available,

small pieces of parietal pleura can be obtained. They are submitted for histologic as well as bacteriologic studies. Biopsy under visual control may be performed with the help of a thoracoscope (pleuroscope). Occasionally open pleural biopsy is considered when simple studies remain inconclusive.

Management. The identification and proper treatment of the cause of pleural effusion are the principles of its successful management. Sometimes, when the pleural effusion is large enough to cause symptoms, removal of part or all of the fluid will be helpful for temporary palliation while waiting for the effect of more specific treatment. Tension hydrothorax should be promptly tapped. When the underlying disease is not effectively treatable, such as in malignant pleural effusion, measures to remove the fluid and cause adhesion of pleural surfaces (**pleurodesis**) will be beneficial. For this purpose, tube drainage will be necessary. Tetracycline is the most commonly used agent to cause pleurodesis by intrapleural administration. In hemothorax, blood should be evacuated by tube drainage in order to assess the blood loss and prevent the development of fibrothorax.

Pleural Empyema

When the pleural fluid is grossly **purulent** or contains pyogenic organisms, it is called empyema. Pathogenic organisms may enter the pleural space from the underlying infectious focus in the lung, such as pneumonia or lung abscess, following thoracic surgery or penetrating chest wound, and rarely from other sources. The common causative organisms are anaerobic bacteria, pneumococcus, staphylococcus, streptococcus, and certain gram-negative bacteria.

In addition to the symptoms and signs of pleural effusion, the patient with empyema usually has fever and other manifestations of bacterial infection. Thoracentesis with demonstration of characteristic fluid and isolation of causative organisms is diagnostic.

Although in its early stage thoracentesis and proper antibiotic therapy may occasionally suffice, most patients with empyema will need tube drainage for successful outcome. When the empyema has been present for some time and there is indication of loculation of pus, thoracotomy with rib resection may be necessary. Rarely, with the development of thick pleural peel, **decortication** will be indicated. The presence of bronchopleural fistula (communication of pleural space with bronchial tree), which is fairly common with postpneumonectomy empyema, requires more prolonged tube drainage and suction. Sometimes extensive surgical procedures may be necessary.

PNEUMOTHORAX

Pneumothorax, or presence of air in the pleural space, is a relatively common clinical condition. It is classified into the two general categories of *spontaneous* and *traumatic*. *Artificial pneumothorax*, which is intentional introduction of air into the pleural space, was commonly used for treatment of pulmonary tuberculosis before the availability of effective chemotherapeutic agents. It is rarely used nowadays and almost exclusively for special diagnositic purpose (pleuroscopy or thoracoscopy). Pneumothorax developing in connection with positive pressure ventilation is included in the traumatic category.

Etiology. Pneumothorax is called spontaneous when it develops without accidental or intentional trauma, regardless of the presence or absence of obvious pleuropulmonary disease. When it occurs in apparently healthy individuals, it is called *idiopathic* spontaneous pneumothorax. This type of spontaneous pneumothorax is predominantly a disease of young males. Most patients are tall and thin and have a long and narrow chest. The underlying pathology, which can be demonstrated in most patients undergoing thoracotomy, is the presence of apical subpleural air cysts or blebs. It is the rupture of one of these superficial bullous lesions that produces pneumothorax.

In the past, pulmonary tuberculosis was considered to be a major cause of spontaneous pneumothorax. It may occur in several diverse pleuropulmonary diseases; however, chronic obstructive lung disease, especially emphysema, is the most common underlying clinically recognizable disorder. Spontaneous pneumothorax is frequently a repeatedly recurring condition.

Traumatic pneumothorax is a common consequence of chest injury. It is a pneumothorax that is usually due to laceration of the visceral pleura, often with a broken rib, or the result of a stab wound of the chest. Chest or neck surgery is another traumatic cause of air entry into the pleural cavity. It may occur following tracheostomy. Several diagnostic and therapeutic procedures may induce pneumothorax by inadvertent or unavoidable perforation or laceration of visceral pleura. Thoracentesis, pleural biopsy, percutaneous or transbronchial lung biopsy, subclavian vein puncture, and some other procedures may be complicated by pneumothorax.

The use of positive pressure breathing, either intermittently or continuously, particularly when higher pressures are required, may result in pneumothorax (**barotrauma**). We would like to emphasize this potential complication of positive pressure respiration to the health professionals involved with such therapeutic interventions.

Pathophysiology. When there is free communication between the pleural space and atmospheric air, the "negative" pressure in the pleural cavity will become atmospheric, and, because of its recoil, the lung will collapse. The ventilation of the collapsed lung will be markedly reduced; as a result, that of the opposite lung will increase. Reduced oxygen and increased carbon dioxide tension, and perhaps other factors, cause diminution of blood flow to the collapsed lung; thus, the contralateral lung will receive a larger share of blood supply. Although this regulatory mechanism is not complete, it will greatly improve the ventilation–perfusion relationship, and thus will prevent severe hypoxemia.

When the communication between the pleural space and the atmosphere is sealed, the trapped air will undergo absorption, resulting in gradual reestablishment of subatmospheric pressure and reexpansion of the lung. As oxygen content of the pneumothorax is absorbed faster, the air in a pneumothorax has higher nitrogen and CO_2 tensions than atmospheric air.

In some instances, the communication behaves as a one-way valve, allowing the air to enter the pleural cavity during elevation of intrathoracic pressure with cough or other expiratory efforts, but preventing its exit. Under this circumstance the pressure in the pneumothorax will become higher than atmospheric. This increased pressure may cause significant shift of the heart and other mediastinal structures to the opposite side, thus impairing the function of the other lung also (Fig. 21–3). Moreover, elevated intrathoracic pressure may impede cardiac function by reducing venous return. This condition is called **tension pneumothorax.** Severe respiratory distress with profound hypoxemia and circulatory collapse are the consequences of this life-threatening event, which necessitates immediate treatment. Tension pneumothorax is more commonly seen when pneumothorax occurs following chest trauma or as a result of ventilator-induced barotrauma.

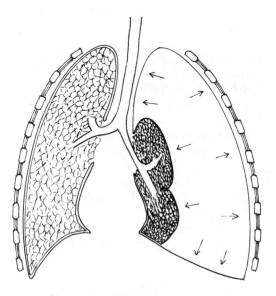

Figure 21–3. Tension pneumothorax.

Clinical Manifestation. The most common presenting symptom of pneumothorax is dyspnea. The severity of dyspnea and its progression depend on the extent of the pneumothorax, presence or absence of underlying pulmonary condition, and tension. In many cases it is more severe at the beginning than several hours later, despite lack of change in the amount of pneumothorax. The combination of sudden onset of sharp chest pain and dyspnea in an otherwise healthy young adult male is highly suggestive of spontaneous pneumothorax. The initial severe sharp pain is usually followed soon by a dull ache. Sudden aggravation of dyspnea in patients with chronic obstructive lung disease, spontaneously or with certain diagnostic or therapeutic interventions mentioned earlier, should arouse suspicion of pneumothorax. Severe dyspnea immediately after an accident frequently is due to pneumothorax, which may be a tension pneumothorax.

Physical examination may show evidence of respiratory distress and cyanosis if the pneumothorax is significant. Reduced to absent breath sounds with resonant percussion note over one hemithorax are the most common physical findings when the pneumothorax is large. In a small pneumothorax, physical examination may be entirely normal. Development of pneumothorax in a patient on a ventilator manifests by an acute deterioration of respiratory mechanics and arterial blood gases. If unrecognized, it may rapidly progress to severe hemodynamic impairment, difficulty with mechanical ventilation, and eventual death.

Radiographic Findings. Radiographic examination is the key to the diagnosis of pneumothorax, assessment of its amount, and evaluation of underlying and associated conditions. X-ray films taken at full expiration accentuate the pneumothorax and, therefore, help in demonstration of a small amount of air in the pleural cavity. With significant pneumothorax, the entire lung seems to have detached from the chest wall, maintaining its connection with the lower half of the mediastinum and medial portion or the diaphragm (Fig. 21–4). Because of reduction of its blood and presence of air around the lung, the density of moderately collapsed lung usually will not be increased. It is the difference between the lung with its markings and air in the pleural space without such markings that helps in detection of pneumothorax. When the lung is completely collapsed, its volume is markedly diminished and its density is increased. Tension pneumothorax results in total collapse of the underlying lung and significant deviation of the heart and mediastinum to the opposite side (Fig. 21–3).

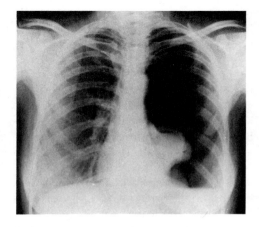

Figure 21–4. Left pneumothorax resulting in complete collapse of the left lung.

Management. Small to moderate asymptomatic pneumothorax, except in association with advanced lung disease or patients on mechanical ventilation, will require no special treatment, but only adequate follow-up until the lung is totally expanded. Once the pleural tear is sealed, which often happens spontaneously, the air in the pleural space will be absorbed, but it may require several days to weeks for completion. Symptomatic patients, those with underlying respiratory insufficiency and those on mechanical ventilation, will need a chest tube for more rapid evacuation of the air. Tension pneumothorax is an emergency and should be immediately relieved by any available means, such as insertion of a needle into the pleural space, which will allow the air under positive pressure to escape. This should be followed by tube thoracostomy or insertion of a Heimlich catheter. The application of excessive negative pressure for evacuation of air from the pleural cavity should be avoided; otherwise, pulmonary edema may develop.

Spontaneous pneumothorax, being a recurrent problem, requires a well-planned follow-up. Most thoracic surgeons recommend thoracotomy in suitable patients when more than one episode of pneumothorax develops spontaneously, at the same or the opposite side, or when there is persistent air leak with a chest tube, preventing the expansion of the lung. The commonly recommended surgical procedures are excision of lung blebs, pleural abrasion, or both. Pleural abrasion results in the adhesion of pleural surfaces. It appears that the simpler methods of pleurodesis with intrapleural sclerosing agents, such as tetracycline and talc, is increasingly replacing surgical methods for prevention of recurrent spontaneous pneumothorax, especially in patients who are poor surgical risks.

BIBLIOGRAPHY

Ali I, Unruh H. Management of empyema thoracis. *Ann Thorac Surg.* 1990; 50:355–359.

Almind M, Lange P, Viskum K. Spontaneous pneumothorax: comparison of simple drainage, talc pleurodesis, and tetracycline pleurodesis. *Thorax.* 1989; 44:627–630.

Grogan DR, Irwin RS, Channick R, et al. Complications associated with thoracentesis. *Arch Intern Med.* 1990; 150:873–871.

Light RW. Parapneumonic effusion and empyema. *Semin Respir Med.* 1987; 9:37–42.

Light RW, O'Hara VS, Moritz TE, et al. Intrapleural tetracycline for the prevention of recurrent spontaneous pneumothorax. *JAMA.* 1990; 264:2224–2230.

Nielsen PH, Jespen SB, Olsen AD. Postoperative pleural effusion following upper abdominal surgery. *Chest.* 1989; 96:1133–1135.

O'Rourke JP, Yee ES. Civilian spontaneous pneumothorax: treatment options and long-term results. *Chest.* 1989; 96:1302–1306.

Pistolesi M, Miniati M, Giuntini C. Pleural liquid and solute exchange. *Am Rev Respir Dis.* 1989; 140:825–847.

Sahn SA. The pathophysiology of pleural effusion. *Annu Rev Med.* 1990; 41:7–13.

Smyrnios NS, Jederlinic PJ, Irwin RS. Pleural effusion in an asymptomatic patient. *Chest.* 1990; 97:192–196.

Wells FC. Empyema thoracis: what is the role of surgery? *Respir Med.* 1990; 84:97–99.

CHAPTER 22

Diseases of Thoracic Wall, and Trauma and Surgery of the Chest

The thoracic wall and diaphragm, which enclose and protect vitally important organs, are essential structures for the production of necessary forces and their effective utilization for respiratory movements (respiratory pump). The ribs, with their characteristic configuration, orientation, and articulation, are the main moving part of the thoracic skeleton. Although each rib has its own range of movement, the ribs' concerted motion, which is powered by various muscles, results in respiratory excursion of the thorax. During inspiration, the thoracic cavity increases its volume vertically, anteroposteriorly, as well as transversally. Because of their higher vertebral ends, the elevation of the ribs by respiratory muscle contraction causes their anterior ends to be thrust forward with the sternum, increasing the anteroposterior diameter of the chest. The transverse increase in the chest diameter is from slight rotation of the ribs at their vertebral points. The vertical diameter is increased by the diaphragmatic contraction. The lower ribs, where the diaphragm is circumferentially attached, are important for its effective function.

Outward movement of these ribs, by increasing the upper abdominal space, also facilitates the action of the diaphragm. A proper interaction between the chest wall and respiratory muscles determines the forces necessary to change the geometry of the thorax, which in turn changes the lung volume for effective ventilation. Therefore, disorders of the chest wall, either congenital or from trauma and surgery, may result in ventilatory impairment more or less similar to one caused by respiratory neuromuscular diseases (see Chapter 23).

DISEASES OF THE CHEST WALL

By far the most important pathologic condition of the bony thorax in this day and age is traumatic injury. Among the various thoracic deformities, funnel chest (**pectus excavatum**) and pigeon breast (**pectus carinatum**) are quite common. In funnel chest, the sternum is depressed while the ribs on each side of it protrude more anteriorly. In pigeon breast deformity, there is abnormal prominence of the sternum due to its forward projection. These deformities, which may be quite remarkable in their physical and radiographic appearances, rarely result in significant respiratory disturbance.

Kyphoscoliosis

Because of the insertion of the ribs to the vertebrae, significant deformity of the thoracic cage may result from abnormal curvature of the dorsal spine. **Kyphosis** is the increased posterior convexity of the thoracic spine; **scoliosis** is the sideway deviation of the spine (Figs. 22–1 and 22–2). For some unknown reason, the convexity of the curvature in scoliosis is toward the right in most cases. Angles of curvature in both scoliosis and kyphosis are inscribed by the straight lines parallel to the upper and lower limbs of the curvature. The

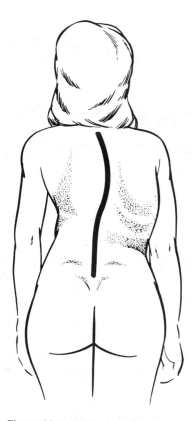

Figure 22–2. Scoliosis of dorsal spine.

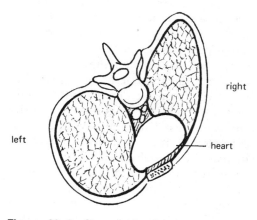

Figure 22–3. Changes in the thorax due to scoliosis. Scoliosis results in rotation of the spine along its longitudinal axis, which in turn causes marked deformity of the rib cage.

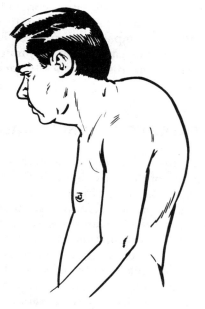

Figure 22–1. Kyphosis of dorsal spine.

combination of these two deformities is referred to as **kyphoscoliosis.**

In scoliosis and kyphoscoliosis, in addition to its abnormal curvature, the spine is usually rotated around its longitudinal axis so that the spinous processes of the vertebrae are directed toward the lateral concavity of the curve (Fig. 22–3). The ribs on the convexity protrude posteriorly; the ribs on the concave side, which are crowded together, are more prominent anteriorly. In severe kyphoscoliosis, the deformity of the chest is, therefore, quite extensive.

Abnormal curvature of the thoracic spine has various causes, such as congenital, traumatic, paralytic, and infectious. Tuberculosis of the spine used to be a very common cause of this deformity. Among neuromuscular disorders, poliomyelitis and syringomyelia are frequently associated with spinal deformity. However, the vast majority of patients with scoliosis or kyphoscoliosis have no known underlying disease. This condition, which is four times more common in females than in males is called *idiopathic* kyphoscoliosis. This deformity may become apparent in childhood or adolescence, and progresses with the patient's growth.

Children and young adults with kyphoscoliosis usually are asymptomatic. In severe cases, the symptoms and signs of cardiorespiratory embarrassment do not ordinarily appear until the fourth or fifth decade of life. Dyspnea, frequent pulmonary infection, progressive respiratory insufficiency, hypoxemia, hypercapnia, and eventual cardiac failure are the common cardiorespiratory manifestations of severe kyphoscoliosis.

Pulmonary function tests show reduced vital capacity and other changes of restrictive ventilatory impairment; however, the residual volume is usually increased. There is uneven ventilation in relation to the blood flow, causing increased dead-space ventilation and hypoxemia. In more advanced disease, alveolar hypoventilation further aggravates the hypoxemia when cor pulmonale also occurs. Severe arterial blood desaturation during sleep is a common problem in advanced kyphoscoliosis. When combined with hypercapnia, nocturnal mechanical ventilation may be necessary.

Alveolar hypoventilation results from the progressive diminution of tidal volume associated with increased physiologic dead-space volume. Both mechanical factors and reduction in the efficiency of respiratory muscles contribute to ventilatory failure. As in other causes of chronic respiratory insufficiency, respiratory infections are major causes of frequent exacerbations.

CHEST TRAUMA

Chest trauma continues to be one of the most common causes of morbidity and mortality among casualties of military conflicts and victims of peacetime accidents and violent crimes. In recent years there has been a steady increase in thoracic surgical procedures, especially coronary artery-bypass operations and pulmonary resection for cancer. Respiratory care providers will be involved in the management of patients with thoracic trauma and surgery, which almost invariably affect respiration. Mechanisms through which respiration is affected in such patients vary and depend on the severity and extent of injury and the structures involved.

Disruption of integrity of the thoracic wall and diaphragm, tear of the pleura with resultant accumulation of air and/or blood in the pleural cavity, and injury to the lung parenchyma and tracheobronchial tree are among the lesions resulting from chest trauma that directly impair respiration. However, because of the presence of other structures in the thorax, such as the heart, pericardium, aorta and other major blood vessels, and the esophagus, chest trauma may involve these organs as well. Moreover, injury to the chest is frequently accompanied by trauma to other areas of the body, such as abdomen, head, neck, spine, and extremities. Respiration, therefore, not only is affected by direct trauma to the chest, but also may be impaired indirectly by injury elsewhere. Severe trauma to the head and the neck may result in upper airway obstruction. Head injury, in addition, may cause respiratory difficulty as a result of loss of consciousness. Spinal cord injury, particularly in the cervical region, affects respiration through respiratory muscle paralysis. Shock due to blood loss, severe trauma, or infection may cause diffuse pulmonary lesion ("shock lung"). Fat embolism is another possible complication of traumatic injury, especially following fractures of large bones. Patients with such injuries are also prone to develop thromboembolic disorders.

Because of the scope of this book, the remaining chapter will be limited to a brief discussion of traumatic injuries to various structures of the chest and thoracic surgery involving the respiratory system.

Simple Rib Fracture

Mild chest-wall injury from blunt trauma usually results in no more than transient pain or tenderness of no significant consequence. Associated rib fracture, however, which is a very common occurrence, may be accompanied or followed by other more significant lesions. Splinting of the chest movement because of severe pain and inability to cough may result in atelectasis or pneumonia, especially in the elderly. Patients with underlying chronic respiratory impairment are particularly susceptible to these complications. Associated pneumothorax or hemothorax should be looked for.

Rib fracture may occur at the point of impact or may result from its excessive bending by indirect forces (Fig. 22–4). Uncomplicated rib fracture is usually treated symptomatically with analgesics. Sometimes injection of a local anesthetic at the fracture site or an intercostal nerve block may be necessary to control the pain and allow the patient to take deep breaths and cough. Multiple broken ribs often indicate the presence of other intrathoracic injuries, especially when the first rib is also fractured.

Flail Chest

Single fracture of a few ribs at one point of their length without separating from their cartilage does not result in mechanical impairment of the chest wall. However, when there are double fractures of three or more adjacent ribs, or fracture of several ribs with separation from their cartilage or fracture of the sternum, a portion of the rib cage will lose its continuity with the rest of the bony thorax (Figs. 22–5 and 22–6). This condition is commonly known as flail chest.

Flail chest is usually the result of severe chest trauma and, therefore, is frequently accompanied by evidence of

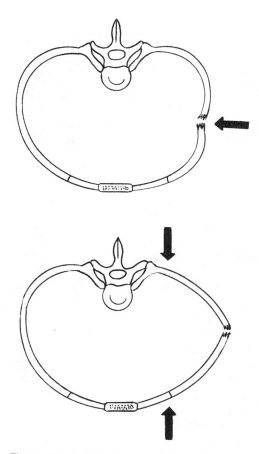

Figure 22–4. Rib fractures due to direct and indirect forces.

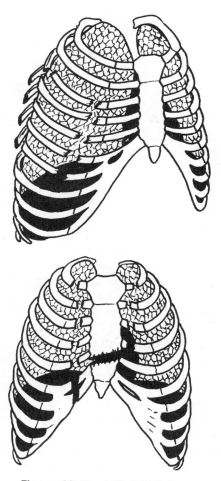

Figures 22–5 and 22–6. Flail chest.

pleural lesion, pulmonary **contusion**, and injury to other structures. Steering wheel injury is a common cause of this condition.

The mechanical effect of flail chest and the resultant ventilatory disturbance are due to **paradoxical movement** of unsupported portion of the chest wall (Fig. 22–7). During inspiration, while the rest of the chest is expanding, the unstable portion moves inward due to more negative intrathoracic pressure. On expiration, par-

ticularly during forced expiration, it bulges outward. If the flail segment is large, the mediastinum swings in the same direction as the unsupported portion. The amplitude of paradoxical movements will depend on the size of the flail segment and pressure changes inside the thorax. As the pressure changes in the chest during the respiratory cycle vary with the compliance of the lungs and thoracic wall, as well as with airway resistance, conditions that

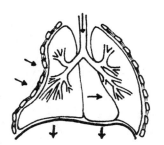 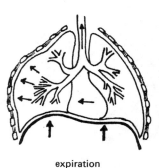

Figure 22–7. Paradoxical movement in flail chest.

inspiration

expiration

result in reduced compliance or increased airway resistance will augment the amplitude of the paradoxical movements. Associated pleuropulmonary lesions due to direct or indirect effect of injury makes the presence of flail chest more evident and its ventilatory effect more manifest. Inefficient ventilation results in increased work of breathing. Ineffective cough and accumulation of secretions result in further ventilatory impairment and eventual respiratory failure.

In the management of patients with flail chest, every effort should be made to correct the conditions that increase airway resistance and/or reduce the compliance. Restoration and maintenance of adequate airway, tracheobronchial toilet, control of infection, treatment of pulmonary congestion, restriction of fluid, and evacuation of air or fluid from the pleural cavity are measures that minimize the deleterious effect of flail chest. Supplemental oxygen is necessary in most patients. Multiple intercostal nerve blocks or epidural block are often used for pain relief. Strapping the chest, especially circumferential adhesive taping, should be avoided as it further compromises ventilation and promotes retention of secretions and atelectasis. Therapeutic success in management of flail

chest will depend more on these measures than preoccupation with stabilization of the flail segment. Many of these patients can be successfully managed without mechanical ventilation or other measures intended to stabilize the chest wall.

The old methods of external chest-wall stabilization, such as traction of the loose segment by various devices, are rarely, if ever, used nowadays. Surgical fixation, however, is occasionally performed when concomitant intrathoracic injury requires open thoracotomy or when, with a large flail segment, more conventional methods fail to improve paradoxical movement in a reasonable amount of time. A simple and quick way in emergency situations is gentle but firm pressure with the palm of the hand against the flail segment, placement of sand bags, or, even, turning the patient on his injured side while being transported to the hospital or waiting for more definitive therapy.

Internal stabilization by mechanical positive pressure ventilation has been much more effective and practical in most situations in need of stabilization. Moreover, associated pulmonary and extrathoracic injury may necessitate assisted ventilation regardless of presence or absence of flail chest. For the purpose of internal fixation, intubation or tracheostomy with a large tube is usually required. It is often necessary, at least initially, to sedate the patient or even paralyze the respiratory muscles for effective ventilation (controlled ventilation) and prevention of excessive movement of the flail segment. In recent years an increasing number of patients with flail chest have been successfully managed by nonventilatory means. With proper respiratory care and prevention of complications that impair the mechanical properties of the lung, the need for prolonged ventilatory support can be lessened. The patients who initially require ventilatory assistance may be weaned off the respirator successfully, even before the chest wall regains stability, provided that other complications are brought under control.

Diaphragmatic Injury

Diaphragmatic injury may result from a perforating wound; but, in civilian practice, it is more commonly due to blunt trauma to the chest and/or abdomen. As with chest-wall injury, automobile accidents are the most frequent causes of diaphragmatic injury. Falls from heights may also result in rupture of the diaphragm. Although diaphragmatic injury is usually indicative of severe trauma, sometimes rupture of the diaphragm may follow a blow to the chest or abdomen that appears to be insignificant. Diaphragmatic rupture from blunt trauma occurs on the left side more frequently than the right side.

Usually, the manifestations of diaphragmatic lesion are overshadowed by those of more obvious injuries to the chest or other organs. It may, therefore, remain unrecognized. Many such lesions are identified during abdominal exploration for treatment of other traumatic injuries, especially laceration of the spleen or the liver. *Herniation* of the abdominal viscera through the diaphragmatic rent may take place immediately or some variable time after the trauma. The symptoms and signs of diaphragmatic injury, which are usually due to herniation, are cardiorespiratory and/or gastrointestinal in nature. Dyspnea, cough, and palpitation are common cardiorespiratory symptoms due to significant herniation. Diminished thoracic excursion, impairment of percussion note, reduction of breath sounds, and presence of bowel sounds in the chest may be detected on physical examination of the thorax. Respiratory embarrassment may be severe in large diaphragmatic ruptures. Gastrointestinal manifestations are usually due to compression and obstruction of stomach and bowels. Nausea, vomiting, and abdominal distension may indicate such complications.

Radiographic studies are essential for diagnosis of diaphragmatic injury. Plain x-ray films may be highly suggestive of diaphragmatic hernia, but examination with contrast material is necessary for definitive diagnosis.

The diaphragmatic rupture is treated surgically when noted during abdominal exploration or after the diagnosis is established by appropriate radiographic studies.

Pleural Injury

Penetrating chest wounds often result in pleural laceration, but blunt chest trauma, which is much more common in civilian medicine, may also cause injury to both parietal and visceral pleurae, especially when accompanied by rib fractures.

Traumatic pleural injury results in accumulation of air and/or blood in the pleural cavity. It is only rarely that air gains access to the pleural space from a chest-wall wound, producing *open pneumothorax* (sucking chest wound). By far the most common mechanism of production of traumatic pneumothorax is the entrance of air through a visceral pleural rent. Pneumothorax is discussed on page 286. It should be emphasized that **tension pneumothorax** is more frequent with traumatic pneumothorax. Moreover, traumatic pneumothorax is commonly associated with the accumulation of blood in the pleural space, which is then called **hemopneumothorax.** The accumulation of air in subcutaneous tissue (subcutaneous emphysema), which may be quite extensive, is common with traumatic pneumothorax.

Hemothorax, with or without pneumothorax, is a common complication of thoracic injury, either penetrating or blunt. Bleeding into the pleural space is mostly due to laceration of the parietal pleura along with a thoracic wall vessel, usually an intercostal artery and sometimes the internal mammary artery. The amount of blood varies from minimal to massive. The immediate problems with hemothorax are related to acute blood loss as well as respiratory embarrassment. Shock and tension hemothorax may result.

Minimal hemothorax requires no treatment except for close observation. When small, blood usually is resolved within a couple of weeks without residue. Moderate hemothorax may be managed by thoracentesis; however, if blood reaccumulates, it should be drained by a chest tube. Accurate measurement of blood loss is important for its replacement by transfusion. The patient's own blood from the pleural cavity may be used (autotransfusion), provided that it is not contaminated and is collected aseptically. Massive hemothorax, which usually indicates rapid and continuous bleeding from a large vessel, is an emergency and should be treated promptly by pleural drainage and restoration of circulating blood volume. Continuation of significant bleeding is an indication for exploratory surgery.

Rarely, as a result of injury to the thoracic duct (the major lymph vessel in the chest), milky effusion, or chylothorax, may develop.

Pulmonary Parenchymal Injury

Lung contusion, or pulmonary bruise, is the most common parenchymal pulmonary injury due to direct chest trauma. It results from the accumulation of edema fluid and blood inside the alveoli, as well as interstitial tissue. The mechanism of its development is thought to be sudden compression and decompression of lung tissue, causing severe pressure changes in the distal airways, alveolar spaces, and interstitium. Pulmonary contusion may be associated with injuries to the chest wall and other parts of the thoracic structures. It is almost always present when chest-wall injury is severe enough to cause flail chest. A small area of lung contusion does not result in significant symptoms referable to the lesion. However, when the contusion is more extensive, respiratory symptoms and signs of dyspnea, cough, hemoptysis, rales, and cyanosis may be present. In more severe cases the clinical picture of adult respiratory distress syndrome will develop. Radiographic examination will show air-space consolidation of patchy or homogeneous pattern, which has no segmental distribution.

The changes become apparent within a few hours following trauma and start to resolve in 24 to 48 hours.

Laceration and **hematoma** of the lung often result from penetrating injury, but it may be secondary to blunt chest trauma. Several alveolar spaces are disrupted, resulting in formation of a cavitary space filled with blood. Sometimes an air-filled cystic lesion may develop. Thoracic CT scanning has shown that lung laceration, often missed by standard chest radiography, is very common in association with pulmonary contusion.

The trachea or bronchi may uncommonly be the site of traumatic injury, which may range from mild laceration of the mucosa to partial or complete fracture, with or without separation of the fragments. These injuries are frequently overlooked because of other associated injuries. Hemoptysis, surprisingly, is not common. Pneumothorax, pneumomediastinum, and subcutaneous emphysema are commonly present. Persistent and progressive pneumo-thorax, despite a chest tube, is highly suggestive of tracheobronchial injury. Complete atelectasis may be the result of separation of fractured bronchial fragments. Bronchoscopy is the key to accurate diagnosis in most cases.

ACUTE TRAUMATIC RESPIRATORY FAILURE

From the foregoing discussion it is evident that acute respiratory failure in patients with severe chest trauma may have various causes that, singly or in combination and by different mechanisms, impair respiratory function. Furthermore, the common association of extrathoracic injury may contribute significantly to respiratory complications. Figure 22–8 schematically demonstrates the various factors involved in causing respiratory failure in patients with severe traumatic injury to the chest and extrathoracic structures. Mechanical effects of flail chest, pneumothorax, hemothorax, diaphragmatic tear, and airway

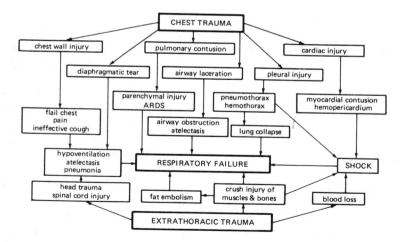

Figure 22–8. Pathogenesis of respiratory failure in thoracic and extrathoracic trauma. Note the multiplicity of factors that cause or contribute to respiratory failure.

laceration with resultant hypoventilation and atelectasis are usually combined with and intensified by pulmonary parenchymal injury from direct trauma as well as indirect causes. Shock may result from both intrathoracic and extrathoracic injuries including hemothorax, cardiac **tamponade** from bleeding inside the pericardial sac, other severe internal hemorrhage, myocardial contusion, and crush injury. As one of the important causes of adult respiratory distress syndrome (ARDS), shock is a major factor in the pathogenesis of acute traumatic respiratory failure (Chapter 25). Pulmonary fat embolism from multiple bone fractures is also known to result in ARDS.

In the management of patients with traumatic respiratory failure, all of the above-mentioned factors should be identified and properly treated. Restoration and maintenance of an adequate airway, optimal oxygenation, and ventilatory support whenever needed are the most important steps in their successful management. The obvious mechanical problems, such as significant pneumothorax or hemothorax, should be corrected immediately. Hypovolemic and cardiogenic shock should be promptly treated, avoiding overhydration. Every effort should be made to prevent avoidable complications, such as atelectasis, aspiration, or infection.

THORACIC SURGERY

Under this heading the commonly performed thoracic surgical procedures, their effect on respiration, and proper respiratory care of patients undergoing such operations are briefly discussed.

Thoracotomy

Thoracotomy means the cutting of the chest wall. Thus any procedure that produces an opening to the pleural cavity is called thoracotomy. An opening through which a tube can be inserted is referred to as *tube* thoracotomy or *closed* thoracotomy; in *open* thoracotomy the pleural cavity or **mediastinum** is exposed. In median **sternotomy,** the mediastinum is exposed without opening the pleural space.

Except for surgical procedures through the lower anterior neck for removal of mediastinal lymph nodes or thymus, or biopsies through bronchoscopy or esophagoscopy, intrathoracic surgery is performed through a thoracotomy. It is done not only for pleuropulmonary surgery, but also for operative procedures on the heart, intrathoracic blood vessels, esophagus, and mediastinal masses. Exploratory thoracotomy is for diagnostic purposes and evaluation for resectability of a lesion. With the availability of excellent diagnostic facilities, nowadays exploratory thoracotomy is rarely performed.

Upon opening the chest and pleural space, the underlying lung will collapse; however, with positive pressure ventilation the lung can be readily expanded. With median sternotomy, or sternal splitting, which is the preferred method for cardiac operations as well as mediastinal surgery, the pleural space need not be entered. In addition to an excellent exposure of the heart and the mediastinal structures, this approach results in less severe postoperative pain and fewer and milder respiratory complications.

Respiratory complications of thoracotomy without lung resection are similar to those of major upper abdominal surgery, and usually are due to general anesthesia and lack of deep breathing and inefficient coughing because of pain, restrictive dressings, use of CNS depressant drugs, and immobility. Atelectasis and pleuropulmonary infection are the most common postoperative pulmonary complications. They are more frequent and more serious among patients with significant underlying bronchopulmonary disease.

Preoperative evaluation of these patients' respiratory status, adequate preparation by thorough tracheobronchial toilet, and treatment of such conditions as infection or heart failure are important in preventing or minimizing postoperative complications. Proper instruction of the patients before surgery about postoperative respiratory care will help significantly in obtaining their cooperation following surgery.

The principles of management of postoperative patients are discussed in Chapter 17. Periodic deep breathing and coughing should be encouraged. Certain mechanical devices such as IPPB, CPPB, or other incentive respiratory gadgets may be used; however, simpler methods of deep-breathing maneuvers are as effective and much cheaper. Cough not only helps to clear the airways but it also improves the distribution of ventilation by opening the distal airways. Tracheobronchial secretions should be removed by postural drainage, gentle chest percussion, and suctioning, if cough is ineffective. Adequate humidity therapy and proper systemic hydration will facilitate bronchial clearing. Overhydration, however, should be avoided for fear of pulmonary congestion and edema. Frequent change of the patient's position

and early ambulation should be encouraged.

Pulmonary Resection

Removal of a lung or a portion of it is done for treatment of various pulmonary diseases. The most common indication for pulmonary resection is the treatment of neoplastic diseases. It is performed occasionally for other conditions such as bronchiectasis, vascular malformation, destructive infectious diseases that do not respond to medical treatment, large emphysematous bullae, and localized diseases that cannot be diagnosed without surgery. A small piece of the lung is sometimes removed for biopsy purposes in certain undiagnosed diffuse lung disease.

Pneumonectomy refers to the resection of a total lung; **lobectomy** indicates removal of a lobe. Bronchial sleeve lobectomy is a modification of a standard lobectomy in which a portion of an adjacent bronchus—usually the mainstem bronchus—is removed along with the resected lobe. The remaining distal bronchus is anastomosed to the proximal stump to preserve the normal lung tissue distal to the resected lobe. When a segment or a small wedge of the lung is excised, the terms *segmental* resection or *wedge* resection are used, respectively. Removal of pulmonary bullae is called **bullectomy.**

Respiratory consequences of resectional surgery will depend on the amount of functioning lung tissue removed and the status of the remaining lung. Pneumonectomy in a young and otherwise healthy person is well tolerated, whereas resection of a smaller lung portion in an elderly individual with diffuse lung disease may result in marked ventilatory impairment. Occasionally, removal of the diseased portion of the lung may result in improved ventilation and gas exchange. For example, resection of a bronchiectatic portion of a lung, excision of a large bullous emphysematous lobe, or removal of the area of the lung with significant arteriovenous malformation frequently improves respiratory function.

In addition to the effect of resection of lung tissue on respiration, the complications of thoracotomy, discussed earlier, may supervene. Evaluation of patients for resectional surgery should include careful studies of pulmonary functions and assessment of pulmonary reserve. In addition, the contribution of the lung, or the portion of it that is considered for resection to the overall pulmonary function, should be estimated. Preoperative evaluation of pulmonary function includes measurement of lung volumes and capacities, flow rates, maximum voluntary ventilation, and arterial blood gases. In an occasional patient, pulmonary artery pressure at rest and with exercise is also measured. Bronchospirometry, which is intended to evaluate the function of the individual lung, is a difficult and tedious task. Similar information can now be obtained by measurement of ventilation and perfusion of different lung regions by radioisotopic studies.

As with thoracotomy, patients undergoing pulmonary resection should be adequately prepared prior to surgery. Preoperative respiratory care will include proper tracheobronchial hygiene, control of infection, correction of circulatory problems, and instruction of the patients regarding deep breathing exercises, effective coughing, and other maneuvers intended to be followed postop-

eratively. Cessation of smoking should be encouraged. Postoperative respiratory problems should be anticipated and measures to prevent their occurrence or to correct them in their early stage should be undertaken. Every effort should be exercised to maintain clear airways and combat infection and atelectasis. Simpler methods of deep breathing maneuvers, effective cough, postural drainage, adequate humidification of airways, and suctioning are most helpful.

Most patients can be extubated following surgery once they wake up from the anesthesia. However, an occasional patient with significant preoperative pulmonary functional impairment, or if the surgery was extensive, may need mechanical ventilation. Management of such a patient is not much different from other patients on a respirator.

With the current methods of anesthesia and postoperative intensive respiratory care, major thoracic operations are performed successfully even in the presence of advanced age and significant respiratory impairment.

Other Thoracic Surgeries

Thoracoplasty is a surgical procedure intended to reduce the volume of a part of the chest by resecting several ribs. This procedure, as well as other methods for collapsing of the underlying lung, was used, prior to the advent of proper antituberculosis drugs, for treatment of pulmonary tuberculosis. Thoracoplasty is rarely used nowadays, and almost exclusively for reduction or obliteration of the thoracic cavity after pneumonectomy. When extensive, thoracoplasty is very deforming, and besides its immediate restrictive effect, it causes gradual additional thoracic and spinal deformity over time. Patients who had thoracoplasty in their early years have significant ventilatory impairment and may suffer from chronic respiratory failure.

Decortication is the removal of the thick pleural peel formed around the lung as a result of infection (empyema) or other fibrosing pleural diseases. This operation is primarily intended to free the lung from an unyielding envelope of thickened visceral pleura and improve its compliance. It is also done for elimination of infected pleura when other therapeutic approaches fail to eradicate the infection. As this operation requires a large thoracotomy, the patient will need intensive preoperative and postoperative respiratory care.

Procedures such as tube drainage of empyema, hemothorax, and pneumothorax; biopsy procedures through mediastinoscopy and bronchoscopy; thoracoscopy or pleuroscopy, pleurodesis, and needle biopsy of the pleura and the lung have been briefly mentioned in appropriate chapters of this book.

Surgery of various other intrathoracic organs, such as the heart, large blood vessels, esophagus, and other mediastinal structures is done through thoracotomy. The respiratory care of these patients, therefore, is not different from that of other thoracotomy patients discussed earlier.

BIBLIOGRAPHY

Bartlett RH, Dechert RE, Mault JR, Clark SF. Metabolic studies in chest trauma. *J Thorac Cardiovasc Surg.* 1984; 87:503–508.

Bollinger CT, Van Eeden SF. Treatment of multiple rib fractures: randomized controlled trial comparing ventilatory with nonventilatory management. *Chest.* 1990; 97:943–948.

Boysen PG. Assessment for lung resection. *Respir Care.* 1984; 29:506–515.

Cagle PT, Thurlbeck WM. Postpneumonectomy compensatory lung growth. *Am Rev Respir Dis.* 1988; 138:1314–1326.

Ellis DG. Chest wall deformities. *Pediatr Rev.* 1989; 11:147–151.

Hodgkin JE. Preoperative assessment of respiratory function. *Respir Care.* 1984; 29:496–503.

Keim HA, Hensinger RN. Spinal deformities: scoliosis and kyphosis. *Clin Symp.* 1989; 41(4):3–32.

Maunder RJ, Pierson DJ, Hudson LD. Subcutaneous and mediastinal emphysema. *Arch Intern Med.* 1984:144–153.

Miller HAB, Taylor GA, Harrison AW, et al. Management of flail chest. *Can Med Assoc J.* 1983; 129:1104–1107.

Pate JW. Chest wall injuries. *Surg Clin North Am.* 1989; 69:59–70.

Pepe PE. Acute post-traumatic physiology and insufficiency. *Surg Clin North Am.* 1989; 69:157–173.

Pinilla JC. Acute respiratory failure in severe blunt chest trauma. *J Trauma.* 1982; 22:221–226.

Richardson JD, Adams L, Flint LM. Selective management of flail chest and pulmonary contusion. *Ann Surg.* 1982; 196:481–487.

Smith TP, Kinasewitz GT, Tucker WY, et al. Exercise capacity as a predictor of postthoracotomy morbidity. *Am Rev Respir Dis.* 1984; 129:730–734.

Symbas PN, Gott JP. Delayed sequelae of thoracic trauma. *Surg Clin North Am.* 1989; 69:135–142.

van der Werken C, Lubbers EJC, Goris RJA. Rupture of the diaphragm by blunt trauma as a marker of injury severity. *Injury.* 1983; 15:149–152.

Wardle EN. Shock lungs: The post-traumatic respiratory distress syndrome. *Q J Med.* 1984; 53:317–329.

Disorders of Respiratory Control

CHAPTER 23

Neuromuscular and CNS Disorders Affecting Respiration

RESPIRATORY MUSCLES

Numerous muscles under various circumstances contribute to mechanical respiratory function. They include the diaphragm, muscles of the rib cage, and the abdominal muscles (Figs. 23–1 and 23–2).

The main respiratory muscles of the rib cage are the *external* and *internal intercostal muscles,* which are arranged in two outer and inner layers between the ribs and differ in their position and the direction of their fibers. It is generally accepted that the external intercostal muscles and interchondral portion of the internal intercostals are inspiratory, while the remaining internal intercostal muscles are expiratory. In addition, the contraction of these muscles serves to stabilize the intercostal spaces, preventing them from being pulled in or pushed out during the respiratory cycle. The innervation of these muscles is by the intercostal nerves, which originate from the spinal cord at corresponding levels of the dorsal spine.

The diaphragm is the principal muscle of inspiration. It is a musculotendinous partition between the abdomen and thorax, anchored all around the circumference of the lower border of the thoracic cage. In its relaxed position it is dome shaped, but upon contraction its central part will move downward, increasing the vertical dimension of the thorax. It also raises the lower ribs, thus enlarging the chest cavity further. In quiet breathing, the diaphragm appears to be the only active inspiratory muscle, but the interchondral and scalene muscles are also active during inspiration. The diaphragm is not indispensable for breathing as long as the thorax and its muscles are normal; respiration can be maintained without the diaphragm participating, as in bilateral diaphragmatic paralysis. With general anesthesia, as the other inspiratory muscles become inactive, the diaphragm remains the only muscle to sustain spontaneous ventilation. The diaphragm is also essential when the intercostal muscles are paralyzed or when the bony thorax becomes rigid and immobile. Each half of the diaphragm is innervated by the **phrenic** nerve, which originates chiefly from the fourth cervical nerve, but is

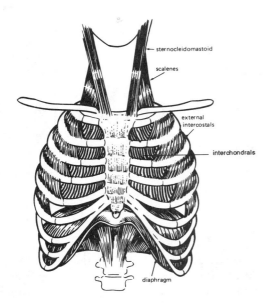

Figure 23–1. Inspiratory muscles. The diaphragm and external intercostals are used with normal breathing. Sternocleidomastoids, scalenes, and other accessory inspiratory muscles are additionally used when the work of breathing is markedly increased. Note that the interchondral portion of the internal intercostals are also inspiratory muscles.

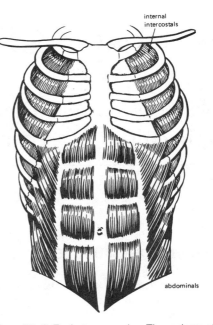

Figure 23–2. Expiratory muscles. The major expiratory muscles are abdominals and internal intercostals except for their interchondral portion.

augmented by fibers from the third and fifth nerves.

In addition to the diaphragm and the intercostal and scalene muscles, other muscles are called into play when there is special need during increased inspiratory effort. Among these, the sternocleidomastoids are the most important. Serratus, trapezius, pectoralis, and others may participate under certain situations.

Expiration is passive with quiet breathing. During the active contraction of the inspiratory muscles, the elastic tissues of the lung and chest wall are stretched, storing potential energy. It is the release of this stored energy by recoil of stretched tissues that engenders expiratory movement. Expiratory muscles, however, actively participate when there is increased ventilation and under certain situations when high expiratory pressures are required, such as with airway obstruction, coughing, sneezing, blowing, straining, and talking. The most important expiratory muscles are the abdominals. Contraction of these muscles reduces the volume of the thoracic cavity by forcing the diaphragm upward with increased abdominal pressure and by depressing the lower ribs. As mentioned above, the internal intercostal muscles, except for the interchondral portion, are also expiratory muscles.

DISEASES OF THE MUSCLES

The diaphragmatic muscle may be the site of certain congenital or acquired defects that may impair its function. *Herniation* through congenital or acquired defects in the diaphragm is common, but rarely causes significant respiratory difficulty. The most common diaphragmatic hernia is that which occurs through an abnormality of the opening in the diaphragm through which the esophagus passes (*hiatus hernia*). Congenital defects in other parts of the diaphragm may result in the entrance of abdominal viscera into the thoracic cavity, sometimes resulting in respiratory symptoms. A rare cause of respiratory distress in newborns is a large diaphragmatic hernia through one of these defects.

Penetrating or blunt trauma to the chest or abdomen may result in a diaphragmatic tear. Herniation through such a rupture may be immediate or may take place some time after the injury. The respiratory difficulty resulting from such a traumatic hernia may be overshadowed or complicated by associated injuries to the chest wall, lungs, and other organs. This is discussed in Chapter 22.

Respiratory muscles may be involved in various generalized muscular disorders of diverse causes. Deficiencies of certain enzymes essential for muscle metabolism are known to cause respiratory difficulty mostly in infants and children, but these may also affect the ventilatory function later in life. *Acid maltase deficiency* is an especially important metabolic cause of **myopathy** in which ventilatory failure may be its predominant manifestation. In its adult form, acid maltase deficiency may manifest as bilateral diaphragmatic paralysis.

The major primary muscular diseases that often involve respiratory function are muscular dystrophies and inflammatory myopathies.

Muscular Dystrophies

Muscular dystrophies are a group of hereditary conditions characterized by progressive degeneration of the striated muscles, resulting in increasingly severe weakness. They have been classified according to certain clinical and genetic features. The most common form is *Duchenne dystrophy*, which because of its genetic characteristics (X-linked recessive) is essentially a disease of males. Becker dystrophy has the genetic and clinical features similar to Duchenne's, but it manifests later and evolves more slowly. Other forms of muscular dystrophy, with an autosomal type of inheritance, are seen equally in both sexes.

The onset of muscular weakness, which is the only presenting symptom in most cases, is quite variable. In Duchenne dystrophy, the weakness starts early in life in the proximal muscles of the extremities. Once the child starts to walk, certain abnormalities can be detected, which become more evident as he grows older. Movements such as getting up from a sitting position or climbing stairs, which require proximal muscle strength, become more and more difficult. In early adolescence, the victim is usually unable to walk. Respiratory muscle weakness can be detected in the early teens, but the diaphragm is usually spared until later. Ventilation, which may be maintained during daytime, becomes impaired during sleep. Progressive increase in severity of respiratory difficulty is aggravated further with each episode of frequently occurring respiratory tract infection. Rarely do patients with Duchenne dystrophy live beyond the age of 20. In other forms of muscular dystrophy, the onset is later, and they are usually designated according to the group of muscles that are primarily involved.

In *myotonic* muscular dystrophy, in addition to progressive muscular weakness, there are certain distinctive features. Difficulty in relaxing the contracted muscles, as in a hand grip, is quite characteristic (myotonia). Early development of cataract, testicular atrophy, and frontal baldness are other associated features. Pulmonary complications are much more common in myotonic dystrophy than other forms.

In muscular dystrophies, in addition to respiratory muscle involvement, there are frequent problems with swallowing and aspiration. Pulmonary function studies in most cases of muscular dystrophy demonstrate some abnormalities. Reduced vital capacity, maximum voluntary ventilation, and maximum expiratory and inspiratory forces are quite common. The severity of these abnormalities depends on the degree of respiratory muscle involvement.

As respiratory failure is the usual cause of death in these unfortunate young patients, their comprehensive management should include a well-planned respiratory-care program.

Inflammatory Myopathies

Polymyositis, which is the major inflammatory muscle disease, is discussed in Chapter 14.

DISORDERS OF THE NEUROMUSCULAR JUNCTION

The junction of the motor nerve endings with the striated muscle (muscle end plate) is the area through which the nerve impulses are transmitted to the muscle (Fig. 23–3). This transmission is accomplished by liberation of **acetylcholine** from the nerve endings and its reaction with the special receptors at the

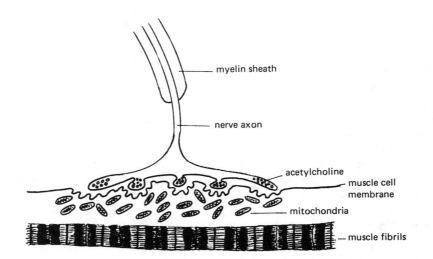

Figure 23–3. Neuromuscular junction.

muscle cell membrane. This interaction results in increased permeability of this membrane to such cations as sodium, potassium, and calcium. The crossing of these ions through the membrane results in the depolarization of muscle and the initiation of its action potential and contraction. An enzyme, called **acetyl-cholinesterase,** inactivates acetylcholine by hydrolysis; thus the muscle is repolarized and becomes ready for reception of another nerve impulse and initiation of another contraction. The proper function of this junctional region is, therefore, essential for orderly muscle activity.

Certain agents are known to disrupt the normal function of the neuromuscular junction. Drugs that interfere with the action of acetylcholinesterase (eg, neostigmine) result in accumulation of acetylcholine in this region, thus facilitating the transmission of impulses through the myoneural junction; however, large doses of these drugs will result in muscle weakness. On the other hand, neuromuscular blocking agents paralyze the muscles by blocking the access of acetylcholine to the motor end plate. Tubocurarine and other curariform drugs, such as pancuronium (Pavulon), act through this mechanism. Succinylcholine (Anectine), another type of paralyzing agent, causes depolarization of muscles as does acetylcholine but is inactivated much more slowly. Repolarization, which is essential for transmission of impulses from the nerve endings, is therefore prevented. These paralyzing agents are used as an adjunct in general anesthesia and for facilitation of management of patients undergoing intubation and mechanical ventilation.

In *botulism,* which is a form of food poisoning from absorption of a toxin produced by a bacterium, *Clostridium botulinum,* paralysis is due to the effect of the toxin on the nerve endings, preventing them from releasing acetylcholine. Rapid ventilatory failure due to respiratory muscle paralysis is the usual cause of death in botulism.

A certain group of antibiotics, known as aminoglycosides (eg, gentamicin, tobramycin), may on rare occasion result in neuromuscular blockade by interference with the release of acetylcholine.

Myasthenia Gravis

Myasthenia gravis is a disease of the neuromuscular junction manifested by muscular weakness and fatigability. It is an acquired autoimmune disorder in which autoantibodies against the acetylcholine receptors are produced. These receptors are located in the muscle-cell membrane, where motor nerve endings meet the muscle fibers. The antibodies cause quantitative and qualitative deficiency of these receptors. The relationship of the thymus gland and myasthenia gravis has long been demonstrated but its pathogenetic role remains undetermined; 70% of the patients have hyperplasia of this gland and another 10% have thymoma (neoplasm of the thymus). The relationship of the thymus gland to myasthenia gravis is probably through its putative role in the production of antiacetylcholine-receptor antibodies.

Most frequently involved in myasthenia gravis are the muscles of the face, eyes, pharynx, and larynx. Every skeletal muscle, however, may be affected. Involvement of the respiratory muscles may result in abrupt development of ventilatory failure. This grave complication is the most common cause of death from this disease.

Myasthenia gravis occurs at all ages; females are affected more often than males. The highest incidence is during the third decade of life in females and sixth decade in males.

Clinical Manifestations. The onset of myasthenia gravis is usually slow and insidious, but, occasionally it may be abrupt. Weakness of the eye muscles, which is the most common manifestation, may result in drooping of the eyelids and double vision. Characteristic facial appearance results from the involvement of the facial muscles. Abnormal speech may be due to weakness of facial, tongue, or laryngeal muscles. These symptoms are more apparent at the end of the day or following repetitive movements of the involved muscles, and they improve with rest. Difficulty with chewing, swallowing, and choking upon eating causes problems with nutrition. Excessive fatigability of muscles of the trunk and extremities can be demonstrated with exercise. Sometimes the weakness may be extreme, and the patient may seem to be totally paralyzed.

Myasthenia crisis refers to the rapid development of weakness to the extent of impairment of respiration. It is usually provoked by infections, especially those involving the respiratory tract. Emotional upset, surgery, discontinuation of medications, or the intake of certain drugs known to increase neuromuscular blockade (such as aminoglycoside antibiotics and institution of high-dose corticosteroids) are other causes of myasthenia crisis. A similar picture may develop in patients who have taken an excessive amount of anticholinesterase drugs (**cholinergic crisis**).

The course of myasthenia gravis is usually unpredictable; it may progress rapidly or slowly, remain unchanged, or remit spontaneously. Certain factors, such as infection, general fatigue, lack of sleep, menstrual period, or other causes of physical or mental stress, may aggravate its course. Respiratory complications as a result of impairment of respiratory muscle function, difficulty with clearing the secretions, aspiration, and frequent respiratory-tract infections are continuous threats to these patients.

A diagnosis of myasthenia gravis is strongly suspected from the characteristic history and usually made by demonstration of muscular weakness and fatigue upon repetitive or sustained contraction of certain muscles, particularly the eye muscles. Regaining of strength after a period of rest further supports the diagnosis. With the administration of anticholinesterase drugs such as neostigmine or, preferably, edrophonium chloride (Tensilon), regaining of strength can be demonstrated in dramatic fashion. This test is also useful in differentiating the weakness of myasthenia from that of excessive anticholinesterase therapy. The characteristic muscle fatigability can also be demonstrated by electric stimulation of muscles and recording their response (electromyography). Determination of circulating antibodies against acetylcholine receptors, present in up to 80% to 90% of patients with myasthenia gravis, is helpful in establishing the diagnosis. Appropriate imaging of the thymus gland, preferably with a CT scanner, is important for detecting thymomas. It is also useful when thymectomy is being considered.

Management. The treatment of patients with myasthenia gravis has undergone significant changes in recent years; however, the principles of management remain essentially the same. These are proper and adequate treatment of acute episodes of severe muscle weakness, including myasthenia crisis, and measures directed to alter the basic pathophysiologic process and to prevent the recurrence of symptoms.

Initially, most patients with myasthenia gravis are hospitalized for further studies, observation of the course of the disease, and evaluation of response to treatment. More severely involved patients are usually put in an intensive care unit. Diligent respiratory care is the most important part of management of these patients during the acute phase of their illness. Unpredictability of the progress of disease requires frequent and regular monitoring of the patients' respiratory function, such as measuring and recording of their vital capacities and maximum inspiratory and expiratory pressures. They should be closely watched for problems such as difficulty with swallowing, aspiration, and effective cough. Infection and other factors known to precipitate myasthenia crisis should be prevented and/or promptly eliminated. Ventilatory failure in myasthenia is the result of increasing weakness of the respiratory pump, usually aggravated by difficulty in handling secretions and aspirations. Repeated measurements of pulmonary mechanics are important in determining the necessity for and proper timing of assisted ventilation. The choice of intubation for mechanical ventilation has been influenced by the advent of endotracheal tubes with low-pressure, high-compliance cuffs. Early tracheostomy is no longer necessary or advisable.

However, as some patients may require prolonged ventilatory support, tracheostomy may be indicated later in the course of such patients.

The main pharmacologic agents in the treatment of acute attacks are anticholinesterase drugs, especially pyridostigmine (Mestinon) or sometimes neostigmine, which result in significant improvement in most cases. Difficulty with arriving at a proper maintenance dosage, variability in response, and occasional development of refractoriness make these agents less than ideal for continuous long-term therapy. Less severe cases, however, can be managed safely with these agents. Mild forms may require no treatment, except during relapse. Corticosteroids, particularly prednisone, given in a large single dose every other day, have been demonstrated to result in remission of cases that responded poorly to other forms of therapy. Therapy with large doses of corticosteroids should be instituted in the hospital while the patient is being closely monitored, as initial worsening before eventual improvement may occur. Other immunosuppressive drugs, especially azathioprine, have also been effective for maintaining remission in myasthenia gravis.

Removal of the thymus gland (thymectomy) is frequently performed, particularly in patients with generalized or rapidly progressive myasthenia gravis. Although the result of surgery for thymus tumor (thymoma) is less than satisfactory, the majority of patients with thymic hyperplasia show long-term benefit from a thymectomy. Because of the seriousness of postoperative complications in myasthenia patients, the necessity for adequate preoperative preparation and proper postoperative care should be emphasized.

Plasma exchange (plasmapheresis) has shown to result in significant, albeit temporary, improvement of some patients with refractory disease. The purpose of this treatment is to remove the circulating acetylcholine-receptor antibodies. It is useful in preparing patients for thymectomy.

DISEASES OF PERIPHERAL MOTOR NERVES

Peripheral nerves may be affected by various toxic agents, metabolic disorders, inflammatory states, vascular disease, trauma, and some unknown causes. Despite the frequency of peripheral nerve disease in clinical practice, involvement of the respiratory motor nerves is uncommon. Many critically ill patients with sepsis and multiple organ failure requiring prolonged mechanical ventilatory support have been recognized who show evidence of polyneuropathy. Involvement of the respiratory muscle nerves is implicated as one of the causes of difficulty in weaning these patients off the respirator.

Unilateral paralysis of the diaphragm is a relatively common occurrence and is often due to invasion or compression of one of the phrenic nerves along its long intrathoracic course by a tumor mass; however, there are other causes of this condition. It may even occur without any apparent cause (idiopathic). Unilateral paralysis of the diaphragm by itself causes no significant symptoms. The physiologic effect, as measured by pulmonary function tests, includes reduction of total lung capacity, particularly when the subject is supine. Radiologic changes are quite characteristic. They include elevation of one hemidiaphragm and its absent or paradoxical movement with respiration. The latter can be more precisely demonstrated fluoroscopically with a rapid inspiratory maneuver, such as sniffing.

Bilateral paralysis of the diaphragm, as an isolated disease, is a rare condition and, as mentioned earlier, is compatible with maintenance of adequate ventilation at rest, and even with a moderate amount of physical activity, provided that other respiratory muscles function normally. Respiration at nighttime does not seem to be affected. Exertional dyspnea and orthopnea, as well as the characteristic physical finding of paradoxical abdominal-thoracic movement (page 12), are the usual manifestations. The chest x-ray film shows marked bilateral elevation of the diaphragm. On fluoroscopy, paradoxical upward movement of the diaphragm on inspiration will be observed. In this condition, there is a significant reduction of vital capacity to less than one-half normal.

Guillain-Barré Syndrome

Guillain-Barré syndrome is the acute form of inflammatory polyneuritis of unknown cause that predominantly affects the peripheral motor nerves and may involve the respiratory muscles. About 20% to 25% of patients require respiratory assistance.

Guillain-Barré syndrome is a relatively common condition, which has its highest incidence in the young and middle-aged. There is frequently a history of preceding upper respiratory tract infection, although the etiology remains unknown. Its association with certain viral diseases, including infectious mononucleosis, influenza, infectious hepatitis, and cytomegalovirus infection, has been demonstated in some cases. Pathologically, there is segmental loss of the myelin sheath of the peripheral nerves and mononuclear cell infiltration. Delayed hypersensitivity against the myelin sheath has been implicated in its pathogenesis. There is also evidence for humoral mechanism with production of antibodies against the peripheral nerve myelin.

Clinical Manifestations.

Typically, the onset is rapid with progressive, more or less symmetrical, weakness that starts in the legs and spreads upward to affect the trunk, arms, and face. It may, however, start in the face or the upper extremities. Respiratory muscles are involved in more severe cases. The paralyzed muscles are flaccid with loss of deep tendon reflexes. Mild sensory changes may also be present. After the establishment of maximum weakness, which is quite variable in individual cases, spontaneous recovery begins. The start of functional recovery is usually expected within 3 to 4 weeks. Delayed onset of remission often results in incomplete recovery. A certain form of the disease may have a chronic relapsing course.

Involvement of the muscles of the pharynx and larynx may result in swallowing difficulty and aspiration. Weakness of abdominal muscles and chest muscles impairs the cough mechanism and, thus, airway clearance, predisposing to respiratory infection and atelectasis. Other respiratory muscles, including the diaphragm, may be affected. Ventilatory failure is expected under these circumstances. As a result of autonomic dysfunction, hemodynamic state may be unstable. Both hypertension and hypotension, especially postural, may occur.

Management.

The management of patients with Guillain-Barré syndrome is primarily *respiratory*. These patients should be hospitalized, preferably in an intensive-care unit, and proper respiratory care given. This includes regular monitoring of the respiratory function, with frequent measurement of vital capacity and maximum inspiratory and expiratory pressures, careful bronchopulmonary toilet, and ventilatory assistance. Recovery will depend on adequate maintenance of patients' respiratory status; therefore, the importance of respiratory care in their management cannot be overstressed. With the proven benefit from plasmapheresis in the early stage of the disease, the importance of early and accurate diagnosis should be emphasized. It has been demonstrated that plasmapheresis, when administered within the first 2 weeks, results in shortening the course of the disease and in reducing its complications.

When there is evidence of respiratory difficulty, as judged by significant reduction in vital capacity and respiratory forces and other signs of ventilatory failure, mechanical ventilatory support should be instituted. Although tracheostomy has been the preferred mode of intubation for ventilatory support in the past, availability of soft cuffs has made endotracheal intubation an acceptable, even preferable, alternative. As the vast majority of patients will eventually recover despite marked impairment of their muscle function, every effort should be made to support their lives until remission takes place. The respiratory therapists and nurses play crucial roles in this rewarding endeavor. An occasional patient may require prolonged mechanical ventilation before any sign of improvement can be demonstrated. Corticosteroids have no proven benefit in Guillain-Barré syndrome; they may even be detrimental.

DISORDERS OF THE SPINAL CORD

Acute anterior poliomyelitis, commonly known as *polio,* used to be the most important cause of ventilatory failure of neuromuscular origin. Fortunately, it is now almost totally eradicated, and its importance has become mostly historical. A catastrophic epidemic of poliomyelitis, which occurred in 1952 in Copenhagen, was an important impetus in the improvement of mechanical ventilators. Some victims of polio, many years after a severe paralytic form of the disease, show evidence of progressive weakness in their already involved muscles. This condition is recognized as *postpolio syndrome.* Ventilatory difficulty from this syndrome occurs in patients in whom the respiratory muscles were affected at the time of their acute polio.

Many other diseases of the spinal cord may occasionally result in respiratory difficulty. Diseases such as **amyotrophic lateral sclerosis,** multiple sclerosis, and various forms of inflammatory or neoplastic diseases of the spinal cord may result in respiratory muscle weakness and ventilatory failure. As the origin of the phrenic nerves is from the high cervical cord, diseases that involve only the lower regions spare the diaphragm, and adequate ventilation is maintained. However, significant weakness of other respiratory muscles, especially abdominals, may result in impairment of effective cough and, thus, cause respiratory problems.

Traumatic injury to the cervical spinal cord below the fourth cervical vertebra results in *quadriplegia* (also known as **tetraplegia**) with maintenance of respiration by the unaffected diaphragm. Injury above this level, however, will result in paralysis of all respiratory muscles except for the **accessory** inspiratory muscle (sternocleidomastoid), which is unable to maintain adequate ventilation. Permanent mechanical ventilatory support is necessary for victims of such an injury. Even with intact diaphragmatic function, quadriplegics are predisposed to respiratory difficulties from frequent bouts of pneumonia and atelectasis as a result of impairment of cough and clearing of the airways, as well as lack of mobility. In addition, these patients are prone to develop thrombophlebitis and repeated pulmonary embolism. Pulmonary functional impairment in the early acute stage following cervical spinal cord injury is more severe than it is during the chronic stage. Most early deaths following acute traumatic quadriplegia are due to pulmonary complications; therefore, the importance of adequate respiratory care in the management of such patients should be stressed. Some of the early complications following acute spinal cord injury are reduced by kinetic therapy, using a rotating bed. Continuous respiratory care should be included in overall chronic management and rehabilitation of these unfortunate patients. Although cough in quadriplegics is generally considered to be a passive process, which results from the elastic recoil of the lungs and abdomen, it has been demonstrated that part of the pectoralis major muscles contributes actively to cough by compressing the upper rib cage. Therefore, appropriate training and strengthening of these muscles should be part of the rehabilitation program of quadriplegics.

RESPIRATORY MUSCLE FATIGUE

In addition to well-defined neuromuscular disorders involving respiration, the respiratory muscles are subject to fatigue under various conditions. Fatigue is defined as the inability of a muscle to continue generating the necessary contractile force to sustain its function. It is different from weakness in that fatigue follows muscular contraction, whereas weakness is loss of force, not due to muscular contraction. A weak muscle, although it tires easily, may not necessarily fatigue if the work demand is small; on the other hand, a strong muscle will fatigue if subjected to a large enough workload. Fatigue, therefore, develops when the demand for energy exceeds the supply of energy by the muscle. Although any of the respiratory muscles may develop fatigue, inspiratory muscles, especially the diaphragm, are most commonly involved and are extensively studied.

Factors predisposing to respiratory muscle fatigue are divided into those that increase energy demand and those that diminish energy supply. High-energy demand is due to increased work of breathing as seen in airway obstruction and reduced thoracic compliance. Other factors include inefficiency of respiratory muscles as in hyperinflation and disturbance in optimal respiratory frequency and tidal volume. Energy supply by the muscle is diminished in various neuromuscular diseases discussed earlier. In addition, reduction in cardiac output and oxygen-carrying capacity of blood results in fatigue of the respiratory muscles. Poor nutrition and marked weight loss are other factors in which energy supply is diminished. Electrolyte disturbances, especially hypokalemia and hypophosphatemia, are known to predispose to muscle fatigue, which may affect the ventilatory function. Hypercapnia also is implicated in impairing diaphragmatic contraction and, together with hypoxemia, may be a significant factor in sustaining respiratory muscle fatigue in respiratory failure.

The development of fatigue is not just a local muscular phenomenon; it may also be the result of reduced motor drive from the central nervous system. It appears that the discomfort of muscular fatigue inhibits the neuronal output to the involved muscle.

In clinical situations in which respiratory muscle fatigue develops, several factors may be simultaneously operative. The ultimate clinical outcome is ventilatory failure (hypercapnia). Respiratory muscle fatigue may develop acutely as in severe asthma and cardiogenic or noncardiogenic pulmonary edema, or it may have an insidious onset as in severe COPD or kyphoscoliosis. Inspiratory muscle fatigue is a common finding in critically ill patients and those on mechanical ventilation, and is the major cause of failure in weaning patients from respirators.

A diagnosis of inspiratory muscle fatigue should be suspected in any patient with respiratory difficulty. It is suggested that fatigue is a common pathway in the development and perpetuation of hypercapnic respiratory failure from many causes. Once suspected, certain clinical manifestations should be looked for. They include an increased respiratory rate, alternating abdominal and rib cage breathing, a paradoxical inward abdominal movement on inspiration, and rising arterial PCO_2. Among these, the paradoxical abdominal motion and alternating abdominal and rib cage breathing are important diagnostic clues. They are easily detected if looked for.

Management. The principles of management of respiratory muscle fatigue are based on the restoration of balance between energy supply and energy demand. Reduction in demand necessitates the correction of underlying pulmonary and extrapulmonary diseases that have increased the mechanical work of breathing. The energy supply may be increased by correcting or eliminating factors known to have reduced it, such as low cardiac output, anemia, or hypoxemia. Aminophylline, as well as caffeine, has been demonstrated to increase the contractility of the fatigued diaphragm. When inspiratory muscle fatigue is severe and there is progressive worsening of spontaneous ventilation with persistent hypercapnia, despite attempts at correcting the underlying causes, resting the muscles by the judicious use of mechanical ventilation is the only effective way that fatigue can be treated. (See "Respiratory Failure," Chapter 25).

RESPIRATION IN DISORDERS OF THE CENTRAL NERVOUS SYSTEM (BRAIN)

Respiration is frequently affected by disorders of the central nervous system. This is understandable considering the particular function of the "respiratory center" and the importance of various reflexes in pulmonary defense, which may be impaired by many diseases involving the brain.

The term "respiratory center" should not impart the notion that it is a compact mass of nerve cells confined to a closely restricted area. It is rather a physiologic center that is concerned with the integration of the activity of muscles of respiration. Although most of the nervous elements for this purpose are collected in the brainstem, especially the medulla, other parts of the central nervous system have influence over this neurologic function.

The center receives impulses not only from various peripheral and central chemoreceptors, stretch lung receptors, and other mechanical receptors, but also from higher cerebral centers. Normally, respiration is readily effected by voluntary control and influenced by such factors as wakefulness or sleep, emotional change, and mental or physical stress. In many diseases of the central nervous system, despite lack of involvement of the brainstem, there is alteration of the respiratory pattern, commonly in the form of hyperventilation, periodic breathing (Cheyne-Stokes respiration) or other abnormal respiratory patterns.

Depression of ventilation in central nervous system (CNS) disorders generally implies reduced activity of the respiratory center. Although there are several causes of respiratory depression of central origin, the most common cause in clinical practice is overdose with CNS depressant drugs, including general anesthetics. Except for rare cases in which the respiratory center is primarily and exclusively depressed, there is always a certain degree of impairment of the other functions of the central nervous system with central hypoventilation. Indeed, in a majority of such conditions, depression of respiration occurs *after* most other CNS functions are suppressed.

In CNS disorders, respiration is not only affected through the influence of the respiratory center, but also altered by derangement of normal mechanisms that ensure airway patency. Impairment or loss of consciousness from any cause may result in respiratory difficulty, even when the respiratory center is not involved. Obstruction of the hypopharynx from relaxation of pharyngeal walls and tongue, with its backward fall; impairment of reflexes that prevent the entry of secretions, vomitus, and foreign matter to and/or help their removal from the air passages; and absence or inadequacy of certain respiratory maneuvers, which normally help to prevent small airway closure and pulmonary atelectasis are some of the problems facing patients with CNS malfunction. Reflexes that are normally operative to close the laryngeal entrance by the epiglottis and vocal cords (glottis) and respiratory maneuvers, such as coughing, sighing, yawning, sneezing, talking, crying, laughing, sniffing, blowing, and straining, are abolished in unconscious patients. Any patient with impaired consciousness is, therefore, highly predisposed to respiratory complications resulting from disturbances of these functions, even though there may be no evidence of ventilatory depression. Lack of mobility and positional change contributes further to these complications. Among them, pulmonary atelectasis, aspiration pneumonitis, bacterial pneumonia, and thromboembolism are quite common. "Neurogenic" pulmonary edema may develop following acute CNS events.

Severe head trauma is known to cause acute hypoxemia immediately after injury without evidence of pulmonary pathology. Patients with underlying chronic pulmonary disease are, obviously, at much higher risk if they develop impaired consciousness.

Acute and transient disturbance of consciousness, such as seen during and for a short time following epileptic seizure, may result in profound respiratory impairment. Marked hypoxemia and respiratory and metabolic acidosis are common during such episodes. In *status epilepticus* (frequent epileptic seizures without restoration of consciousness between them), the most feared fatal complication is respiratory, which may be due to seizures, as well as the large amount of sedatives necessary for their control.

In the management of patients with impairment of CNS function, especially when they are unconscious, respiratory care plays a major role. Pulmonary complication is the most common cause of death in most such situations.

DRUG OVERDOSE

The subject of drug overdose is selected for discussion with more detail because of its common occurrence and the frequency of respiratory complications. Drug overdose is a leading cause of unconsciousness among patients admitted to critical care units. The principles of respiratory management of this condition are applicable equally well to any comatose or stuporous patient from other causes. Although overdose from any drug may have deleterious and even fatal effects, the more frequently encountered drug overdose in clinical practice is due to accidental or, more commonly, suicidal intake of large amounts of CNS depressant drugs. These include sedatives, hypnotics, tranquilizers, narcotics, alcohol, and numerous other drugs used in the treatment of psychiatric disorders. Discussion of common clinical features and principles of management of overdoses by CNS-depressant drugs will be followed by a brief outline of individual characteristics of commonly occurring specific drug overdoses that affect respiration.

Clinical Manifestations. The most common clinical manifestation of overdose by drugs is depression of CNS function. Variable degrees of impairment of consciousness, from sleepiness to deep coma, may be observed depending on the nature and the amount of drug and the time that it has been ingested. Various classifications, including Glasgow Coma Scale, are used for staging the level of responsiveness. However, for descriptive purposes, the following classification is widely used for staging the severity of intoxication from CNS depressant drugs.

- *Stage 0.* Sleepy state from which the patient can be aroused and can answer questions.
- *Stage I.* Comatose state, but the patient responds to painful stimuli by withdrawal. Respiration and blood pressure are normal and the deep tendon reflexes are intact.
- *Stage II.* Comatose and no response to pain. Most reflexes are intact and there is no respiratory or circulatory depression.
- *Stage III.* Comatose, most or all reflexes are absent; there is no

response to pain, but respiration and blood pressure are maintained.
- *Stage IV.* Comatose, most reflexes are absent and there is depression of respiration and/or decreased blood pressure.

This classification is not intended for narcotic overdose in which respiration may be markedly depressed *before* total loss of consciousness or changes in reflexes. Indeed, respiratory depression out of proportion to the severity of coma is strongly suggestive of narcotic drug overdose.

In addition to ventilatory depression, unconscious patients with drug overdose, like other comatose patients, are prone to respiratory complications from multiple causes. *Aspiration* is a common complication in drug overdose. It may be spontaneous or secondary to therapeutic procedures such as induced vomiting, gastric lavage, or tracheal intubation. Pulmonary *atelectasis* and maldistribution of ventilation are frequent and result from retained secretions, lack of intermittent deep breaths, and immobility. Widening of the alveolar-arterial PO_2 difference and, even, clinically significant hypoxemia may be observed without hypoventilation.

Many overdosed patients will have some fever with or without transient infiltration on the chest radiograph, probably as a result of pulmonary atelectasis, aspiration, or infection. Some patients may develop frank pneumonia, lung abscess, or empyema. Aspiration of contaminated upper airway secretion is often the cause of these infectious complications. Sometimes contaminated respiratory therapy equipment may be the culprit.

Circulatory impairment is common in severe overdose from many centrally acting drugs. Reduction in effective circulatory volume from decreased vascular tone and myocardial depression are usual causes. Hypotension and reduced tissue perfusion may complicate the direct toxic effects of drugs on many organs, including the brain. Anoxic brain damage may result from hypoxemia and reduced cerebral perfusion.

Patients with shock or severe hypoxemia may develop pulmonary edema from alveolar capillary damage, which would be enhanced by cardiac failure and made worse by overzealous fluid infusion. Pulmonary edema is more common in narcotic drug overdose.

Management. Patients with mild intoxication are usually managed by close observation and monitoring of the vital signs, level of consciousness, reflexes, and urinary output. The removal of unabsorbed drug from the gastrointestinal tract by such measures as gastric lavage and use of cathartics is usually tried. However, if the patient is poorly responsive or comatose, attempt at gastric lavage should only be made after adequate airway with cuffed endotracheal tube has been established.

The most important aspect of management of patients with drug overdose is supportive therapy, particularly the maintenance of cardiovascular and respiratory functions. Respiratory care includes establishment and maintenance of adequate airway, tracheobronchial toilet, adequate oxygenation, and ventilatory assistance. The establishment of adequate airway is the first priority in any comatose patient. The assurance of an adequate IV access is mandatory, and the status of urine output should be monitored by an indwelling bladder catheter. Blood, urine, and gastric lavage samples should be obtained for toxicological analysis. When there is deep coma (Stage II and higher), signs of respiratory depression, risk of vomiting and aspiration, or evidence of significant hypoxemia, endotracheal tube should be inserted. Patients with drug overdose will need proper bronchial toilet by adequate humidification, frequent change of position, postural drainage, and tracheobronchial suctioning. A variable degree of hypoxemia is common in these patients due to atelectasis or aspiration. Severe hypoxemia is strongly suggestive of pulmonary edema or aspiration pneumonitis. An adequate amount of oxygen should be administered to combat hypoxemia. Change of position, bronchial toilet, and intermittent positive pressure breathing or periodic bagging will help to prevent atelectasis.

Mechanical ventilation should be instituted when there is any indication of inadequate ventilation, severe hypoxemia, or risk of worsening of the respiratory state. We prefer to put deeply comatose patients on respirator, regardless of their ventilatory states as they may change quite unpredictably. Large tidal volumes (10–15 mL/kg) at a respiratory rate necessary to maintain adequate alveolar ventilation are recommended. In patients with pulmonary edema, as may occur with narcotic overdose or severe aspiration pneumonitis, addition of positive end-expiratory pressure will assure more satisfactory oxygenation, and will obviate the necessity for administration of a toxic concentration of oxygen.

Hemodynamic status should be

closely monitored by frequent examination of blood pressure, pulse, and peripheral perfusion. Determination of hourly urinary output is important as an indicator of adequacy of tissue perfusion. In certain situations, especially when there is evidence of myocardial depression, poor tissue perfusion, unstable blood pressure, or pulmonary edema, direct hemodynamic monitoring with a Swan-Ganz catheter may be helpful as a guide for proper fluid therapy and administration of inotropic and vasoactive drugs.

Except for narcotic overdose, there is no effective "antidote" for CNS depressant drugs. If narcotic drug intoxication is suspected, a narcotic antagonist such as naloxone hydrochloride (Narcan) is administered. Response to the proper dose of this agent in the case of narcotic overdose is rapid and often dramatic.

The measures to prevent the absorption of the drug after its ingestion are effective when they are employed within a few hours of the time of its intake. They include induction of vomiting, gastric lavage, and the administration of activated charcoal and cathartics. Protection of airways should always be carried out whenever there is a chance of aspiration resulting from any of these therapeutic measures. Activated charcoal is considered to be the most effective for the purpose of prevention of absorption in most common drug overdoses. Removal of the drug after its absorption may be enhanced by various methods, depending on the pharmacokinetics of the drug and the necessity and usefulness of its faster removal. In most situations of overdose by CNS depressant drugs, it is neither effective nor significantly beneficial toward eventual clinical outcome. Forced diuresis, hemodialysis, hemoperfusion, and multiple-dose activated charcoal administration are some of the methods used for enhancing drug elimination.

The emphasis in management of CNS depressant drug overdose should be placed on *supportive measures,* especially a proper and diligent respiratory care and maintenance of adequate circulatory state. With such measures, patients with drug overdose are expected to survive. The rare fatal cases in the hospital are seen among patients with severe cardiac depression unresponsive to optimal therapeutic measures, advanced anoxic brain damage, or severe infectious complications.

SPECIFIC DRUG OVERDOSE

Narcotics
Narcotic drugs with a significant overdose potential include heroin, methadone, codeine, meperidine (Demerol), pentazocine (Talwin), and propoxyphene (Darvon). With a few exceptions, the clinical picture of acute poisoning and its management are similar for overdose from any of these drugs. They are notorious for their ventilatory-depressant action through their direct effect on the respiratory center. Both the rate and volume of ventilation are depressed, and Cheyne-Stokes respiration is common. Except for meperidine, narcotics result in constriction of pupils, unless there is extreme hypoxemia. The well-known triad of coma, respiratory depression, and pinpoint pupils is highly suggestive of narcotic drug overdose. Noncardiac pulmonary edema, especially with heroin and codeine poisoning, is another fairly common feature of narcotic overdose. Most of the

fatal cases of narcotic overdose are caused by or associated with pulmonary edema with or without concomitant aspiration. Pulmonary edema may develop even after the CNS effect has improved. The exact mechanism of pulmonary edema in narcotic intoxication is not clear, although increased alveolar capillary permeability resulting from severe hypoxia and hypotension seems likely. Other possible causes are aspiration of acid gastric content, neurogenic effect on pulmonary vessels, and hypersensitivity reaction.

Other complications of overdose from narcotics include hypotension and hypothermia. Convulsive seizures may also occur, especially in overdose with meperidine and propoxyphene. Poisoning from the latter drug is also known to cause cardiac arrhythmias.

Principles of management of poisoning from CNS depressant drugs in general are applicable to narcotic overdose. In addition, the highly specific narcotic antagonist naloxone (Narcan) is very effective in reversing the CNS effect, including respiratory depression, of narcotic drugs. Because of its shorter half-life than that of many narcotics, especially methadone, repeated administration or continuous infusion of Narcan may be necessary. This drug has both a diagnostic and a therapeutic use for coma of unknown cause. A rapid response is diagnostic of narcotic drug poisoning. Naloxone has no effect on pulmonary edema from narcotic overdose.

Sedative-Hypnotic Drugs

Overdose from sedative-hypnotic drugs—which include barbiturates; benzodiazepines, such as diazepam (Valium) and alprazolam (Xanax); meprobamates; and other "tranquilizers" and "sleeping pills"—results primarily in CNS depression ranging from mild sedation to deep coma. In combination with alcohol and other CNS depressants, the toxic effect of these drugs is markedly enhanced. With severe toxicity, respiratory depression and hypotension may develop. The management principles outlined earlier are best applicable to overdose from these drugs. Rarely are measures such as dialysis for the drugs' increased elimination necessary or advisable. Because of a significant difference in the metabolism and excretion of these drugs, the duration of coma from their overdose varies. With proper supportive care, barring rare fatal complications, survival from sedative-hypnotic drug overdose is the rule.

Antidepressant drugs

Tricyclics, the most commonly used antidepressants, are the leading cause of serious and potentially lethal drug overdose. The early manifestations of toxicity from these drugs are the result of their anticholinergic effects, which include tachycardia, dry mucous membranes, blurred vision, and dilated pupils. The early CNS symptoms of agitation, restlessness, confusion, and hallucination may be rapidly followed by coma, with or without convulsions. The cardiovascular toxic effects include sinus tachycardia, various forms of arrhythmia and other electrocardiographic abnormalities, and hypotension. Pulmonary edema may occur in some patients, especially when there is hypotension. Among other pulmonary complications of tricyclic antidepressant overdose, respiratory center depression, pulmonary aspiration, atelectasis, and pneumonia are fairly common.

Hypoxemia and marked increase in alveolar-arterial oxygen tension gradient occur in most patients even in those without clinical or radiographic evidence of pulmonary involvement. Acidosis from various causes, including hypotension and convulsive seizures, increases the toxicity of these drugs. Lower blood pH increases the proportion of free (not bound to proteins) drug concentration. Most of the toxic effects on the cardiovascular system are especially enhanced with acidosis.

In management of patients with tricyclic antidepressant overdose, in addition to proper respiratory care and other supportive measures for coma, cardiovascular abnormalities should be adequately evaluated and treated. Acidosis should be appropriately corrected by adequate ventilation, control of seizures, treatment of hypotension, and the administration of sodium bicarbonate. Most of the toxic effects of tricyclics, especially cardiac arrhythmias and hypotension, are ameliorated by correction of acidosis and alkalinization of blood. Hypotension often responds to fluid administration and correction of acidosis, but may also require vasopressor drugs. Seizures and arrhythmias should be controlled with specific drugs as needed. Although physostigmine has been used as an "antidote" for tricyclic drug toxicity, it is rarely recommended because of its unpredictable side effects.

Aspirin

An important cause of accidental drug overdose in children is aspirin. In adults, in addition to suicidal ingestion, aspirin overdose may occur as a result of cumulative effects of its regular chronic use, especially in the elderly. As there is significant individual variation in its

pharmacodynamics, a toxic effect may develop even with a usual daily "therapeutic" dose if taken for a long period. In very high blood level, aspirin has CNS-depressant effects including respiratory suppression. However, with moderate toxicity and early in the course of severe toxicity, it is a strong respiratory center stimulant, resulting in hyperventilation and respiratory alkalosis. Metabolic acidosis, especially in children, further complicates the acid-base status. With acute aspirin poisoning, vomiting is very common. CNS effects of aspirin poisoning include confusion, delirium, convulsion, and coma. Aspirin at normal blood pH is mostly ionized and thus difficult to penetrate the cells of various tissues including the CNS. However, in acidemia, the non-ionized portion is increased, which enhances its toxicity. A serious complication of aspirin poisoning is the development of pulmonary edema, which occurs mostly in elderly patients. A high index of suspicion is necessary for the diagnosis of aspirin poisoning, which is readily confirmed by the determination of blood aspirin levels.

In treatment of aspirin poisoning, measures to inhibit its further absorption and increase its elimination should be combined with the correction of fluid, electrolytes, and acid-base abnormalities. Activated charcoal not only inhibits the absorption of aspirin, but also, when given in repeated doses, reduces its plasma half-life (increases its removal). Sodium bicarbonate is given to correct metabolic acidosis and, by so doing, to reduce the toxic effect of aspirin. By alkalinizing the urine, bicarbonate also increases its renal excretion. Mechanical ventilation may be necessary in unconscious patients, when pulmonary edema develops, or when there is evidence of respiratory depression. Peritoneal dialysis or hemodialysis may be necessary in severe aspirin intoxication.

BIBLIOGRAPHY

Baydur A. Respiratory muscle function in systemic disorders. *Sem Respir Med.* 1988; 9:223–238.

Bennett DA, Bleck TP. Diagnosis and treatment of neuromuscular causes of acute respiratory failure. *Clin Neuropharmacol.* 1988; 11:303–347.

Braun SR, Giovannoni R, O'Connor M. Improving the cough in patients with spinal cord injury. *Am J Phys Med.* 1984; 63(1):1–10.

Celli BR. Clinical and physiologic evaluation of respiratory muscle function. *Clin Chest Med.* 1989; 10:199–214.

Colice GL, Bernat JL. Neurologic disorders and respiration. *Clin Chest Med.* 1989; 10:521–543.

Cooper KR, Morrow CF. Pulmonary complications associated with head injury. *Respir Care.* 1984; 29:263–269.

Coronel B, Mercatello A, Couturier JC, et al. Polyneuropathy: potential cause of difficult weaning. *Crit Care Med.* 1990; 18:486–489.

Dec GW, Stern TA. Tricyclic antidepressants in the intensive care unit. *J Intensive Care Med* 1990; 5:69–81.

DeTroyer A, Estenne M. Coordination between rib cage muscles and diaphragm during quiet breathing in humans. *J Appl Physiol.* 1984; 57:899–906.

England JD. Guillain-Barré syndrome. *Annu Rev Med.* 1990; 41:1–6.

Estenne M, DeTroyer A. Cough in tetraplegic subjects: an active process. *Ann Intern Med.* 1990; 112:22–28.

Finley JC, Pascuzzi RM. Rational therapy of myasthenia gravis. *Semin Neurol.* 1990; 10(1):70–82.

Gibson GJ. Diaphragmatic paresis: patho-physiology, clinical features, and investigation. *Thorax.* 1989; 44:960–970.

Gilgoff I, Prentice W, Baydur A. Patient and family participation in the management of respiratory failure in Duchenne's muscular dystrophy. *Chest.* 1989; 95:519–524.

Glenn WWL, Hogan JF, Loke JSO, et al. Ventilatory support by pacing of the conditioned diaphragm in quadriplegia. *N Engl J Med.* 1984; 310:1150–1155.

Gracey DR, Divertie MB, Howard FM Jr. Mechanical ventilation for respiratory failure in myasthenia gravis. *Mayo Clin Proc.* 1983; 58:597–602.

Gracey DR, Divertie MB, Howard FM Jr, Payne WS. Postoperative respiratory care after transsternal thymectomy in myasthenia gravis. *Chest.* 1984; 86:67–71.

Gracey DR, Howland FM Jr, Divertie MB. Plasmapheresis in the treatment of ventilator-dependent myasthenia gravis patients. *Chest.* 1984; 85:739–743.

Grassino A, Macklem PT. Respiratory muscle fatigue and ventilatory failure. *Annu Rev Med.* 1984; 35:625–647.

Hedemark LL, Kronenberg RS. Chemical regulation of respiration. *Chest.* 1982; 82:488–494.

Heffner JE, Sahn SA. Salicylate-induced pulmonary edema. *Ann Intern Med.* 1981; 95:405–409.

Jay SJ, Johanson WG Jr, Pierce AK. Respiratory complications of overdose with sedative drugs. *Am Rev Respir Dis.* 1975; 112:591–598.

Juan G, Calverley P, Talamo C, et al. Effect of carbon dioxide on diaphragmatic function in human beings. *N Engl J Med.* 1984; 310:874–879.

Kreitzer SM, Saunders NA, Tyler HR, Ingram RH Jr. Respiratory muscle function in amyotrophic lateral sclerosis. *Am Rev Respir Dis.* 1978; 117:437–447.

Laroche CM, Carroll N, Moxham J, Green M. Clinical significance of severe isolated diaphragm weakness. *Am Rev Respir Dis.* 1988; 138:862–866.

Linton DM, Philcox D. Myasthenia gravis. *Dis Mon.* 1990; 36:599–637.

Mansel JK, Norman JR. Respiratory complications and management of spinal cord injuries. *Chest.* 1990; 97:1446–1452.

McGuigan MA. Treatment of poisoning. *Clin Symp.* 1984; 36(5):3–32.

Mier A. Respiratory muscle weakness. *Respir Med.* 1990; 84:351–359.

Mulder DG, Graves M, Herrmann C. Thymectomy for myasthenia gravis: recent observation and comparison with past experience. *Ann Thorac Surg.* 1989; 48:551–555.

NHLBI. Workshop Summary. Respiratory muscle fatigue. *Am Rev Respir Dis.* 1990; 142:474–480.

Nicholson DP. The immediate management of overdose. *Med Clin North Am.* 1983; 67(6):1279–1293.

Reines HD, Harris RC. Pulmonary complications of acute spinal cord injuries. *Neurosurgery.* 1987; 21:193–196.

Rochester DF, Arora NS. Respiratory muscle failure. *Med Clin North Am.* 1983; 67(3):573–597.

Rochester DF, Esau SA. Malnutrition and the respiratory system. *Chest.* 1984; 85:411–415.

Roussos C. Respiratory muscle fatigue and ventilatory failure. *Chest.* 1990; 97(suppl): 89S–96S.

Roussos C, Macklem PT. The respiratory muscles. *N Engl J Med.* 1982; 307:786–797.

Roy TM, Ossorio MA, Cipolla LM, et al. Pulmonary complications after tricyclic antidepressant overdose. *Chest.* 1989; 96:852–856.

Scanlon PD, Loring SH, Pichurko BM, et al. Respiratory mechanics in acute quadriplegia. *Am Rev Respir Dis.* 1989; 139:615–620.

Smith PEM, Edwards RHT, Calverley PMA. Ventilation and breathing pattern during sleep in Duchenne muscular dystrophy. *Chest.* 1989; 96:1346–1351.

Steinhart CM, Pearson-Shaver AL. Poisoning. *Crit Care Clin.* 1988; 4:845–872.

Steljes DG, Kryger MH, Kirk BW, Millar TW. Sleep in postpolio syndrome. *Chest.* 1990; 98:133–140.

Strumpf DA, Millman RP, Hill NS. The management of chronic hypoventilation. *Chest.* 1990; 98:474–480.

Supinski GS, Deal EC Jr, Kelsen SG. The effects of caffeine and theophylline on diaphragmatic contractility. *Am Rev Respir Dis.* 1984:130:429–433.

Treatment of acute drug abuse reactions. *Med Lett Drugs Ther.* 1987; 29:83–86.

Vale A, Meredith T, Brendan B. Eliminating poisons. *Brit Med J.* 1984; 289:366–369.

CHAPTER 24

Sleep-Related Breathing Disorders

The effect of sleep on breathing and its role in various respiratory disorders have been extensively studied in recent years. Both basic research and clinical investigation have resulted in significant advances in knowledge and understanding of this important but hitherto neglected area of pulmonary medicine. It has been realized that sleep-related disorders of respiration are quite common and may be the cause of significant mortality and morbidity. The clinical entity known as Pickwickian or obesity-hypoventilation syndrome is recognized to be only a part of the wide spectrum of these disorders.

RESPIRATION DURING SLEEP

The effects of sleep on respiration vary according to the state and the stage of sleep. There are two entirely different states of sleep: non-rapid eye movement (NREM) and rapid eye movement (REM). They occur cyclically at about 90-minute intervals. NREM sleep, with its four successive stages, is referred to as quiet sleep and is characterized by progressive deepening of sleep and slowing of brain waves (EEG). With the onset of sleep, there is gradual re-

duction of sympathetic activity during NREM sleep; unopposed parasympathetic activity causes slowing of the heart rate. Systemic blood pressure also diminishes with the progression of NREM sleep. During drowsiness and early stages of NREM sleep, the pattern of breathing may be periodic, with cyclic waxing and waning of respiratory rate and tidal volume. In older individuals, true Cheyne-Stokes respiration may occur. With deeper NREM sleep, breathing becomes regular and steady. In healthy persons, minute ventilation at the later stages of NREM sleep is somewhat less than during resting but wakeful state; as a result the arterial PCO_2 rises and PO_2 decreases by about 5 torr.

REM sleep is characterized by bursts of rapid eye movements and changes in the EEG, indicative of increased neuronal activity. Dreaming occurs in this sleeping period and, if awakened, the subject recalls vividly the content of his or her dream. Changes in autonomic nervous system activity result in fluctuation of the heart rate and the blood pressure. Skeletal muscle tone is markedly diminished during REM sleep. Intercostal muscle activity is also decreased, resulting in paradoxical motion of the rib cage with breathing. During REM sleep, respiration is characteristically irregular and may even be interrupted by short periods of apnea. Up to 30 apneic episodes in a 7-hour sleep period is considered to be normal. Alteration in rate, rhythm, and depth of breathing causes fluctuation in the state of alveolar ventilation during REM sleep.

In addition to changes characteristic of each sleep period, there are certain alterations in pulmonary defense and ventilatory control mechanisms with sleep. Mucociliary clearance, protective reflexes of the airways, and arousal responses to noxious stimuli are decreased during REM and late stages of NREM sleep. As a result, small amounts of upper airway secretions may be aspirated during sleep. Ventilatory and arousal responses to both hypercapnia and hypoxemia are also diminished to variable degrees dependent on the sleep state. Activity of the upper airway muscles is important in maintaining the patency of its muscular portion (pharynx). Active pharyngeal muscle contraction with each inspiration plays a significant role in preventing the airway from collapsing, which otherwise would occur as a result of negative pressure of inspiration. It has been demonstrated that pharyngeal muscle activity is reduced during sleep.

SLEEP APNEA SYNDROME

Apnea is defined as the cessation of airflow (at the level of both the nostrils and the mouth) lasting for at least 10 seconds. *Sleep apnea syndrome* refers to a pathologic condition in which the number of apneic episodes exceed 5 per hour of sleep (8 in the elderly), and it results in arterial blood desaturation, sleep disruption, and daytime somnolence. Sleep apnea syndrome, therefore, comprises disturbances of both sleep and respiration.

Classification and Mechanism. Conventionally, sleep apnea is classified into three types:

1. The **central** type is an apnea in which cessation of airflow is the result of absence of ventilatory effort.
2. The **obstructive** or occlusive type is characterized by cessation of airflow despite the presence of chest and abdominal movements.
3. The **mixed** type is a combination of central and obstructive apnea in which the initial cessation of ventilatory effort is followed by its resumption without airflow because of upper airway obstruction.

In the majority of patients, apneic episodes are a variable combination of central, obstructive, or mixed apneas suggesting that a functional defect in the central respiratory drive during sleep affects both inspiratory muscle contraction and upper airway muscle activity. Central apnea without obstructive component is very uncommon, except for brief and infrequent episodes during REM sleep. Diminished respiratory center output may on rare occasions occur in patients with CNS lesions involving the respiratory control system. In central apnea, the inspiratory drive ceases, as manifested by the lack of diaphragmatic and intercostal muscle activity.

In the obstructive type, intermittent closure of the upper airway at the level of the oropharynx prevents the airflow despite inspiratory muscle contractions. Several structural abnormalities predispose to obstructive apnea, such as hypertrophic tonsils and adenoids, large tongue, and recessed jaw. In most patients, however, no clinically apparent anatomical abnormality of the upper airway can be identified.

As most patients with obstructive sleep apnea are overweight, it appears that obesity contributes to pharyngeal obstruction during sleep. Studies of the upper airways by various means, including computed tomography (CT), have shown that in these patients the upper airway at the level of the oropharynx has smaller than normal dimensions and is more collapsible. The soft palate (including the uvula), base of the tongue, and loose pharyngeal wall contribute to airway narrowing. It is readily apparent (Fig. 24–1) that lack of muscle tone in this region would result in further narrowing of the oropharynx.

Genioglossus is the most important muscle of the tongue, whose active contraction with inspiration prevents the closure of the airway at this level. Whenever the negative pressure during inspiration, which tends to collapse the pharynx, cannot be overcome by dilating muscular force, airway occlusion occurs. As was mentioned earlier, the inspiratory activity of the pharyngeal muscles is normally diminished during sleep. In obstructive sleep apnea, the inspiratory activity of these muscles, particularly the genioglossus, has been shown to be absent during apnea; as a result, the base of the tongue touches the soft palate and the uvula, pushing

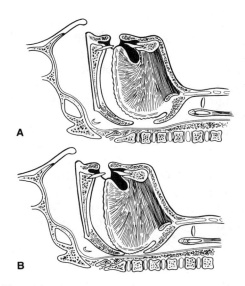

Figure 24–1. Upper airway in obstructive sleep apnea. (A), during wakefulness. (B), during sleep. Note that during sleep the relaxation of the genioglossus muscle results in backward displacement of the base of the tongue, which touches the soft palate, uvula, and posterior pharyngeal wall, causing upper airway obstruction.

them against the posterior pharyngeal wall. With the inspiratory effort, the intraluminal negative pressure of the upper airway completes its obstruction. Thus in obstructive apnea, both anatomic abnormality of the upper airway and functional impairment of its musculature from lack of inspiratory neural drive are involved in airway obstruction during sleep. Progressive increase in hypoxemia, hypercapnia, and inspiratory muscle effort results in arousal and subsequent reactivation of upper airway dilating muscles and resumption of ventilation. The cycle repeats throughout the sleeping hours with varying frequency and duration, depending on the stage of sleep and arousability.

REM sleep, in which arousability is reduced, is associated with more frequent and more severe apneic episodes. It should be noted that loud snoring, an invariable feature of this disorder, is the result of vibration of the palate and the uvula between the tongue and the pharyngeal wall when the air passage is incompletely obstructed. Habitual snoring is considered to be an important risk factor for the development of obstructive sleep apnea. It has been demonstrated that the upper airway in snorers is narrower and flabbier than in non-snorers. It seems that from both temporal and pathophysiologic standpoints, snoring represents an intermediate stage between a normal upper airway function and airway obstruction of sleep apnea.

Pathophysiology. The major physiologic consequence of sleep apnea is the development of hypoxemia, which depends not only on the frequency and duration of apneic episodes, but also on the baseline arterial oxygen content and lung volume. Cessation of ventilation, as expected, results in both hypoxemia and hypercapnia; however, the severity of hypoxemia during apneic episodes is out of proportion to the degree of alveolar hypoventilation indicated by the rising $PaCO_2$. Reduced FRC, which may be less than closing volume, results

in a significant abnormality of gas transport and, therefore, contributes to hypoxemia. Oxygen desaturation is usually more pronounced with obstructive apnea than with central apnea.

Repeated interruption of sleep during the night results from frequent arousals when hypoxemia and hypercapnia are severe enough at the end of apneic episodes. The resumption of respiration signifies arousal or change in the state of sleep from a deeper to a lighter stage. Fragmented and restless sleep is the major cause of daytime somnolence, which is one of the characteristic features of sleep apnea syndrome. Severe hypoxemia in association with altered autonomic nervous system function causes cardiac arrhythmia and elevation of blood pressure. In the advanced stage of the syndrome, repeated episodes of nocturnal hypoxemia and hypercapnia over several years may result in pulmonary hypertension, polycythemia, and eventual heart failure. It seems that with progression of this syndrome, there is further impairment of ventilatory control due to changes in blood gases as well as sleep deprivation; thus, a vicious circle develops (Fig. 24–2). Sleep apnea syndrome in association with severe obesity, if untreated, often advances to a state of

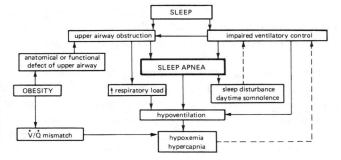

Figure 24–2. Schematic demonstration of pathogenesis of sleep apnea syndrome. Note that the abnormalities of both the upper airway and ventilatory control mechanisms are involved.

persistent hypoventilation throughout the day, and the characteristic picture of Pickwickian syndrome develops.

Clinical Manifestations. Patients with infrequent and short apneic episodes usually have no significant symptoms. Most patients with sleep apnea syndrome are middle-aged males. Excessive daytime sleepiness and nocturnal insomnia are the most common complaints. In the most prevalent obstructive type, loud snoring, silence of cessation of breathing, and its resumption with a blasting snort are invariably present and reported by the distraught spouse. Restlessness and abnormal motor activities, such as flinging the arms and the legs around, are common. Patients usually wake up in the morning tired and often with a headache. Alcohol intake and sleeping medications make the matter worse. Daytime somnolence may occur at any time, even during physical activity. Personality changes and decreased intellectual function have been reported. Systemic hypertension is a frequently associated condition.

The findings on the physical examination may be normal, but most patients with this disorder are obese. In severe cases, patients may fall asleep during the interview or the physical examination. In a minority of patients, gross abnormalities of the upper airway (such as nasal obstruction, large tonsils and adenoids, enlarged tongue, or recessed lower jaw) may be detected. Pickwickian syndrome is characterized by extreme obesity, cyanosis, and signs of right-side heart failure.

Diagnosis. A diagnosis of sleep apnea syndrome should be suspected in patients presenting with the above-mentioned symptoms and physical findings. Although careful observation of the patient during sleep gives important clues to the diagnosis, study in a sleep laboratory is necessary not only to establish the diagnosis but also to assess its severity and the mechanism of its production. **Polysomnography** is the simultaneous recordings of CNS, respiratory, and cardiac functions during sleep (p. 56). Recording of the airflow at the mouth and the nostrils, and of the thoracic and abdominal movement shows the number and the duration of apneas and identifies their type. Ear oximetry, which monitors oxygen saturation, is important in assessing the clinical significance of apneic episodes. The state and the stage of sleep are determined by EEG and EOG (**electrooculogram**). The electrocardiographic tracing shows changes in the heart rate and rhythm in association with apnea. Cardiac arrhythmia is a frequent finding with severe sleep apnea and is the cause of significant morbidity and even mortality. The presence of over 30 apneic episodes during a night's sleep, especially when they occur during the NREM sleep, is abnormal. Most patients with sleep apnea syndrome will have up to 200 to 300 such episodes during a 7-hour sleep. They may spend over half the sleeping time without ventilation. Oxygen desaturation to critically low levels is not unusual.

Functional and anatomic studies of the upper airways by different methods may demonstrate abnormalities. The maximum flow-volume loop and the CT scan are most informative in this regard.

Management. The proper management of patients with sleep apnea syndrome necessitates an accurate diagnosis of its presence, severity, and cause. In less severe cases, simpler measures, such as weight reduction and avoidance of alcohol and other CNS depressants, may suffice. Such patients, however, should be followed closely as they may progress to more severe stages of the disease. Administration of oxygen during sleep should be considered for nocturnal hypoxemia after cardiopulmonary sleep study with adequate monitoring. No uniformly effective therapy exists for predominantly central sleep apnea; respiratory stimulants, a rocking bed, a negative pressure ventilator such as the chest cuirass, and, occasionally, a positive pressure ventilator may be used. Electrical pacing of the diaphragm has been used in a few patients with some success.

In predominantly obstructive or mixed apneas, bypassing the obstructing site with a tracheostomy is considered to be the most effective therapeutic measure. However, technical difficulty in some patients, the potential complications, and lack of its acceptability by most patients are its main drawbacks. Methods that can maintain upper airway patency have proven successful in numerous instances. One such method is the application of continuous positive airway pressure (CPAP) through the nose. Acting as an internal pneumatic splint, nasal CPAP prevents upper airway collapse during inspiration. Its beneficial effect is almost as dramatic as the tracheostomy. With the restoration of a consolidated sleep pattern, daytime somnolence improves rapidly. After nightly application of nasal CPAP for several weeks, most patients will not need it every night. Its periodic use, however, will be necessary for prevention of relapse. Expiratory positive air-

way pressure (EPAP) may also be effective. Its beneficial effect is by increasing the FRC, which in turn improves gas exchange.

Reconstructive surgery of the pharynx and the palate and the application of various prosthetic devices in selected patients appear to be effective in relieving the obstruction, but more studies and longer follow-up are necessary before their role in treatment of this disorder is established. The benefit of surgery in patients with well-defined anatomic lesions is obvious.

EFFECT OF SLEEP ON CHRONIC RESPIRATORY DISORDERS

Sleep apnea syndrome may also occur in a setting of chronic respiratory disorders. Because of the presence of an already recognized underlying condition, sleep apnea syndrome in patients with these disorders is usually not suspected. Many patients with COPD, kyphoscoliosis, and various neuromuscular disorders are identified by sleep study to also have obstructive sleep apnea.

Other sleep-related respiratory dysfunctions, discussed at the beginning of this chapter, are known to contribute to the symptoms and the complications in patients with chronic pulmonary or ventilatory disorders. The worsening of arterial oxygen desaturation during sleep, especially in the REM state, is commonly observed. The severity of the disturbance of blood gases during sleep cannot reliably be predicted from the abnormality of pulmonary function tests or arterial blood studies during wakefulness. However, it has been demonstrated that in COPD, **blue bloaters** tend to have more severe nocturnal oxygen desaturation than **pink puffers.**

Certain features should alert the respiratory care provider to the possibility of sleep-related disturbances in patients with chronic respiratory disease. These include insomnia, sudden awakening with a choking sensation, and severe morning headaches. Pulmonary hypertension and cor pulmonale out of proportion to the degree of pulmonary functional impairment and awake blood gas values are other manifestations. When sleep-related disorders are suspected, the monitoring of oxygen saturation by pulse oximetry and electrocardiography during a night's sleep are indicated. Selected patients may require polysomnography. Patients with chest wall deformity and chronic neuromuscular disorders who demonstrate evidence of chronic hypoventilation, polycythemia, pulmonary hypertension, and daytime somnolence and fatigue should be considered for sleep studies. It is important to identify the subjects who will benefit from nocturnal oxygen therapy.

Patients with other chronic respiratory problems may likewise have sleep-related worsening of their conditions. In congestive heart failure, in addition to well-known Cheyne-Stokes respiration, recurrent apneas may occur during sleep. Some of these patients may benefit from nasal CPAP. Many asthmatics are known to have nocturnal exacerbation of their asthma (See Chapter 9).

BIBLIOGRAPHY

American Thoracic Society. Indications and standards for cardiopulmonary sleep studies. *Am Rev Respir Dis.* 1989; 139:559–568.

Berthon-Jones M, Sullivan CE. Ventilatory and arousal responses to hypoxia in sleeping humans. *Am Rev Respir Dis.* 1982; 125:632–639.

Block AJ, Faulkner JA, Hughes RL, et al. Factors influencing upper airway closure. *Chest.* 1984; 86:114–122.

Borowiecki BD, Sassin JF. Surgical treatment of sleep apnea. *Arch Otolaryngol.* 1983; 109:508–512.

Collop NA, Block AJ, Hellard D. The effect of nightly nasal CPAP treatment on underlying obstructive sleep apnea and pharyngeal size. *Chest.* 1991; 99:85–860.

Culver BH. Pulmonary responses to sleep. *Respir Care.* 1989; 34:510–515.

Douglas NJ, Flenley DC. Breathing during sleep in patients with obstructive lung disease. *Am Rev Respir Dis.* 1990; 141:1055–1070.

Douglas NJ, White DP, Weil JV, et al. Hypercapnic ventilatory response in sleeping adults. *Am Rev Respir Dis.* 1982; 126:758–762.

Funsten AW, Suratt PM. Evaluation of respiratory disorders during sleep. *Clin Chest Med.* 1989; 10:265–276.

Guilleminault C. Obstructive sleep apnea. *Med Clin North Am.* 1985; 69:1187–1203.

Guilleminault C, Stoohs R, Duncan S. Snoring: daytime sleepiness in regular heavy snorers. *Chest.* 1991; 99:40–48.

Hudgel DW, Harasick T, Katz RL, et al. Uvulopalatopharyngoplasty in obstructive apnea. *Am Rev Respir Dis.* 1991; 143:942–946.

Kuna ST, Bedi DG, Ryckman C. Effect of nasal airway positive pressure on upper airway size and configuration. *Am Rev Respir Dis.* 1988; 138:969–975.

Midgren B. Oxygen desaturation during sleep as a function of the underlying respiratory disease. *Am Rev Respir Dis.* 1990; 141:43–46.

Parish JM, Shepard JW Jr. Cardiovascular effects of sleep disorders. *Chest.* 1990; 97:1220–1226.

Remmers JE. Sleeping and breathing. *Chest.* 1990; 93(3 suppl):77S–80S.

Sanders MH, Kern N. Obstructive sleep apnea treated by independently adjusted inspiratory and expiratory positive airway pressure via nasal mask: physiologic and clinical implications. *Chest.* 1990; 98:317–324.

Shepard JW Jr. Cardiopulmonary consequences of obstructive sleep apnea. *Mayo Clin Proc.* 1990; 65:1250–1259.

Staats BA, Bonekat HW, Harris CD, Offord KP. Chest wall motion in sleep apnea. *Am Rev Respir Dis.* 1984; 130:59–63.

Strohl KP, Cherniack NS, Gothe B. Physiologic basis of therapy for sleep apnea. *Am Rev Respir Dis.* 1986; 134:791–802.

Sullivan CE, Issa FG, Berthon-Jones M, Eves L. Reversal of obstructive sleep apnea by continuous positive airway pressure applied through the nares. *Lancet.* 1981; 1:862–865.

Waldhorn RE, Herrick TW, Nguyen MC, et al. Long-term compliance with nasal continuous positive airway pressure therapy of obstructive sleep apnea. *Chest.* 1990; 97:33–38.

Wiggins RV, Schmidt-Nowara WW. Treatment of the obstructive sleep apnea syndrome. *West J Med.* 1987; 147:561–568.

Respiratory Failure

CHAPTER 25

Respiratory Failure

Throughout this book, the effect of various diseases on respiratory function and its disturbance by different mechanisms have been discussed. Impairment of respiratory function may be minimal and only detectable by very sensitive laboratory tests, or it may be severe enough to result in symptoms and easily detectable abnormalities on physical examination and routine laboratory studies. As the respiratory system fails to maintain its principal functions, that is, adequate oxygenation of arterial blood and/or proper elimination of carbon dioxide with normal activities, it is no more *sufficient*. This state of functional impairment is, thus, termed *respiratory insufficiency* or *failure*.

Respiratory insufficiency may be acute, chronic, or both. In *chronic respiratory insufficiency,* slow development and long duration of disturbances of lung function will allow for intervention of various *compensatory mechanisms,* which prevent, or at least diminish, the harmful effect on the body homeostasis. These compensatory mechanisms include changes in respiratory pattern and utilization of accessory respiratory muscles to overcome the increased airway resistance and reduced compliance; hyperventilation to increase carbon diox-

ide elimination and alveolar oxygen tension; circulatory adjustment to improve oxygen transport, particularly to more vital organs; alteration in blood to facilitate oxygen delivery to tissues; and renal compensation to ameliorate acid-base derangement. Reduction in physical activity, which is a major mechanism to cope with respiratory insufficiency, determines the degree of disability that results.

In *acute respiratory insufficiency* or *failure,* because of rapidity of development of respiratory impairment, the compensatory mechanisms will be inadequate for prevention of serious consequences. Inadequate tissue oxygenation and/or severe acid-base disturbance will ensue unless appropriate measures are undertaken. It is now customary to define acute respiratory failure on the basis of arterial blood gas abnormalities, that is, acute reduction of arterial blood PO_2 below 60 torr (at sea level) and/or acute elevation of arterial blood PCO_2 above 50 torr as a consequence of impaired respiratory function.

It should be emphasized that the above definition is valid only in cases in which baseline arterial blood gases are known, or assumed, to be normal. In patients with established chronic hypoxemia and/or hypercapnia, it is the *acute deterioration* of blood gases, rather than their absolute values, that characterizes acute respiratory failure. In other situations, although the acuteness of hypercapnia can be inferred from the expected reduction in arterial blood pH, the acuteness of hypoxemia can only be ascertained retrospectively by its clinical course.

Classification. In addition to its division into acute and chronic forms, respiratory failure has also been classified according to the predominance of the mechanism involved in its pathogenesis. When the primary abnormality involves the respiratory pump, with or without significant lung disease, inadequate alveolar ventilation manifested by hypercapnia is appropriately referred to as *ventilatory failure*. Hypoxemia in this setting is the result of low alveolar oxygen tension and is proportional to the increase in arterial carbon dioxide tension. On the other hand, when the primary abnormality is an impairment of oxygen transport because of pulmonary parenchymal injury, the term *hypoxemic respiratory failure* applies. In this type, alveolar ventilation is increased or at least normal. Adult respiratory distress syndrome (ARDS) is the prototype of hypoxemic respiratory failure. With hypercapnia, when the severity of hypoxemia is out of proportion to CO_2 retention, respiratory failure results from a combination of inadequate ventilation and abnormal pulmonary gas transport. This type, which is known as *hypoxemic-hypercapnic respiratory failure,* is usually indicative of a markedly deranged ventilation-perfusion relationship and is characteristically seen in chronic airway disease.

Pathogenesis and Etiology. For understanding of the pathogenesis of respiratory failure, it is imperative that the reader be familiar with the mechanisms by which arterial oxygen and carbon dioxide tensions are maintained within physiologic range despite continuous variation of metabolic activity. Although oxygenation of arterial blood and elimination of carbon dioxide are interrelated, the mechanisms of their regulations are quite different.

The *control of carbon dioxide*, being part of a delicate hydrogen ion regulation, is much more precise. It is accomplished by ventilatory response through various sensitive receptors. The level of alveolar ventilation is so well adjusted to the metabolic rate that normally the arterial blood pH is maintained within a remarkably narrow range (7.4 ± 0.04) by elimination of carbon dioxide, the byproduct of tissue metabolism. Thus the arterial blood carbon dioxide tension is also held within normal range. The dependency of carbon dioxide regulation on hydrogen ion metabolism is evident by the fact that chemoreceptors are primarily sensitive to the hydrogen ion concentration and that their apparent sensitivity to CO_2 is probably mediated through local production of H^+.

The stimuli from chemoreceptors as well as from other sources are integrated in the *respiratory center*, which sends nerve impulses to the *respiratory muscles*. The orderly contraction of these muscles performs the work necessary for rhythmic expansion of thoracic cavity. The increase of thoracic volume results in lowering the intrathoracic and, therefore, intraalveolar pressure. Air flow is the result of the pressure difference between two areas. During inspiration the pressure in the alveoli is below atmospheric pressure and flow is toward the alveoli; during expiration, recoil of lungs and thoracic wall increases the intrathoracic and intraalveolar pressures and air flow is directed to the outside. The amount of inspired or expired air during the cycle (tidal volume) and the rate of breathing determine the minute ventilation. Normally, about 70% of ventilation is effective in gas exchange, which is known as alveolar ventilation. It is the alveolar ventilation that eliminates the carbon dioxide accumulated in alveoli, thus maintaining its tension at normal range. Because of its ready diffusibility, carbon dioxide tension in the alveoli is practically the same as in the blood leaving them (ie, arterial blood). The integrity of this sensitive ventilatory control system ensures the elimination of the exact amount of carbon dioxide produced with the body metabolism, and thus maintains the arterial blood pH and PCO_2 within the normal range.

The mechanism of *regulation of oxygen intake* is not that precise, and the ventilatory response to O_2 lack is less sensitive and less effective. In health, the control of oxygen uptake is operative, at least partly, through carbon dioxide and H^+ regulation. There is only a small ventilatory response to low arterial blood PO_2 per se until it has fallen to below 50 torr. The increased tissue requirement of O_2 is mostly met by circulatory response to various stimuli. The ventilatory response to CO_2 and H^+ regulation along with increased blood flow provides the necessary supply of oxygen. Other factors, including change of affinity of hemoglobin, also facilitate oxygen delivery.

In respiratory failure there is derangement of these regulatory mechanisms at various parts of ventilatory control system and/or marked abnormality of pulmonary gas transport. Respiratory failure may, therefore, result from malfunction of the respiratory center, abnormal respiratory neuromuscular system, diseases of the chest wall, airway obstruction, or parenchymal lung disorders. The important disorders leading to respiratory failure, classified according to the major areas of involvement of respiratory control system, are as follows:

I. Intrinsic lung and airway diseases
   A. Large airway obstruction
      1. Congenital deformities
      2. Acute laryngitis
      3. Foreign bodies
      4. Intrinsic tumors
      5. Extrinsic pressure
      6. Traumatic injury
      7. Enlarged tonsils and adenoids
      8. Obstructive sleep apnea
   B. Bronchial diseases
      1. Chronic bronchitis
      2. Asthma
      3. Acute bronchiolitis
   C. Parenchymal diseases
      1. Pulmonary emphysema
      2. Pulmonary fibrosis and other chronic diffuse infiltrative diseases
      3. Severe pneumonia
      4. Acute lung injury from various causes (ARDS)
   D. Cardiovascular disease
      1. Cardiac pulmonary edema
      2. Massive or recurrent pulmonary embolism
      3. Vasculitis, pulmonary
II. Extrapulmonary disorders
   A. Diseases of pleura and chest wall

1. Pneumothorax
2. Pleural effusion
3. Fibrothorax
4. Thoracic wall deformity
5. Traumatic injury to the chest wall: flail chest
6. Obesity

B. Disorders of respiratory muscles and neuromuscular junction
    1. Myasthenia gravis and myasthenia-like disorders
    2. Muscular dystrophies
    3. Polymyositis
    4. Botulism
    5. Muscle-paralyzing drugs
    6. Severe hypokalemia and hypophosphatemia

C. Disorders of peripheral nerves and spinal cord
    1. Poliomyelitis
    2. Guillain-Barré syndrome
    3. Spinal cord trauma (quadriplegia)
    4. Amyotrophic lateral sclerosis
    5. Tetanus
    6. Multiple sclerosis

D. Disorders of central nervous system
    1. Sedative and narcotic drug overdose
    2. Head trauma
    3. Cerebral hypoxia
    4. Cerebrovascular accident
    5. Central nervous system infection
    6. Epileptic seizure: status epilepticus
    7. Metabolic and endocrine disorders
    8. Bulbar poliomyelitis
    9. Primary alveolar hypoventilation
    10. Sleep apnea syndrome

Many of these disorders have been discussed in appropriate chapters of this book.

In addition to the basic disease leading to respiratory failure, certain precipitating or exacerbating factors are operative, such as the following:

1. Changes of tracheobronchial secretions
2. Infection: viral or bacterial
3. Disturbance of tracheobronchial clearance
4. Drugs: sedatives, narcotics, anesthesia, oxygen
5. Inhalation or aspiration of irritants, vomitus, foreign body
6. Cardiovascular disorders: heart failure, pulmonary embolism, shock
7. Mechanical factors: pneumothorax, pleural effusion, abdominal distension
8. Trauma, including surgery
9. Neuromuscular abnormalities
10. Allergic disorders: bronchospasm
11. Increased oxygen demand: fever, infection
12. Inspiratory muscle fatigue

These precipitating factors play a very important role in exacerbation of preexisting respiratory insufficiency. In practically every case of acute respiratory failure superimposed on chronic pulmonary disease, one or more of these factors can be identified. Because of their reversibility, their early detection and prompt treatment are essential in proper management of acute respiratory failure. Respiratory muscle fatigue has been demonstrated to be an important factor in precipitating as well as in perpetuating respiratory failure.

Certain factors associated with respiratory failure are considered both among leading causes and precipitating causes. Pulmonary infection may be the major or even the only cause of acute respiratory failure in widespread pneumonia, whereas it is a frequent precipitating factor in chronic obstructive lung disease. The ingestion of large amounts of narcotic and sedative drugs is a common cause of acute respiratory failure in otherwise normal individuals, but in patients with chronic lung disease, even a small amount of such drugs may precipitate an episode of respiratory failure. This is also true for heart failure, pulmonary embolism, aspiration, surgery, pneumothorax, and many others.

Pathophysiology. Abnormal gas exchange is the dominating physiologic alteration in respiratory failure. Hypoxemia, common to all forms of respiratory failure, may be caused by any of the following basic mechanisms, singly or in various combinations:

1. **Alveolar hypoventilation** results in an increase in the alveolar PCO_2, which in turn is the cause of low alveolar PO_2. Even with a normal alveolar-arterial PO_2 gradient, low alveolar PO_2 results in arterial hypoxemia. Hypoxemia in ventilatory failure is due to this mechanism.

2. **Impairment of diffusion,** although present in emphysema and other diffuse lung injury, has only an insignificant role in the hypoxemia of acute respiratory failure. The alveolar-arterial oxygen tension gradient solely from a diffusion defect is usually small and readily compensated by even a small increase in the fractional concentration of inspired oxygen (FIO_2).

3. **Ventilation-perfusion mismatching** is the most common cause of hypoxemia in clinical situations. Disorders involving the airways result in uneven ventilation of various lung regions and units whose perfusion frequently fails to match the changes of ventilation (Fig. 25–1). Both chronic lung diseases and most acute leading or precipitating causes of respiratory failure are known to be associated with ventilation-perfusion inequality.

4. **Right-to-left shunt** as a cause of hypoxemia in acute respiratory failure is the result of continuous perfusion of nonventilated regions of the lung (Fig. 25–2). It almost always indicates the closure of air passages, especially the distal airways and alveoli, by various causes so common in acute respiratory failure.

5. **Reduced oxygen in mixed venous blood.** In addition to the above basic mechanisms, extrapulmonary factors such as cardiac output and metabolic rate are known to affect arterial PO_2 tension, particularly in association with abnormal pulmonary gas exchange. Increased oxygen extraction from the arterial blood in these clinical situations results in reduced mixed-venous blood PO_2. Any degree of hypoxemia from pulmonary causes, especially with a right-to-left shunt and ventilation-perfusion mismatching, is aggravated by this extrapulmonary

mechanism, which is almost invariably present in critically ill patients.

Hypercapnia, the hallmark of ventilatory failure, is indicative of an alveolar ventilation that is inadequate for the proper elimination of carbon dioxide. Ventilation-perfusion mismatching, when not compensated by increased ventilation of well-perfused regions, is a significant cause of hypercapnia in chronic obstructive pulmonary disease. The clinical type of hypercapnic-hypoxemic respiratory failure most characteristically occurs in this setting.

In acute hypercapnia, as expected, arterial blood pH will be reduced, indicating acute respiratory acidosis. It should, however, be mentioned that the superimposition of metabolic acidosis on preexistent chronic respiratory alkalosis produces an arterial blood-gas picture indistinguishable from that of acute respiratory acidosis. With chronic hypercapnia, as seen in advanced cases of COPD, the onset of acute respiratory failure is indicated by a further increase of arterial PCO_2 to a very high level and a reduction of blood pH. Serum bicarbonate levels will be significantly increased.

In hypoxemic respiratory failure, arterial blood pH is usually alkalotic as a result of hyperventilation, unless it is offset by concomitant metabolic acidosis of tissue hypoxia. The combination of acute hypercapnia in ventilatory failure and metabolic acidosis causes a more severe reduction in pH (mixed respiratory and metabolic acidosis).

The major impact of respiratory failure on various organs is through hypoxemia and disturbance in acid-base balance mainly from hypercapnia. However, it should be emphasized that hypoxemia usually has more disastrous consequences and its effect on vital organs is more damaging than hypercapnia. Practically every organ and tissue may suffer from hypoxemia, and acidosis is known to impair many cellular functions. Both hypoxemia and acidosis result in increased pulmonary vascular resistance. Preexistent cor pulmonale in patients with chronic lung disease is aggravated by acute respiratory failure.

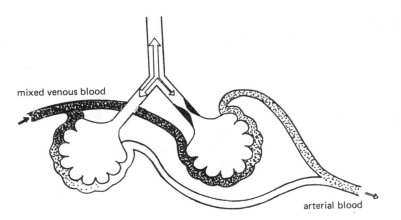

mixed venous blood

arterial blood

Figure 25–1. Mismatching of ventilation with perfusion. Perfusion in excess of ventilation resulting in arterial hypoxemia.

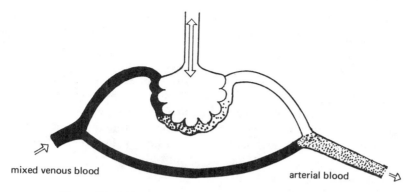

Figure 25–2. Hypoxemia resulting from venoarterial shunting.

The effect of hypoxemia on the myocardium not only is an additional cause of right-side heart failure, but left ventricular function is also impaired. Reduced cardiac output and cardiogenic pulmonary edema exacerbate hypoxemia. Respiratory muscles are also known to be affected by both hypoxemia and hypercapnia. Diaphragmatic fatigue, which can occur as a result of increased work load, may be precipitated by hypoxemia, reduced perfusion, and hypercapnia. It appears, therefore, that acute respiratory failure may reach a point when a positive feedback mechanism is established. This vicious circle results in the precipitous deterioration of respiratory failure and death unless appropriate treatment is instituted.

Clinical Manifestations. The clinical presentation of acute respiratory failure is a combination of clinical features of underlying disease and precipitating factor(s) and manifestations of hypoxemia and/or hypercapnia. As numerous pulmonary and extrapulmonary disorders may lead to acute respiratory failure and various factors may precipitate it, the clinical picture will be quite variable. Moreover, the presence or absence of preceding chronic respiratory insufficiency and predominance of hypoxemia or hypercapnia will further change the clinical manifestations.

The commonly mentioned symptom of dyspnea, which is the hallmark of hypoxemic respiratory failure, may be entirely absent in ventilatory failure resulting from depression of the respiratory center. The rate of respiration, likewise, will be quite variable; it is generally increased in hypoxemic respiratory failure and decreased in ventilatory failure due to respiratory-center depression. Although inadequacy of alveolar ventilation is **pathognomonic** for ventilatory failure, its bedside detection is often difficult if not impossible in most instances. It is not uncommon to make an assumption of adequacy of alveolar ventilation from the respiratory rate and apparent depth of breathing that turns out to be quite inaccurate by arterial blood gas analysis. Use of accessory muscles of respiration and intercostal or supraclavicular retraction are indicative of significant mechanical impediment to respiration and increased ventilatory effort. As with dyspnea, these signs may be totally absent in central hypoventilation. In diaphragmatic weakness or fatigue, paradoxical abdominal movement is a characteristic finding.

Cyanosis, although not very sensitive, is a common feature of hypoxemic respiratory failure. Lack of improvement of cyanosis on breathing oxygen usually signifies severe gas transport abnormality, shunting, or poor tissue perfusion.

Other respiratory symptoms and physical findings on examination of the chest will depend on underlying chronic or acute pulmonary disease leading to or aggravating respiratory failure. These have been discussed in appropriate chapters dealing with specific disease states. Signs of right-side heart failure (cor pulmonale), including peripheral edema, engorged neck veins, and enlarged liver, are usually indicative of chronic underlying pulmonary condition.

Clinical manifestations of hypoxemia and hypercapnia are discussed in Chapter 1. It should be emphasized that most of these manifestations are common for both hypoxemia and acidosis from hypercapnia. They include change in mental state, headaches, weakness, lassitude, and muscle tremor or twitching. Drowsiness, confusion, somnolence, irritability, agitation, and coma are some of the usual mental changes due to severe hypoxemia with or without hypercapnia. Increased intracranial pressure, sometimes manifested by changes in the eyeground, is fairly common in both of these conditions. Cardiac arrhythmias are common manifestations of acute respiratory failure. Bronchodilators, including aminophylline and beta-adrenergics, are known to cause or aggravate cardiac arrhythmias, especially in patients with hypoxemia and/or acidosis.

Radiographic Findings. Radiographic examination of the chest is essential for the diagnosis of underlying, as well as precipitating, causes of respiratory failure. As with symptoms and physical findings, chest x-ray changes in respiratory failure will vary with underlying disease. It may be entirely normal in ventilatory failure due to extrapulmonary disorders. Changes of COPD or diffuse fibrosis, with or without superimposed acute changes due to infection or other complicating and precipitating pulmonary events, are common radiographic findings in chronic cases. Most cases of acute hypoxemic respiratory failure without underlying chronic lung disease manifest with bilateral diffuse interstitial and air-space densities suggesting pulmonary edema (p 364).

Radiographic studies are important for the proper follow-up of patients with acute respiratory failure and for the early detection of complications, such as superinfection, atelectasis, pneumothorax, and other mishaps of intubation and mechanical ventilation.

Diagnosis. Although the history, physical examination, and radiographic findings are very important for the diagnosis of respiratory failure, it can be conclusively established only by determination of the blood gases and pH. These tests are essential not only for the diagnosis, classification, and assessment of the severity of respiratory failure, but are also indispensable for the evaluation of its progress and response to therapeutic measures. With a diagnosis of respiratory failure, the identification of its underlying cause and the recognition of the precipitating event(s) are crucial for an appropriate management plan.

The presence and the extent of

parenchymal lung disease, particularly acute lung injury and inflammation, are best assessed by radiographic examination. Infection, being one of the most common causes of respiratory failure, should always be suspected and properly evaluated. Examination of the sputum, among other bacteriologic studies, is essential for its detection. Airway obstruction should be confirmed and its severity gauged by flow studies such as measurement of peak expiratory flow. Other variables of respiratory mechanics are evaluated by determining tidal volume, minute ventilation, vital capacity, and maximum inspiratory and expiratory pressures. Determination of the latter is essential for the diagnosis of disorders of the respiratory pump resulting in ventilatory failure or contributing to other forms of respiratory failure.

As will be discussed later in this chapter, one of the important differentiations in respiratory failure is between cardiogenic pulmonary edema and adult respiratory distress syndrome (ARDS). Pulmonary artery catheterization with a balloon-flotation catheter is useful for this purpose. It may also give valuable information for the proper management of patients with acute respiratory failure in whom concomitant cardiac impairment and fluid imbalance are quite common.

MANAGEMENT OF RESPIRATORY FAILURE

General Principles

Principles of management are applicable to all forms of acute respiratory failure, although the therapeutic approach will vary according to the particular underlying disease, predisposing factor(s),

and pathophysiologic abnormalities. Establishment and maintenance of an adequate airway, proper oxygenation, correction of acid-base disturbance, restoration of water and electrolyte balance, improvement of circulatory status, treatment of underlying correctable conditions and precipitating causes, and prevention of potential complications are measures that should be followed in every patient with respiratory failure.

Management of patients with acute respiratory failure superimposed on chronic pulmonary disease is somewhat different from management of patients whose respiratory failure is due to acute pulmonary injury or extrapulmonary conditions. This distinction is especially important in deciding for tracheal intubation and mechanical ventilation.

Treatment of the underlying disease and precipitating conditions should be combined with measures intended for correction of *pathophysiologic* changes of acute respiratory failure.

Although the following steps in the management of respiratory failure are discussed separately, in most clinical settings they are carried out more or less concurrently. Moreover, certain measures are effective in correcting more than one abnormality.

Establishment and Maintenance of Adequate Airway. It is essential that an adequate airway be provided at all times for a patient with respiratory failure. In patients with upper airway obstruction as the cause of respiratory failure, the establishment of a patent airway will immediately restore ventilation. This is discussed in Chapter 7. Use of simple devices, such as oropharyngeal or nasopharyngeal tubes, will suffice in certain situations (eg, during transient loss of consciousness). In many instances, particularly when there is a need for ventilatory support, tracheal intubation is necessary (page 352).

In addition to providing an appropriate airway for mechanical ventilation, tracheal intubation may be indicated for protecting the lung from aspiration, for maintenance of airway patency, and for effective suctioning.

As secretions and other materials in the airways are frequent causes of airway obstruction, the importance of adequate tracheobronchial toilet, with or without tracheal intubation, cannot be overstressed. Deep breathing and coughing, postural drainage and other physiotherapeutic maneuvers, and tracheobronchial suctioning should be considered in every patient with respiratory failure. Many times, the success or failure of therapy will depend on adequacy and proper application of these measures. The presence of a tracheal tube makes its care, as well as tracheobronchial hygiene, even more important.

Oxygenation. The proper supply of oxygen to the tissues is the major concern in the management of patients with respiratory failure, as the lack of adequate tissue oxygenation is the most important deleterious consequence of this condition.

In addition to the arterial blood oxygen content, tissue oxygenation depends on its blood supply. For an adequate tissue oxygen delivery, cardiac output and tissue perfusion are at least as important as the arterial blood oxygen level.

Chronic hypoxemia, sometimes to a severe degree, is usually well tolerated. Certain adaptive mechanisms, including changes in blood perfusion, shift of the oxyhemoglobin dissociation curve, reduced metabolic activities, and perhaps more efficient oxygen extraction by the tissues, are operative in chronic hypoxemia. On the other hand, *acute* hypoxemia usually results in significant tissue hypoxia because of the lack of adaptive mechanisms. Obviously, the easiest way of improving the arterial oxygen tension is to increase the inspired oxygen concentration. It should be emphasized, however, that the maneuvers which improve alveolar ventilation and gas distribution will also result in enhancement of arterial blood oxygenation.

In acute respiratory failure, oxygen may be administered by various means to increase the arterial oxygen tension to a satisfactory level, which varies according to the duration of hypoxemia and other circumstances of respiratory failure. In hypoxemia without ventilatory failure (normal or low PCO_2), the administration of oxygen usually restores an adequate arterial PO_2 and, unless the FIO_2 exceeds 0.5 for a prolonged period of time, it is quite safe.

In hypercapnic states, however, oxygen should be given more judiciously. As many patients with hypercapnia have decreased ventilatory response to PCO_2 and H^+, hypoxemia is their major remaining respiratory stimulus. In addition, by eliminating hypoxic pulmonary vasoconstriction, oxygen administration may enhance ventilation-perfusion mismatching. This mechanism may be even more important than inhibition of hypoxic ventilatory drive. Regardless of the mechanism involved, inappropriate oxygen administration in hypercapnic patients may result in further CO_2 retention and respiratory acidosis. Fortunately, in most instances of hypoxemia with ventilatory impairment, a small increment in concentration of inspired oxygen is sufficient for a clinically significant improvement in oxygenation. Because of the steepness of the oxyhemoglobin dissociation curve in hypoxemic range, a modest increase in the arterial oxygen tension results in a significant improvement of the oxygen content.

For example, raising the arterial oxygen tension from 30 to 50 torr results in an increase in its saturation from 57% to 83.5% (Fig. 25–3). This is the rationale for *controlled oxygen therapy* in patients with acute respiratory failure due to chronic obstructive pulmonary disease. It is conveniently accomplished by administration of oxygen via a Venturi mask or judicious use of nasal O_2, which, along with monitoring arterial blood gases, will allow one to manage the acute and critical reduction of the arterial PO_2 in these patients, without aggravating their respiratory acidosis.

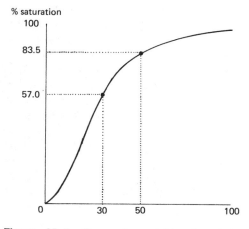

Figure 25–3. Oxygen-hemoglobin dissociation curve. At hypoxemic level, small rise in arterial PO_2 results in significant improvement of its oxygen content.

In practice there is no significant advantage in increasing the arterial PO_2 to over 60 torr; and, in many cases, PO_2 levels in the low 50s are acceptable. Continuous monitoring of arterial oxygen saturation with pulse oximetry is an important addition to a safer way of oxygen therapy.

In addition to increasing the arterial PO_2, tissue oxygenation is also improved by correcting anemia, restoring adequate cardiac output, and controlling fever.

In hypoxemic respiratory failure, such as adult respiratory distress syndrome, it is often difficult to adequately oxygenate the patients by simply increasing their FIO_2. In certain selected patients, especially when they are alert and cooperative, the addition of continuous positive airway pressure (CPAP) or expiratory positive airway pressure (EPAP) by a nasal or facial mask with a soft, tight seal helps oxygenation and may obviate the necessity for intubation and mechanical ventilation. In more severe cases with refractory and progressive hypoxemia, mechanical ventilatory support will be necessary.

Correction of Acid-Base Disturbance. As discussed earlier, respiratory failure is almost always accompanied by certain degrees of acid-base abnormalities. In *ventilatory* failure and hypoxic-hypercapnic respiratory failure, an increase in PCO_2 results in reduction of pH (acidosis), unless renal compensation increases the serum bicarbonate level. Renal compensation at very high PCO_2 levels is usually not complete, and the resultant pH will be somewhat acidotic. In acute ventilatory failure, renal compensation, which requires a certain time to take place, will be lacking; therefore, acute respiratory acidosis is always present. Furthermore, superimposition of metabolic acidosis, which is a fairly common occurrence, results in further reduction of the pH. In hypoxemic respiratory failure, on the other hand, hyperventilation and, thus, respiratory alkalosis may be evident. Severe tissue hypoxia may result in anaerobic metabolism, production of lactic acid, and hence metabolic acidosis.

Because in acute respiratory failure pH abnormality is more deleterious to the proper functions of vital organs than changes of PCO_2, emphasis should be placed on correction of pH and its maintenance rather than PCO_2. Metabolic acidosis is usually treated by administration of bicarbonate; however, correction of causes of metabolic derangement, such as severe hypoxemia, is essential for successful outcome. In acute hypercapnia with significant acidosis, improving the alveolar ventilation is the most logical approach. This can be accomplished by various means. In addition to mechanical ventilatory support (see below), simpler measures intended for improvement of alveolar ventilation, such as establishment and maintenance of an adequate airway, treating bronchospasm, controlling heart failure, and eliminating other precipitating factors discussed below should be undertaken. Controlling fever, sepsis, and other hypermetabolic states results in reduced CO_2 production and improvement of hypercapnia. Dietary adjustment (see below) is known to alter the respiratory exchange ratio and thus may also be helpful in reducing carbon dioxide production. Often times such measures will obviate the necessity for mechanical ventilation. The use of "respiratory center stimulants," except for aminophyl-

line and occasionally other drugs, has not shown significant therapeutic benefit. The use of depressant drugs, including indiscriminate oxygen administration, should be avoided. The use of bicarbonate in acute respiratory acidosis is controversial but may be considered in certain unusual circumstances.

Restoration of Cardiac Function and Fluid Balance. An injured lung tends to contain more extravascular water because of loss of integrity of the alveolar-capillary membrane. Moreover, cardiac malfunction is common in respiratory disease, particularly in acute respiratory failure. Cardiac decompensation may result in further accumulation of fluid in the lung and/or pleural space. It is, therefore, essential to control the fluid balance by monitoring fluid intake and output and the body weight to avoid excessive fluid administration and positive fluid balance. Cardiac abnormality should also be treated properly, keeping in mind that significant hypoxemia and acid-base imbalance impair cardiac function. Conversely, the function of respiratory muscles may be impaired by their inadequate blood flow as a result of low cardiac output. For proper management of combined respiratory and cardiac failure, hemodynamic monitoring, preferably with a pulmonary artery catheter, is advisable.

Treatment of Underlying Disease and Precipitating Factors. While patients with acute respiratory failure are being managed for the abnormalities of blood gases, disturbances of fluid and acid-base balance, and **hemodynamic** derangements, every effort should be made to identify and properly treat the underlying disease and precipitating factors. Management of various pulmonary or extrapulmonary disorders leading to respiratory failure has been discussed in appropriate chapters and will not be repeated here.

The factors that precipitate or contribute to acute respiratory failure are numerous (see page 340). Many of these disorders are treatable and, often, preventable. Respiratory tract infection seems to be the common culprit in this regard. It may be viral, bacterial, or rarely fungal in origin. Its prevention, early diagnosis, and treatment are crucial in management of respiratory failure.

Increased tracheobronchial secretions, changes in their characteristics, and difficulty in their elimination due to various factors may result in airway obstruction, particularly in patients with chronic obstructive pulmonary disease. As was emphasized before, proper tracheobronchial hygiene is one of the most important measures in management of these patients.

Congestive heart failure and other circulatory disorders are common precipitating events; they should be identified and appropriately treated. Bronchospasm, particularly in patients with a background of asthma, may be a significant reversible factor contributing to respiratory failure, which will respond to bronchodilators. Corticosteroids are often used in this and other situations in which the anti-inflammatory effects of these drugs are considered to be beneficial.

Organic or metabolic disorders affecting the central nervous system or neuromuscular function should always be considered when investigating the precipitating causes of respiratory decompensation. Sedative, hypnotic, and particularly narcotic drugs are poorly tolerated by patients with chronic ventilatory insufficiency, and may precipitate an acute episode of respiratory failure. The use of these agents should be discontinued, and, in case of narcotic drug intake, a proper antidote should be administered. Indiscriminate use of oxygen, which may aggravate CO_2 retention or even result in CO_2 narcosis, should be avoided.

The presence of air or fluid in the pleural cavity may significantly impair the ventilation; their removal may result in dramatic improvement in some patients. Abdominal distention, which may cause compression of the lung bases and interference with diaphragmatic movement, should be adequately treated and prevented from recurring. Use of respirator bags without a tracheal tube frequently results in distention of the stomach with air; this should be emptied by a nasogastric tube.

Respiratory impairment due to trauma and surgery, which may lead to or precipitate a bout of acute respiratory failure, is discussed in Chapter 22. Limitation of the thoracic wall movement, ineffective cough, immobility, and lack of deep breathing are among factors that contribute to respiratory difficulty under these circumstances.

Fever and other causes of heightened metabolism, which by increasing oxygen demand and carbon dioxide production contribute to respiratory failure, should be properly treated.

Fatigue of the respiratory muscles, especially the diaphragm, has been recognized as an important contributory factor in almost all forms of ventilatory failure. Its early recognition and treatment are essential parts of management of respiratory failure. Resting these muscles by mechanical ventilatory support is the most effective measure in restoring their contractility. Aminophylline and beta-adrenergic agonists are known to improve the contractile force of the diaphragm and delay its fatigue. Among disorders of electrolyte balance, deficiencies of serum phosphates, potassium, and calcium are known to impair respiratory muscle function. They should be properly identified and adequately corrected.

Nutritional Support. Nutritional deficiency is known to contribute to respiratory failure through different mechanisms. They include the impairment of respiratory muscle function, reduction of ventilatory drive, and weakening of pulmonary defenses. Malnourished patients usually have a reduced diaphragmatic muscle mass. Ventilatory response to hypoxemia is diminished following inadequate nutrition. Impaired immunologic defenses, especially from an alteration of cell-mediated immunity, in malnourished patients predisposes them further to various infections including nosocomial pneumonia. Poorly nourished subjects have significant difficulty in being weaned off mechanical ventilatory support necessitating prolonged and complicated hospitalization in critical care units. It is, therefore, essential that in the management of patients in respiratory failure, proper nutritional assessment and adequate nutritional support be steadfastly pursued. In most patients, enteral alimentation is preferred over parenteral feeding.

As most calories in usual nutritional formulas are derived from carbohydrates, patients receiving them have a high respiratory quotient (ratio of CO_2 production to O_2 consumption). The increased CO_2 production may contribute to hypercapnic respiratory failure and may become an obstacle against a successful weaning from mechanical ventilation. High lipid formulas, on the other hand, result in lower respiratory quotient and, therefore, may be more suitable for the nutritional support of patients in hypercapnic respiratory failure.

MECHANICAL VENTILATION

The following section focuses on the most commonly used conventional positive pressure ventilation. Discussion of the much less frequently used methods of negative pressure ventilation and the recently introduced, but still mostly experimental, high-frequency ventilation, is beyond the scope of this book.

Indications. The decision to institute tracheal intubation and mechanical ventilation is made by considering several factors that are quite variable from patient to patient. Although it is easy to decide in situations with obvious indication for ventilatory support, such as cardiopulmonary resuscitation, deeply comatose patients, respiratory muscle paralysis, postoperative or posttraumatic respiratory insufficiency, severe intractable asthma, refractory hypoxemia, and severe acute respiratory acidosis, the indication for mechanical ventilation in most other cases of respiratory failure is less precise. Generally, patients with *acute* and *reversible* underlying cause for respiratory failure, in whom artificial ventilation will not be prolonged, are more suitable candidates.

The decision to ventilate patients in respiratory failure with underlying chronic irreversible pulmonary or extrapulmonary disorders should be made with great care, in view of the fact that many such patients can be successfully managed without ventilatory support, and that intubation and mechanical ventilation are fraught with significant complications in these patients. In such patients, the result of conservative management with controlled oxygen therapy, adequate tracheobronchial toilet, elimination of infection, control of heart failure, and proper treatment of other precipitating conditions is usually better than the outcome with mechanical ventilation. Obviously, patients who are in advanced respiratory failure with severe respiratory acidosis, who are stuporous or comatose, who do not respond to proper and adequate conservative care, who show progressive deterioration of respiratory failure, or who demonstrate evidence of exhaustion should be intubated and ventilated. A critical level of hypoxemia that cannot be improved by controlled oxygen therapy without causing significant carbon dioxide retention and acidosis is generally considered an indication for ventilatory support.

As mechanical ventilation is intended to maintain the patient and tide him over the acute episode, it should be considered more seriously in situations where there are certain correctable and reversible disorders. On the other hand, patients with end-stage chronic destructive lung diseases or progressive degenerative neuromuscular conditions developing respiratory failure *without* a treatable precipitating cause are considered for mechanical ventilatory support only if the intention is to continue it indefinitely or until the very end.

The necessity for mechanical ventilation should be judged individually, taking several factors into consideration; however, certain guidelines have been proposed that help in deciding for ventilatory support in patients with acute respiratory failure. The most widely used criteria are as follows:

1. Vital capacity less than 10 mL/kg "ideal" body weight.
2. Minute ventilation less than 3 or more than 20 L.
3. Maximum inspiratory pressure less than 20 cm of H_2O.
4. P_aO_2, while on 50% oxygen by mask, less than 55 torr.
5. $P(A-aDO_2)$ on 100% oxygen, more than 450 torr.
6. P_aCO_2 more than 55 torr *and* pH less than 7.25.
7. V_D/V_T ratio more than 0.6.
8. Respiratory rate more than 35/min.

These guidelines should be used along with several other individual factors, including associated nonrespiratory conditions. Mechanical ventilatory support is often initiated when there is a good indication that the increased work of breathing necessary for adequate gas exchange cannot be sustained much longer, even with satisfactory arterial blood gases. In rapidly progressive respiratory insufficiency, such as seen in posttraumatic cases, the decision for institution of ventilatory support is made before the above parameters deteriorate to such abnormal levels, otherwise the patient may rapidly reach a moribund stage. Similarly, patients with CNS-depressant drug overdose are usually ventilated with no, or only minimal, deterioration of their respiratory function. On the other hand, in acute respiratory failure superimposed on chronic pulmonary disease, although several of the above criteria are met, conservative management (without mechanical ventilation) is often preferred.

The question of mechanical ventilation, as well as cardiopulmonary resuscitation (CPR), of patients with terminal and incurable disease is a difficult one, and cannot be answered without consideration of ethical, legal, socioeconomical, *and* medical issues. As the decision to discontinue ventilatory support is much more difficult and complicated, a great deal of circumspection should be exercised in deciding for the institution of artificial ventilation and/or CPR in such patients.

Intubation. Once it is determined that a patient needs mechanical ventilation, a proper method of *tracheal intubation* should be selected. Translaryngeal intubation with an orotracheal or nasotracheal tube is the method of choice, with the notable exception of certain types of upper airway obstruction and preexisting tracheostomy. Speed and ease of translaryngeal tube insertion make it very practical in emergency situations. Moreover, with the improvement of endotracheal tubes, particularly the adoption of soft and low-pressure cuffs, complications of prolonged endotracheal intubation are markedly reduced. It is now feasible to continue translaryngeal intubation for periods up to 3 or more weeks. For longer ventilatory support, tracheostomy is usually performed while the translaryngeal tube is in place and the patient is being properly ventilated.

Tracheostomy is indicated not only when prolonged mechanical ventilation is anticipated, but also when, because of increased tracheobronchial secretions and the patient's inability to clear them, frequent suctioning after the discontinuation of ventilatory support will be necessary. The choice between orotracheal and nasotracheal intubation is less essential. The experience of the operator, ease of intubation, patient's acceptance and tolerance, and differences in sizes between the two tubes may influence their selection. Orotracheal intubation with a large tube is more desirable when secretions are troublesome and if bronchoscopy is anticipated. In cardiopulmonary resuscitation, because of necessity for speed in securing an airway, oral intubation is the procedure of choice. It is also preferred in patients with nasal obstruction or bleeding disorders.

In recent years, a specially designed nasal mask is being used in certain situations for administering mechanical ventilation. It may be used both on a short-term basis in acute respiratory failure and on a long-term basis for prolonged, mostly nocturnal, ventilatory support.

Artificial airway requires particular care to keep it safe and properly functioning. Securing the tube to prevent its slipping in or out, avoiding its unnecessary movement, appropriate inflation of the cuff, its cleaning or occasional changing, and adequate humidification are some of the measures for its care.

Ventilation Modes

The method by which a ventilator delivers a desired tidal volume is referred to as *ventilation mode*. Many of the modern positive-pressure ventilators have the capability of providing the following ventilatory modes (Fig. 25–4).

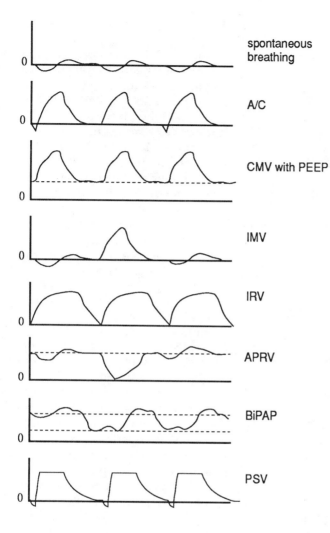

spontaneous
breathing

A/C

CMV with PEEP

IMV

IRV

APRV

BiPAP

PSV

Figure 25–4. Airway pressures in various ventilation modes.

1. **Controlled mechanical ventilation (CMV)** is a mode in which a preset tidal volume is delivered at a predetermined rate. It is primarily intended for anesthetized and comatose patients. Awake patients, especially when confused and uncooperative, require adequate sedation and even muscle-paralyzing medication for an effective ventilation with this mode.

2. In **assisted mechanical ventila-** tion **(AMV),** a preset volume is delivered only when the patient triggers the ventilator by his or her spontaneous inspiratory effort. This mode is now routinely combined with a backup controlled ventilation. This combination, known as *assist/controlled* (A/C) mode, ensures a minimum minute ventilation in the event that the patient makes no inspiratory effort, or when the level of inspiratory effort is less than

adequate for triggering an assist breath. A/C mode of ventilation usually results in a satisfactory patient-ventilator interaction and provides the needed ventilatory support. However, it may cause a significant fluctuation in the level of alveolar ventilation when the spontaneous respiratory rate changes as a result of an alteration of central respiratory drive or changes in pulmonary mechanoreceptor activity.

3. **Intermittent mandatory ventilation (IMV)** mode allows the patient to breathe spontaneously between the "mandatory" ventilator breaths whose rate and volume are preset. In contrast to the A/C mode, in which the tidal volume delivered by the patient's inspiratory effort during the assist breath is the same as the controlled tidal volume, the tidal volume between IMV breaths is determined by the strength of the patient's inspiratory effort. The IMV was originally intended as a method of weaning from mechanical ventilation (p. 360), but it has now become the preferred ventilation mode in most centers for the management of respiratory failure. Its advantages, especially if synchronized (SIMV), include better patient acceptance, ventilation with lower mean airway pressure, reduced need for sedation, and less wide fluctuation of the level of alveolar ventilation.

   Mandatory minute ventilation (MMV) may be used with IMV to ensure a minimum minute ventilation with low IMV rates in case the spontaneous ventilation becomes inadequate.

4. **Inverse ratio ventilation (IRV),** in which the inspiratory to expiratory (I:E) ratio is usually 2:1 or greater, is intended to keep the alveolar units open by not allowing enough time for them to collapse during the brief expiratory time. As an alternative to positive end-expiratory pressure (PEEP) discussed below, IRV has the advantage of raising the mean airway pressure without increasing the peak inspiratory pressure. It usually necessitates a ventilator that can be pressure controlled and time cycled; and because of its poor patient tolerance, sedation and muscle paralysis are required.

5. **Airway pressure release ventilation (APRV)** is a mode of mechanical ventilation of patients on continuous positive airway pressure (CPAP) in which intermittent and prompt discontinuation of positive airway pressure for a short time results in passive exhalation. This mode is intended to enhance alveolar ventilation in patients on CPAP when there is evidence of inadequate ventilation. It occurs without an increase in airway pressure above the CPAP. APRV may be considered as a variant of IRV, except that during inflation the patient on APRV continues to ventilate spontaneously and sedation or muscle paralysis is not necessary. APRV may be applied by a CPAP mask.

6. **Pressure   support   ventilation**

(PSV) is basically the addition of a set amount of positive pressure to the spontaneous breaths during inspiration. It differs from the intermittent positive pressure breathing (IPPB) in that the pressure in PSV is maintained at a plateau as long as an inspiratory flow is occurring. Low-level pressure support may be used to overcome the artificial airway resistance—and, thus, to improve patient comfort—and to reduce the added respiratory work load of the spontaneously breathing patient with or without IMV. With higher pressures, PSV plays the role of conventional ventilatory support. It has the advantage of a better patient–ventilator synchrony. PSV is also used as a weaning method (see page 360).

7. **Independent lung ventilation** (ILV) is a rare mode of ventilatory support in which two ventilators with different settings are used to ventilate each lung independently. It requires a special double-lumen endotracheal tube. ILV allows a better ventilation and oxygenation when there is predominantly unilateral severe lung disease.

Bi-level positive airway pressure (BIPAP) is a relatively simple method of ventilatory assistance that is used with a nasal mask. It is intended for periodic (mostly nocturnal) ventilatory support for patients suffering from chronic ventilatory insufficiency resulting mainly from thoracic deformity or neuromuscular disorders. Alternating levels (bi-level) of airway pressure, generated by a CPAP machine modified with a time-cycling device, results in a form of intermittent positive pressure ventilation.

PEEP. The improvement of oxygen transport upon addition of positive pressure during expiration, commonly known as *positive end-expiratory pressure* (PEEP), is primarily due to prevention of early closure of the distal airways and alveoli; thus FRC will become larger than closing volume. It also helps recruit collapsed lung units, thus improving pulmonary compliance and further enhancing gas exchange. PEEP is primarily used in respiratory failure from acute lung injury (ARDS) in which reduced functional residual capacity, microatelectasis, and intrapulmonary shunting are characteristic features. The use of PEEP allows oxygenation with a lower FIO_2, thus reducing the risk of oxygen toxicity. It is not effective in the treatment of acute respiratory failure in which lung volumes are already increased, as in asthma or emphysema.

The benefit of PEEP may be at least partly offset by its effect on cardiac output and the added risk of lung injury from excessive airway and alveolar pressure (barotrauma). A reduction in cardiac output is quite common following the application of PEEP; it is mainly the result of reduced venous blood return to the right ventricle. It is more pronounced in patients with inadequate circulating volume. Reduction in cardiac output improves with time and can be overcome by volume expansion. Restoration of blood volume is therefore important in preventing as well as correcting this complication. As tissue oxygenation depends also on its perfusion, an improvement in arterial oxygenation may not enhance tissue oxygenation if blood flow is diminished as a result of PEEP. Moreover, the response of arterial blood oxygenation to PEEP is not always predictable; it may occasionally fail to improve, or even worsen, the hypoxemia. This occurs when the effect of PEEP on nonuniform pathologic changes of the lungs causes the blood flow to shift from the healthier lung units to the less ventilated diseased areas. Therefore, the decision for the application of PEEP and the selection of its level is made on an individual basis and with proper assessment of its benefit and risk.

Ventilator Settings

The optimal mechanical ventilatory pattern is quite variable depending on the nature of the underlying disease and the characteristics of respiratory mechanics. In initiating mechanical ventilation, either A/C or IMV mode is usually employed. The choice is often an individual preference. Tachypneic patients, however, are more satisfactorily ventilated with IMV mode. The argument that A/C mode by reducing the work of breathing is conducive to more respiratory muscle rest is not tenable, as IMV at high enough rates is equally effective for this purpose.

Although primarily determined by effective alveolar ventilation (determined by arterial PCO_2), tidal volumes preferably should be high enough to prevent the collapse of the distal airways and alveoli. Usually a tidal volume of 10 to 15 mL/kg ideal body weight is well tolerated, and obviates the necessity for intermittent hyperinflation (sighing). A minute ventilation of about 10 L/min is often required, which can be achieved with a backup respiratory rate of 12 and tidal volume

of 800 mL. As the level of minute ventilation necessary for adequate alveolar ventilation (normal $PaCO_2$) is determined by physiologic dead space and CO_2 production, it may vary significantly from one patient to the next. Overventilation and resultant hypocapnia can be corrected by reducing respiratory rate or addition of artificial dead space. However, the tidal volume setting may need downward adjustment if pressure requirement is excessive. In ventilating patients with chronic hypercapnia whose serum bicarbonate levels are high, rapid reduction of the arterial PCO_2 should be avoided; otherwise, alkalosis would develop rapidly resulting in cardiac and cerebral complications. Close monitoring of blood gases during the first few hours of mechanical ventilation cannot be overstressed. In A/C mode, *trigger sensitivity* is usually set at 1 to 3 cm H_2O.

The *peak inspiratory flow rate* should be set to maintain a proper *inspiratory to expiratory time ratio* (I:E). It should allow the tidal volume to be delivered quickly enough to leave sufficient time for complete exhalation. By listening with a stethoscope over the suprasternal notch, one can verify the completion of expiration *before* the next positive pressure inspiration if the I:E ratio is proper. A ratio of 1:2 is preferable; it should not be allowed to be more than 1, except when inverse ratio ventilation (IRV) is intended. In patients with severe airway obstruction, as in asthma or COPD, who need more time for exhalation, a ratio of 1:3 to 1:4 may be indicated. This necessitates a higher inspiratory flow rate. Flow rate is usually set at 40 L/min. Optimal selection of a mechanical ventilatory pattern is not only essential for proper CO_2 elimination, but also important in regard to its mechanical effects on the lungs, gas distribution, oxygen transport, and cardiovascular function.

An effective tissue oxygenation is the most important immediate goal of mechanical ventilation. Selection of *inspiratory oxygen concentration* (FIO_2) is often arbitrary at the beginning of artificial ventilation. However, the initial FIO_2 should preferably be set at 100% if there is uncertainty about oxygenation with a lesser concentration. After the arterial blood PO_2 is determined, the FIO_2 is then titrated downward to a level that maintains adequate arterial blood oxygenation (P_aO_2 60 torr). The optimal FIO_2 will depend on the severity of the gas-transport abnormality. Measures directed to improve pulmonary oxygen transport reduce the need for high, and potentially toxic, oxygen concentrations. Certain adjustments of the ventilatory pattern (eg, inspiratory plateau) is also known to improve oxygenation. More significant improvement of oxygen transport occurs when the lung volume is increased throughout the respiratory cycle, which is accomplished by adding positive pressure during expiration (PEEP).

Among the criteria for the application of PEEP, the most important one is the inability to maintain a P_aO_2 of at least 60 torr on an FIO_2 of 0.5 with intermittent positive pressure ventilation. The proper amount of added expiratory pressure is decided by a trial method, starting with a small amount of PEEP, eg, 5 cm H_2O. As guides for determination of an optimal or "best" PEEP, several variables are followed. They include pulmonary oxygen transport (P_aO_2, shunt fraction, A-aDO$_2$), respiratory system compliance, and oxygen

delivery to the tissues. Frequently with application of PEEP, the total respiratory system compliance (determined by dividing the tidal volume into the inspiratory plateau pressure minus end-expiratory pressure) improves and reaches a maximum at variable PEEP levels. This usually coincides with an improvement of arterial blood oxygenation as a result of a reduction in the fraction of the intrapulmonary shunt. Tissue oxygen transport is the product of cardiac output and arterial oxygen content. Although there are indications that improvement of compliance with PEEP coincides with the enhancement of oxygen delivery, this effect is not always predictable. For a more accurate evaluation of tissue oxygenation, measurements of cardiac output or mixed venous blood PO_2 may be necessary. A level of PEEP of about 10 cm H_2O that results in an arterial blood PO_2 of 60 torr or higher with an FIO_2 of 0.6 or less is usually safe and may be optimal in most instances. PEEP levels greater than 15 cm are rarely recommended as the incidence of barotrauma increases sharply beyond this level. Patients with ARDS who have very low FRCs and have recruitable collapsed alveoli usually benefit from PEEP the most.

When it is determined that despite maximum safe PEEP, FIO_2, and peak inspiratory pressure, arterial oxygenation is still inadequate (P_aO_2 60), inverse ratio ventilation (page 354) may be tried. In an occasional patient with severe unilateral lung disease and difficult oxygenation, positioning the patient with the healthy lung down may enhance oxygenation by improving ventilation/perfusion mismatch. Rarely, independent lung ventilation (page 355) may be employed.

WEANING FROM MECHANICAL VENTILATION

In many clinical situations, mechanical ventilation is necessary only for a short period of time when the underlying causes of respiratory failure are readily reversible. General anesthesia, drug overdose, and many postresuscitation cases are examples in which ventilatory support can be uneventfully terminated once the patients become alert. Such patients are extubated soon after mechanical ventilation is discontinued. The term *weaning* should be applied only when the withdrawal from mechanical ventilation is done in a gradual and stepwise fashion in order for the patient to become *accustomed* to decreasing levels of ventilatory support until it is completely discontinued. Duration of weaning process depends, among other factors, on the length of time that the patient has been on ventilatory support.

The plan for weaning the patient from the ventilator starts at, or even precedes, the initiation of mechanical ventilation. One important consideration in deciding for artificial ventilation is the question of feasibility of its eventual discontinuation. Successful weaning will primarily depend on how well the underlying conditions leading to respiratory failure, and its precipitating factors, are controlled. The same causes of respiratory failure that compel the institution of mechanical ventilatory support will also prevent its successful withdrawal. Moreover, the very nature of prolonged artificial ventilation—which may cause disuse and discoordination of the respiratory muscles, alteration of sensitivity of the respiratory center, psychological dependency, malnutrition, and other complications—

may contribute to the difficulty in weaning. A vicious circle between prolonged ventilation and difficult weaning may thus be established: the more prolonged the ventilation, the more difficult the weaning and vice versa.

Discontinuation of mechanical ventilation will be feasible in patients with a stable clinical condition if the following interrelated basic respiratory derangements are corrected or ameliorated:

1. Increased work of breathing due to reduced pulmonary and/or thoracic compliance, elevated airway resistance, increased wasted ventilation, and high metabolic requirement.
2. Decreased respiratory muscle strength resulting from poor nutrition, disuse, neuromuscular disease, use of certain drugs, and, most important, respiratory muscle fatigue.
3. Depressed respiratory center due to CNS lesions, metabolic abnormalities, and depressant drugs.
4. Marked $\dot{V}/\dot{Q}$ abnormality and intrapulmonary shunting from severe pulmonary pathology.

Evaluation of these abnormalities by various methods, as in deciding for the institution of mechanical ventilation, will determine the suitable time and proper way for weaning. Criteria often used in deciding whether to wean are the measurements that usually predict successful weaning in most patients. These are indicated in Table 25–1. These criteria are only guidelines and should be used in conjunction with other factors specific for individual cases.

Meeting the criteria does not always result in successful weaning, and they need not be satisfied in every case.

TABLE 25–1. MEASUREMENTS THAT PREDICT SUCCESSFUL WEANING IN MOST PATIENTS (SPONTANEOUS RESPIRATION)

Respiratory rate	$\leq$ 25/min
Tidal volume	$\geq$ 5 mL/kg
Vital capacity	$\geq$ 10 mL/kg
Minute ventilation	$\leq$ 10 L
Maximum inspiratory pressure	$\geq$ 25 cm H_2O
PaO_2 with $FIO_2 \leq 0.5$	$\geq$ 60 torr

They are more useful in deciding to wean the patient whose overall condition has been stabilized, the functions of other organs are under control, and ventilatory support has not been very long (under 7 days). Patients with poor control of their underlying disease process, unstable cardiorespiratory status, significant metabolic derangement, high fever, and failing of other organs should not be considered for weaning from ventilatory support until they are properly treated. It should also be noted that the criteria may never be met in some patients with prolonged mechanical ventilation, especially in severe COPD, and they still could be successfully weaned. Therefore, the weaning is often a clinical experiment, and is accomplished by trial and error.

Weaning Methods

Although there are different methods of weaning from mechanical ventilation, they are all based on the principle of allowing the patient to assume progressively increasing ventilatory work until he or she is able to carry it out without mechanical support. In *T-tube* or *T-piece* weaning, the patient is allowed to breathe spontaneously for a variable length of time determined by the clinical situation. Ventilators with a built-in CPAP capacity may be set to function as a T-tube system by using a CPAP setting

at 0. However, it has the disadvantage of interposing an added resistance of the tubings. An adequately humidified oxygen mixture is administered at a concentration slightly higher than what the patient was receiving immediately before the initiation of weaning. The patient's cardiorespiratory status is closely and carefully monitored with special attention to the heart rate and rhythm, blood pressure, respiratory rate, and signs of respiratory muscle fatigue. The use of pulse oximetry during the weaning trial facilitates monitoring. With the development of significant changes in respiratory or cardiac status, such as tachypnea, increasing paradoxical abdominal-thoracic movement, tachycardia, cardiac arrhythmias, change in blood pressure, alteration of mental status, and occurrence of hypoxemia, the patient is returned to full ventilatory support without delay.

Lacking any of these changes, the patient is allowed to breathe unassisted with the continuation of monitoring. A moderate rise in respiratory rate and transient paradoxical abdominal-thoracic movement immediately following the assumption of spontaneous breathing are common and should not be construed as evidence for respiratory muscle fatigue and indication of weaning failure. Depending on the underlying cause of respiratory failure, the length of ventilatory support, and the patient's tolerance of unassisted breathing trial, the weaning process may vary from being fairly rapid and uncomplicated to being most difficult and protracted. A patient with hypoxemic respiratory failure requiring short-term ventilatory support (under 7 days) usually tolerates spontaneous breathing better and can often be weaned successfully with little difficulty. If the patient appears comfortable off the respirator without evidence of significant cardiac or respiratory alteration for about a half hour, and the arterial blood gases remain satisfactory, he or she is usually ready for extubation.

On the other hand, in a patient with ventilatory failure requiring prolonged mechanical support, weaning becomes a challenging task, necessitating a much slower and more gradual approach. Initial short, spontaneous daytime breathing periods of 5 to 15 minutes between long rest periods are slowly increased in duration and frequency. In such a patient, a complete rest of respiratory muscles between unassisted breathing is essential. At night, the patient is put on uninterrupted ventilatory support for a restful sleep until he or she is able to tolerate spontaneous breathing throughout the day. By that time, the patient is usually able to assume spontaneous respiration at night as well, and may be considered for extubation after 24 hours off the respirator.

Intermittent mandatory ventilation (IMV) has been increasingly used for gradual weaning from mechanical ventilation. This method allows the patient to breathe spontaneously between gradually decreasing rates of periodic, controlled mechanical ventilation with eventual resumption of the entire respiration. Because an increasing number of patients are being ventilated with an IMV mode (page 354), weaning with IMV has become the most commonly employed method. Although its superiority over a well-planned and properly executed T-piece weaning has not been convincingly proven, it appears to be a convenient, safe, and more comfortable method of achieving a smooth transition from artificial to spontaneous respiration. The IMV method, however, does not seem to accelerate the weaning process. At the start of weaning, the IMV rate is determined by the amount of ventilatory assistance necessary to sustain an adequate alveolar ventilation. The rate is then progressively reduced at intervals decided by the above-mentioned factors, as well as the patient's tolerance. The complete weaning may be achieved within a short period of time if spontaneous respiratory efforts remain adequate while the IMV rate is being decreased. With satisfactory blood gases at the IMV rate of 0, the patient may be extubated. In weaning from a prolonged mechanical ventilation and difficult-to-wean patients, the IMV rate is reduced much more slowly, beginning once every 24 hours. As with T-tube weaning, it is recommended that the patient be returned to full ventilatory support during the night until he or she is able to breathe unassisted throughout the day.

Pressure support ventilation (PSV) as a weaning method may be useful in situations in which respiratory muscle fatigue prevails and prevents successful weaning by conventional methods. To initiate weaning by this method, a level of pressure support just enough to maintain adequate alveolar ventilation is used. Gradual reduction of pressure levels is undertaken in a way that would result in increasing the activity of respiratory muscles while avoiding their fatigue. Minimum minute ventilation (MMV) may be added to assure an adequate ventilation with PSV, which is also used in conjunction with T-piece or IMV weaning.

COMPLICATIONS OF RESPIRATORY FAILURE AND MECHANICAL VENTILATION

A host of complications may arise during acute respiratory failure from several causes. Despite improvement in prognosis of acute respiratory failure in recent years, these complications continue to be major causes of significant mortality and morbidity. Many of these complications are directly related to therapeutic procedures, particularly mechanical ventilation, although the combination of several factors, including various underlying diseases, is responsible. Any sudden or unexpected changes in the patient's condition or ventilator mechanics are important warning signs for possible complications. Necessary measures for prevention of such complications, and their early recognition and treatment, are essential for the proper management of patients in respiratory failure.

Complications Due to Tracheal Intubation. Difficult and traumatic endotracheal intubation, intubation of the right main stem bronchus, excessive bleeding with tracheostomy, pneumomediastinum, and pneumothorax are complications that occur at the start of intubation or tracheostomy. Later in the course of intubated patients, insecure fixation of tubes results in their excessive movement and consequent injury to the larynx and the trachea. Self-extubation is a common occurrence, which may result in significant morbidity and even mortality. Kinking of the tube or mucous plugging can cause acute occlusion. Necrosis of the nose and sinusitis from lack of drainage of the paranasal sinuses are complications of prolonged nasotracheal intubation. Improper inflation or dislocation of the cuff, significant air leak from inability to seal around the tube, tracheal dilatation and **tracheomalacia,** and stomal infection of the tracheostomy are some other known complications that may occur while the tube is in place. The proper care of artificial airways is an important aspect of the management of patients on mechanical ventilators.

Immediate complications following extubation of the endotracheal tube include difficulty with phonation accompanied by laryngeal edema; the latter may be severe enough to cause stridor. Late complications are related to scarring of traumatic injury from the tube and/or its cuff and tracheostomy, which may cause significant stricture several weeks, or even months, after extubation. The use of low-pressure, soft cuffs has significantly diminished the complications due to excessive cuff pressure.

Complications Related to Ventilator Malfunction. Machine disconnection is fairly common, but easily noticeable with a properly functioning alarm system. Alarm failure, therefore, is one of the most serious mishaps, which may result in a fatal outcome. Inadequate humidification may result from defective ventilator humidifying system. Occasionally, overheating of the inspired air may occur. Other mechanical malfunctions are readily recognized by various monitoring and alarm devices.

Complications Related to Improper Machine Setup. The two major consequences of improper machine setup are alveolar hypoventilation and hyperventilation. There is a certain tendency to overventilate patients with hypercapnia to normalize the arterial blood PCO_2, despite elevated serum bicarbonate. This may result in serious alkalosis.

Pulmonary oxygen toxicity may be caused by either inadvertent or intentional administration of high oxygen concentrations. With inappropriate settings of flow rates, air trappings or inordinately high airway pressures may result. Intrinsic or auto-PEEP, in which the alveolar pressure at the end of expiration remains elevated from air trapping, occurs frequently in patients with predominantly obstructive airways disease, even with proper ventilator settings. It can be demonstrated and measured by the positive pressure reading on the ventilator monometer when the expiratory port is occluded at the end of expiration (when the monometer shows 0 pressure). If significant, auto-PEEP may result in reduction of cardiac output and adversely affect the ventilation. Application of small amounts of external PEEP may help in preventing premature closure of small airways and in reducing auto-PEEP effect.

Barotrauma. Barotrauma is defined as the injury from mechanically induced positive airway pressure that results in air entry into the extraalveolar tissues and spaces. Air can enter and dissect the interstitial tissue of the lung, causing **interstitial emphysema.** From there, it tracks its way along the perivascular and peribronchial tissue and enters the mediastinum, resulting in **pneumomediastinum. Subcutaneous emphysema** develops when the air, usually from the mediastinum, enters the subcutaneous tissue. In rare instances, the air may find its way to the peritoneal space

(pneumoperitoneum). However, the most common and serious complication of mechanical ventilation related to barotrauma is **pneumothorax.** As it is usually progressive and markedly impairs ventilation, its early recognition and prompt treatment are essential for effective management of these patients. Otherwise it may rapidly progress into a tension pneumothorax. There is fairly good correlation between the airway pressures (both peak inspiratory pressure and mean airway pressure) and the occurrence of barotrauma. One of the disadvantages of PEEP is its association with this complication, although the underlying pulmonary disease for which PEEP is used is probably a more important predisposing factor.

Measures that result in the improvement of airway resistance and pulmonary compliance and proper ventilation settings will reduce the need for the use of high inflation pressures and, thus, diminish the incidence of barotrauma. More careful selection of patients for institution of PEEP and determination of optimal expiratory pressures will also be helpful in prevention of this complication.

Infectious Complication. Pulmonary infection not only plays a major role in causing respiratory failure, but also is a common complication in patients on prolonged ventilatory support. The factors predisposing to this complication are numerous and include inadequate tracheobronchial toilet, ready colonization of the respiratory tract by pathogenic organisms, contaminated respiratory therapy equipment, presence of foreign materials in the airways, impaired local and systemic defense mechanisms, and use of antibiotics.

The diagnosis of nosocomial pneumonia in mechanically ventilated patients is a challenging problem because of difficulty in differentiating it from various other pulmonary lesions and identifying its cause by usual methods. The use of protected specimen brush with bronchoscopy and/or bronchoalveolar lavage may be necessary for its definitive diagnosis and isolation of offending organisms. The incidence of infectious complications is much higher in ARDS with a very high mortality.

Cardiovascular Complications. Cardiac arrhythmias due to changes in acid-base and electrolyte balance and hypoxemia are common in patients with respiratory failure. A hemodynamic effect of positive pressure ventilation, particularly with the addition of PEEP, such as reduced cardiac output, may be observed. Overhydration, fluid retention, and cardiac failure are not uncommon, but frequently overlooked. Patients on prolonged mechanical ventilatory support are prone to develop venous thrombosis and pulmonary embolism.

Gastrointestinal Complications. Distention of the stomach and intestines is common in patients on mechanical ventilators; it may be due to massive air swallowing and/or inhibition of gastrointestinal motility (ileus) Diarrhea from different causes may become a vexing problem in these patients. Significant abdominal distention may be a cause of restriction of proper ventilation. One of the common and serious complications of patients in respiratory failure, especially when on a mechanical ventilator, is the development of stress ulcers and subsequent upper GI bleeding. These patients should be prophylactically treated with an antiulcer medication. Because of the colonization of the stomach with microorganisms as a result of increased gastric pH from antacids or H_2 antagonists, the antiulcer drug sucralfate, which does not change the pH, is preferred in such patients. Enteral alimentation appears to decrease the incidence of gastrointestinal bleeding in this setting.

Nutritional Deficiency. As discussed earlier (page 350), most critically ill patients on mechanical ventilation are known to suffer from inadequate and improper nutrition, which results in prolongation of their hospitalization and increased complications. One important cause of failure in weaning patients from mechanical ventilation is malnutrition, which is known to affect respiratory muscles.

Psychiatric Complications. It is understandable that many critically ill patients on respirators will develop psychiatric problems. Inability to communicate, complex ICU environment, sleep disturbances, sensory deprivation, and the use of various medications are among the factors that contribute to the development of such complications.

Other Complications. No body organ is spared from potential complications in patients with respiratory failure who require prolonged hospitalization on mechanical ventilation and who are subject to various diagnostic and therapeutic interventions. Renal, hematologic, endocrine, dermatologic, and neurologic complications are not uncommon in these vulnerable patients. Physicians and others involved in the care of these patients should always be aware of such possibilities and should make every necessary effort toward their prevention, early detection, and proper treatment.

ADULT RESPIRATORY DISTRESS SYNDROME

Adult respiratory distress syndrome (ARDS) has been described as a distinct form of acute respiratory failure resulting from diffuse pulmonary injury of various causes, characterized by rapidly progressive dyspnea, tachypnea, refractory hypoxemia, diffuse pulmonary infiltration, and reduced lung volumes and compliance. Pathologic changes are a collection of atelectasis, interstitial and alveolar edema and hemorrhage, and, sometimes, **hyaline** membrane formation. Because of these common clinical, radiographic, pathologic, and physiologic changes and their similarity in therapeutic requirement and response, several clinical entities have been gathered together under the designation of adult respiratory distress syndrome. They include *shock lung, posttraumatic pulmonary insufficiency, severe aspiration pneumonia, massive fat embolism, pulmonary edema due to narcotic overdose, smoke inhalation, near drowning, severe viral pneumonia,* and several other similar conditions. It should be emphasized that the diagnosis of acute respiratory distress syndrome is just the recognition of this particular form of respiratory failure; therefore, the identification of its underlying specific cause is essential for proper management.

Etiology. Adult respiratory distress syndrome, despite its name, can affect patients of all age groups including children. Respiratory distress syndrome of the newborn is, however, a distinct entity resulting from primary surfactant deficiency (Chapter 26), whereas surfactant deficiency in ARDS is secondary to acute diffuse lung injury. Among numerous conditions known to be associated with ARDS, many have a definite and direct causal relationship, while the others affect the lungs indirectly and with less precise mechanisms. However, they all have the common denominator of diffuse parenchymal injury of the lungs. What follows is a partial list of these etiologic conditions:

- Sepsis syndrome
- Thoracic trauma, pulmonary contusion
- Severe extrathoracic trauma, including head injury
- Extensive burns
- Pulmonary aspiration
- Inhalation of toxic fumes or gases
- Diffuse pulmonary infection (viral pneumonias, *pneumocystis carinii* pneumonia)
- Oxygen toxicity
- Fat embolism
- Transfusion of massive amount of banked blood
- Prolonged cardiopulmonary bypass
- Acute severe pancreatitis
- Disseminated intravascular coagulation
- Near drowning
- Narcotic drug overdose
- Ionizing radiation
- Acute paraquat poisoning

Although any of these causes can result in lung injury on preexistent pulmonary disease, most patients have no prior cardiorespiratory disorders.

Pathology. Although the underlying etiologic factors are quite varied, pathologic changes are almost similar. Diffuse alveolar damage with resultant changes secondary to alveolar-capillary leak and inflammatory reaction are the bases of morphologic abnormalities seen in the lungs of patients with ARDS. Early acute changes include destructive lesions and loss of endothelial and type I alveolar epithelial cells, edema, hemorrhage, infiltration with inflammatory cells, microatelectasis, and hyaline membrane formation. Persistence of lung injury beyond 7 to 10 days usually results in chronic changes of organizing stage, in which type II alveolar cells proliferate. Increased number of fibroblasts denote beginning of fibrosis that may develop rapidly. Bronchoalveolar lavage (BAL) fluid recovered from patients with ARDS contains large numbers of polymorphonuclear leukocytes. BAL fluid surfactant is deficient in its surface-tension lowering activity as a result of the alteration of its chemical composition.

Pathogenesis and Pathophysiology. The lungs may be injured directly from a variety of causes, such as pulmonary contusion, aspiration of acid gastric content, and smoke inhalation. However, the mechanism of acute pulmonary injury in seriously ill patients without direct involvement of the lungs, as in sepsis syndrome, is not entirely known. Several more or less interrelated factors have been proposed as playing a part in initiating and maintaining the lung injury as well as inflammatory changes characteristic of ARDS. In different mechanisms considered in pathogenesis of ARDS, the importance of blood neutrophils has been increasingly recognized. Among various mediators released from macrophages in response to bacterial toxins and other stimuli, tumor necrosis factor (TNF) appears to play a central role. This factor by affecting the endothelial cells of microvasculatures and by stimulating the neutrophils results in their interaction, promoting their adherence and eventual migration of neutrophils across the endothelium. The release of toxic oxygen radicals and proteolytic enzymes from neutrophils causes the diffuse injury of the lungs and their capillaries. Endotoxins and TNF may also cause tissue damage directly. In addition, the activation of complement and coagulation systems, the release of numerous other mediators, and involvement of other inflammatory cells have been considered to participate in pathogenesis of ARDS.

As a result of diffuse pulmonary injury, the alveolar capillary membrane becomes leaky; thus the extracellular lung fluid increases, causing noncardiogenic pulmonary edema. The accumulation of fluid in the interstitial space, alveoli, and distal airways, together with reduction and inactivation of surfactant, results in airway closure and alveolar collapse. The lungs become stiff and lose their volumes; in an advanced form, they become almost airless.

Maldistribution of ventilation and perfusion is usually very pronounced; many lung units cease to have any ventilation, causing intrapulmonary shunting. Severe hypoxemia is due to both ventilation-perfusion mismatch and right-to-left shunting. Because of increased sensitivity of the lung receptors, alveolar hyperventilation (hypocapnia) is a common feature unless there is such a marked reduction in functioning lung units that maintenance of adequate ventilation is not possible. Pulmonary hypertension from vascular injury and occlusion, a common occurrence in ARDS, is further enhanced by severe hypoxemia.

As many patients with ARDS have significant abnormality of other organ systems, the pathophysiologic alteration resulting from lung injury is further intensified. Supply-dependency of oxygen consumption, a pathophysiologic abnormality in which the tissue oxygen uptake depends on its delivery, may result from improper regulation of systemic blood flow and/or from endothelial injury of organs besides the lungs. It appears that the same pathogenic mechanisms of tissue injury involving the lungs may also affect other organs,

albeit in a less dramatic fashion. Indeed, multiple organ failure is the cause of death in many patients with ARDS, especially when it results from sepsis syndrome. Impairment of renal, cardiac, and hepatic functions enhances fluid accumulation in an already damaged lung. Protein loss through the gastrointestinal tract and into the extravascular spaces results in reduction of plasma oncotic pressure, which in turn contributes to pulmonary edema. Figure 25–5 schematically shows the pathogenesis and pathophysiologic changes that occur in ARDS.

Clinical Manifestations. The clinical manifestations of many of the causes of acute pulmonary injury leading to adult respiratory distress syndrome have been

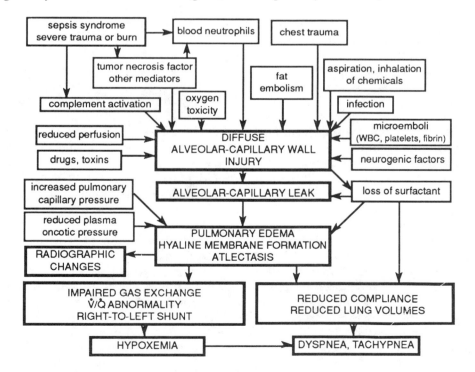

Figure 25–5. Pathogenesis and pathophysiology of adult respiratory distress syndrome.

discussed in the appropriate chapters of this book. The onset of the syndrome, which usually occurs within 24 to 48 hours following serious injury or illness, is heralded by progressively severe dyspnea, tachypnea, and grunting respiration. Cyanosis and intercostal and suprasternal retraction are evident in the advanced stage. Cough, with or without frothy and blood-tinged sputum, is common. Physical findings on examination of the chest are surprisingly scant. Bronchial breath sounds and occasional rales may be heard. Respiration is rapid, and the minute ventilation is markedly increased.

As the clinical settings for the development of ARDS are different, a variety of associated disorders will be present. Systemic hypotension, fever, changes of CNS function, evidence of sepsis, signs of trauma to various sites, or manifestations of failure of other organs may be evident.

The most consistent laboratory finding in ARDS is arterial hypoxemia refractory to the administration of high oxygen concentrations. P_aO_2/FIO_2 ratio, often used as an index of severity of hypoxemia, is less than 100 in severe cases. Radiographic finding of bilateral diffuse interstitial and airspace infiltration is characteristic (Fig. 25–6). Normal heart size, absent pleural effusion, and lack of enlarged vessels differentiate ARDS from cardiogenic pulmonary edema.

Diagnosis. The diagnosis of ARDS with full-blown clinical, radiographic, and laboratory pictures is not difficult. A history of catastrophic event in a patient without chronic cardiopulmonary disorders is usually obtained. Diffuse, progressive, and bilateral pulmonary infil-

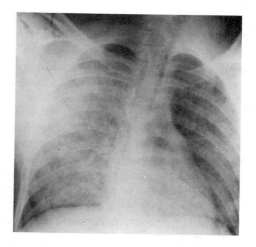

Figure 25–6. Pulmonary edema in adult respiratory distress syndrome.

tration on chest x-ray film; refractory hypoxemia ($P_aO_2 < 50$ torr when $FIO_2 > 0.6$); and reduced total respiratory system compliance are among the essential criteria for the diagnosis of ARDS. The important differential diagnosis is with cardiogenic pulmonary edema. Although usually the clinical presentation and radiographic picture in heart failure are quite distinctive, in critically ill complicated patients with multiple-organ system failure, the distinction is not always easy. A flow-directed pulmonary artery catheter is very helpful in differentiating noncardiogenic from cardiogenic pulmonary edema and may also help in proper management of some patients with ARDS.

Management. The principles of management of adult respiratory distress syndrome are the same as those of acute respiratory failure in general. In view of the severity of hypoxemia and difficulty of its treatment, every effort should be made to improve oxygenation without resorting to the administration of a toxic concentration of oxygen. Although in the early stage, conservative treatment with oxygen, without intubation and mechanical ventilation, may succeed, progressive hypoxemia and failure to respond to this approach are indications for tracheal intubation. CPAP or application of PEEP without mechanical ventilation (EPAP) may be tried in less severe cases. The treatment of choice, however, is the use of a volume respirator, employing adequate tidal volumes (10 to 15 mL/kg ideal body weight). The need for application of positive expiratory pressure can be judged by the results of arterial blood gas analysis; failure to oxygenate adequately with an FIO_2 of 0.5 on intermittent positive pressure ventilation is a distinct indication for application of PEEP. The mechanism of action and the proper use of PEEP and other aspects of mechanical ventilation, including its weaning and complications, are discussed in the management of acute respiratory failure.

Measures known to improve oxygen transport should be a major part of the respiratory management of this syndrome. Treatment of the underlying disease, clearing of secretions, maintaining good cardiac output and normal hemoglobin level, control of infection, and correction of other complications are some of the therapeutic measures that improve oxygenation. The control of fever and other causes of increased metabolism reduces oxygen consumption. The correction of anemia with transfusion of packed red cells enhances oxygen delivery. Fluid balance is very important in the management of these patients. Because of the leakiness of the alveolar-capillary membrane in this condition, any degree of overhydration

may result in further pulmonary edema. The administration of diuretics, with or without infusion of albumin or other colloids, is generally recommended. Monitoring the pulmonary capillary pressure by a Swan-Ganz catheter is helpful for this purpose. Pulmonary artery catheterization, in addition, is used for the measurement of other hemodynamic variables, including cardiac output and for the determination of proper PEEP levels. The use of corticosteroids and other anti-inflammatory drugs in management of established adult respiratory distress syndrome is controversial. If given early, these drugs may reduce lung injury in some patients.

With maximum respiratory support, hypoxemia usually will improve without resorting to a toxic level of oxygen. Unfortunately, in certain situations, hypoxemia remains refractory and may reach a dangerously severe degree, even with very high and potentially toxic oxygen concentrations.

Almitrine is a drug known for its improvement of ventilation/perfusion matching by increasing pulmonary vascular response to regional hypoxia. This drug is not yet approved for clinical use in the United States. From the European studies, almitrine seems to improve arterial blood PO_2 in ARDS as well as in COPD.

Course and Prognosis. Despite remarkable advances in the knowledge and the understanding of ARDS and the availability of sophisticated therapeutic modalities, the survival rate of patients with this condition who require mechanical ventilation is only about 50%.

Generally, patients whose P_aO_2 improves early in the course of their disease have a much better prognosis. Survivors from ARDS usually recover completely and have no significant pulmonary sequelae or abnormal respiratory function. ARDS secondary to sepsis syndrome has a worse prognosis. Death is usually due to multiple organ failure and intercurrent infection. With appropriate intensive care, death from respiratory cause is much less common.

BIBLIOGRAPHY

ACCP/SCCM Consensus Panel. Ethical and moral guidelines for the initiation, continuation, and withdrawal of intensive care. *Chest.* 1990; 97:949–958.

Ashworth LJ. Pressure support ventilation. *Crit Care Nurse.* 1990; 10(7):20–25.

Bach JB, Alba AS. Management of chronic alveolar hypoventilation of nasal ventilation. *Chest.* 1990; 97:52–57.

Bégin P, Grassino A. Inspiratory muscle dysfunction and chronic hypercapnia in chronic obstructive pulmonary disease. *Am Rev Respir Dis.* 1991; 143: 905–912.

Bell RC, Coalson JJ, Smith JD, Johanson WG Jr. Multiple organ system failure and infection in adult respiratory distress syndrome. *Ann Intern Med.* 1983; 99:293–298.

Bennett DA, Bleck TP, Diagnosis and treatment of neuromuscular causes of acute respiratory failure. *Clin Neuropharmacol.* 1988; 11:303–347.

Benotti PN, Bistrian B. Metabolic and nutritional aspects of weaning from mechanical ventilation. *Crit Care Med.* 1989; 17:181–185.

Bone RC, Eubanks DH. The basis and basics of mechanical ventilation. *Dis Mon.* 1991; 37:327–406.

Bronchard L, Harf A, Lorino H, Lemaire F. Inspiratory pressure support prevents diaphragmatic fatigue during weaning from mechanical ventilation. *Am Rev Respir Dis.* 1989; 139:513–521.

Bronchard L, Isabey D, Piquet J, et al.

Reversal of acute exacerbations of chronic obstructive lung disease by inspiratory assistance with a face mask. *N Engl J Med.* 1990; 323:1523–1530.

Cerra FB. The multiple organ failure syndrome. *Hosp Pract.* 1990; 25(8):169–176.

Cohen CA, Zagelbaum G, Gross D, et al. Clinical manifestations of inspiratory muscle fatigue. *Am J Med.* 1982; 73:308–316.

Colice GL, Stukel TA, Dain B. Laryngeal complications of prolonged intubation. *Chest.* 1989; 96:877–884.

Consensus conference on artificial airways in patients receiving mechanical ventilation. *Chest.* 1990; 96:178–180.

Coronel B, Mercatello A, Couturier JC, et al. Polyneuropathy: potential cause of difficult weaning. *Crit Care Med.* 1990; 18:486–489.

Craven DE, Steger KA. Nosocomial pneumonia in the intubated patient: new concepts on pathogenesis and prevention. *Inf Dis Clin North Am.* 1989; 3:843–866.

Dorinsky PM, Gadek JE. Mechanisms of multiple nonpulmonary organ failure in ARDS. *Chest.* 1989; 96:885–892.

Downs JB, Stock MC. Airway pressure release ventilation: a new concept in ventilatory support. *Crit Care Med.* 1987; 15:459–461.

Dunham CM, LaMonica C. Prolonged tracheal intubation in the trauma patient. *J Trauma.* 1984; 24:120–124.

Elliott MW, Steven MH, Phillips GD, Branthwaite MA. Non-invasive mechanical ventilation for acute respiratory failure. *Br Med J.* 1990; 300:358–360.

Glauser FL, Polatty RC, Sessler CN. Worsening oxygenation in the mechanically ventilated patient: causes, mechanisms, and early detection. *Am Rev Respir Dis.* 1988; 138:458–465.

Goldstone J, Moxham J. Weaning from mechanical ventilation. *Thorax.* 1991; 46:56–62.

Grassino A, Macklem PT. Respiratory muscle fatigue and ventilatory failure. *Annu Rev Med.* 1984; 35:625–647.

Groeger JS, Levinson MR, Carlon GC. Assist control versus synchronized intermittent mandatory ventilation during acute respiratory failure. *Crit Care Med.* 1989; 17:607–612.

Grum CM, Chauncey JB. Conventional mechanical ventilation. *Clin Chest Med.* 1988; 9:37–46.

Halevy A, Sirik Z, Adam YG, Lewinsohn G. Long-term evaluation of patients following the adult respiratory distress syndrome. *Respir Care.* 1984; 29:132–137.

Hamilton-Farrell MR, Hanson GC. General care of the ventilated patient in the intensive care unit. *Thorax.* 1990; 45:962–969.

Heffner JE. Airway management in the critically ill patient. *Crit Care Clin.* 1990; 6:533–550.

Heffner JE, Repine JE. Pulmonary strategies of antioxidant defense. *Am Rev Respir Dis* 1989; 140:531–554.

Hubmayer RD, Abel MD, Rehder K. Physiologic approach to mechanical ventilation. *Crit Care Med.* 1990; 18:103–113.

Hudson LD. The prediction and prevention of ARDS. *Respir Care.* 1990; 35:161–173.

Johnson MM, Sexton DL. Distress during mechanical ventilation: patient's perception. *Crit Care Nurse.* 1990: 10(7):48–57.

Juan G, Calverley P, Talamo C, et al. Effect of carbon dioxide on diaphragmatic function in human beings. *N Engl J Med.* 1984; 310:874–879.

Kacmarek RM, Meklaus GJ. The new generation of mechanical ventilators. *Crit Care Clin.* 1990; 6:551–578.

Lain DC, DiBenedetto R, Morris SL, et al. Pressure control inverse ratio ventilation as a method to reduce peak inspiratory pressure and provide adequate ventilation and oxygenation. *Chest.* 1989; 95:1081–1088.

Larca L, Greenbaum DM. Effectiveness of intensive nutritional regimes in patients who fail to wean from mechanical ventilation. *Crit Care Med.* 1982; 10:297–300.

Ludwigs UG, Baehrendtz S, Wanecek M, Matell G. Mechanical ventilation in medical and neurological diseases: 11 years of experience. *J Intern Med.* 1991; 222:117–124.

Marsh HM, Gillespie DJ, Baumgartner AE. Timing of tracheostomy in the critically ill patient. *Chest.* 1989; 96:190–193.

Maunder RJ, Hudson LD. Pharmacologic strategies for treating the adult respiratory distress syndrome. *Respir Care.* 1990; 35:241–246.

Meduri GU. Ventilator-associated pneumonia in patients with respiratory failure: a diagnostic approach. *Chest.* 1990; 97:1208–1219.

Morganroth ML, Grum CM. Weaning from mechanical ventilation. *J Intensive Care Med* 1988; 3:109–120.

Murray JF, Matthay MA, Luce JM, Flick MR. An expanded definition of the adult respiratory distress syndrome. *Am Rev Respir Dis.* 1988; 138:720–723.

Niederman MS, Fein AM. Sepsis syndrome, the adult respiratory distress syndrome, and nosocomial pneumonia: a common clinical sequence. *Clin Chest Med.* 1990; 11:633–656.

NIH workshop on withholding and withdrawing mechanical ventilation. *Am Rev Respir Dis.* 1989; 140(2 part 2):S1–S46.

Pepe PE, Thomas RG, Stager MA, et al. Early prediction of the adult respiratory distress syndrome by a simple scoring method. *Ann Emerg Med.* 1983; 12:749–755.

Petty TL. Acute respiratory distress syndrome. *Dis Mon.* 1990; 36:7–58.

Pierson DJ. Complications associated with mechanical ventilation. *Crit Care Clin.* 1990; 6:711–724.

Pingleton SK. Complications of acute respiratory failure. *Am Rev Respir Dis.* 1988; 137:1463–1493.

Ponte J. Indications for mechanical ventilation. *Thorax.* 1990; 45:885–890.

Prewitt RM, Matthay MA, Ghignone M. Hemodynamic management in the adult respiratory distress syndrome. *Clin Chest Med.* 1983; 4:251–268.

Pugin J, Auckenthaler R, Lew DP, Suter

PM. Oropharyngeal decontamination decreases incidence of ventilator-associated pneumonia. *JAMA*. 1991; 265:2704–2710.

Reines HD. Manifestations of barotrauma in acute respiratory failure. *Am Surg*. 1981; 47:421–425.

Rinaldo JE, Rogers RM. Adult respiratory distress syndrome: changing concepts of lung injury and repair. *N Engl J Med*. 1982; 306:900–909.

Rochester DF, Esau SA. Malnutrition and the respiratory system. *Chest*. 1984; 85:411–415.

Roussos C. Respiratory muscle fatigue and ventilatory failure. *Chest*. 1990; 97(3 suppl):89S–96S.

Sassoon CSH, Mahutte CK, Light RW. Ventilator modes: old and new. *Crit Care Clin*. 1990; 6:605–634.

Schlichtig R, Sargent SC. Nutritional support of the mechanically ventilated patient. *Crit Care Clin*. 1990; 6:767–784.

Schuster DP. A physiologic approach to initiating, maintaining, and withdrawing mechanical ventilatory support during acute respiratory failure. *Am J Med*. 1990; 88:268–278.

Stock MC, Downs JB, Frolicher DA. Airway pressure release ventilation. *Crit Care Med*. 1987; 15:462–466.

Swank DW, Moore SB. Role of neutrophils and other mediators in adult respiratory distress syndrome. *Mayo Clin Proc*. 1989; 64:1118–1132.

Tobin MJ. Respiratory monitoring during mechanical ventilation. *Crit Care Clin*. 1990; 6:679–709.

Tobin MJ, Yang K. Weaning from mechanical ventilation. *Crit Care Clin*. 1990; 6:725–747.

Tomlinson JR, Miller KS, Lorch DG. A prospective comparison of IMV and T-piece weaning from mechanical ventilation. *Chest*. 1989; 96:348–352.

Trouillet JL, Guiguet M, Gilbert C, et al. Fiberoptic bronchoscopy in ventilated patients. *Chest*. 1990; 97:927–933.

Viires N, Aubier M, Murciano D, et al. Effects of aminophylline on diaphragmatic fatigue during acute respiratory failure. *Am Rev Resp Dis*. 1984; 129:396–402.

Weg JG. Oxygen transport in adult respiratory distress syndrome and other acute circulatory problems: relationship of oxygen delivery and oxygen consumption. *Crit Care Med*. 1991; 19:650–657.

Weinberger SE, Schwartzstein RM, Weiss JW. Hypercapnia. *N Engl J Med*. 1989; 321:1223–1231.

Weisman IM, Rinaldo JE, Rogers RM. Positive end-expiratory pressure in adult respiratory failure. *N Engl J Med*. 1982; 307:1381–1384.

Weisman IM, Rinaldo JE, Rogers RM, Sanders MH. Intermittent mandatory ventilation. *Am Rev Respir Dis*. 1983; 127:641–647.

Zucker AR. Therapeutic strategies for acute hypoxemic respiratory failure. *Crit Care Med*. 1988; 4:813–830.

CHAPTER 26

Respiratory Distress Syndrome of the Newborn

Newborn infants may suffer from breathing difficulty as a result of a variety of causes, but respiratory distress syndrome (RDS) also known as hyaline membrane disease, is by far the most common acute pulmonary disorder of the newborn. RDS is characterized by respiratory failure following premature birth and is associated with severe atelectasis. *Deficiency of surfactant* is the fundamental abnormality. RDS is the leading cause of death in the neonatal period.

ETIOLOGY AND PATHOGENESIS OF RDS

Although respiratory distress syndrome is occasionally referred to as "idiopathic," it is now securely established that it is due to lack of maturity of the lung and its unpreparedness to assume an adequate respiratory role. RDS is primarily a disease of premature infants with a direct relationship between its incidence and the degree of prematurity, whether indicated by gestational age or birth weight. While it occurs in about 60% of infants less than 28 weeks of gestational age, it is rarely seen in babies born at term. The severity of respiratory distress and mortality from it are also proportional to the degree of prematurity. Maternal diabetes, delivery by Cesarean section, and complicated pregnancy are added risk factors for the development of RDS.

Inadequate development prior to birth affects the respiratory function at birth through several mechanisms, which include a lack of growth of the respiratory units and a weak and compliant rib cage. However, the most important factor is the presence of a high surface tension in the alveoli from a deficiency or an absence of surfactant. Surfactant, made up of a mixture of phospholipids (mostly lecithin) and proteins, is synthesized by and stored in the type II alveolar cells prior to its release into the alveoli during the last few weeks of a normal gestation. During this time, surfactant continues to fill the alveoli and the airways, partly spilling into the amniotic fluid. Its presence in this fluid is therefore an indication of its formation and release in the lung. Premature birth and defects in biosynthesis or lack of secretion of surfactant from other causes prevent its adequate accumulation in the alveoli.

Once the alveoli are filled with air following the baby's first breath, surfactant, by coating the alveoli and reducing their surface tension, is essential in preventing their collapse during expiration. The need for the surface tension-lowering effect of surfactant is greatest when the alveolar volume is small and thus the potential for its collapse is increased. Normally the presence of surfactant on the alveolar lining lowers its surface tension further when the alveolar volume is decreased during expiration (Chapter 18). Therefore, this surface-active material is a potent anti-atelectatic factor, and has the dual function of decreasing the pressure needed to distend the lung and of maintaining the alveolar stability. The lung that possesses this ability is considered as mature and ready to assume its role of ventilation and gas exchange.

The lack of adequate amounts of surfactant in RDS is the major cause of failure of the respiratory system to adapt to the postnatal air-breathing state. Inadequate expansion of the lungs and *diffuse atelectasis* are basic mechanisms of this failure. In addition to atelectasis, pulmonary edema and hyaline membrane formation result in a marked reduction of pulmonary compliance. The pressure necessary to expand the lungs will be too great for small, poorly developed immature infants to muster. Because of their supple and yielding chest wall, the amount of intrathoracic pressure that they can generate will be limited, causing further atelectasis.

Inadequate ventilation and gas exchange cause severe hypoxemia, hypercapnia, and acidosis, which increase the pulmonary vascular resistance. Elevated pressures in the right heart chambers and pulmonary artery keep the fetal communication between the two sides of circulation open (foramen ovale between the atria and ductus arteriosus between the pulmonary artery and aorta), resulting in right-to-left shunt, further hypoxemia, and reduced pulmonary perfusion. **Ischemic** injury to the alveolar capillary membrane causes leaking of fluid into the interstitial and alveolar spaces and formation of hyaline membrane. Injury to the surfactant-producing cells further impairs their function (Fig. 26–1).

On pathologic examination, the lungs look purplish red and liver-like, with extensive atelectasis, exudate, and hemorrhage. Hyaline membrane is seen in cases in which death occurs less rapidly. In many cases, death occurs so fast that there is no time for hyaline membrane formation.

Clinical Manifestations. The breathing difficulty is usually evident from the time of birth, most often requiring resuscitative measures. The high inflating pressure necessary to open the alveoli for the first breath is also required for subsequent breaths; because of the inability of the lungs to hold residual air on expiration, they collapse with each expiration. Very immature infants (born between 26th and 30th weeks of gestation) develop the syndrome immediately. In some cases, when the lungs are more mature, they may function normally for a brief period of time, and then fail. Rapid and shallow respiration heralds the onset of respiratory distress

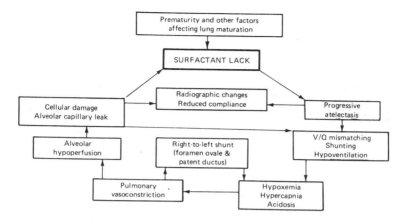

Figure 26–1. Pathogenesis and pathophysiology of respiratory distress syndrome of the newborn. The central abnormality is the lack of surfactant. Note several vicious circles in the scheme.

syndrome. The respiratory rate reaches 60 to 120 per minute, from a normal of 40 to 50 per minute. Expiratory grunting or whining is the result of breathing against a partially closed larynx, which is a feeble effort at preventing alveolar closure during expiration. Subcostal, intercostal, and suprasternal retraction signifies large intrathoracic pressure changes necessary for ventilation. The baby has a dusky color, and cyanosis may be severe and unresponsive to oxygen administration. Breath sounds are usually diminished; rales may be heard, but are not common. Infants with severe hypoxemia show evidence of circulatory collapse and are hypothermic.

The chest x-ray has diffuse granular appearance; air bronchogram is readily visible (Fig. 26–2). Arterial blood gas analysis shows marked hypoxemia; PCO_2 is usually elevated. Mixed respiratory and metabolic acidosis is common.

Most deaths from acute respiratory distress syndrome occur in the first 3 to 4 days; in severe cases, they may occur within a few hours.

Diagnosis. The diagnosis of RDS is made from the characteristic clinical presentation, chest roentgenogram, and arterial blood studies in infants born prematurely. Other causes of respiratory distress, such as pneumothorax,

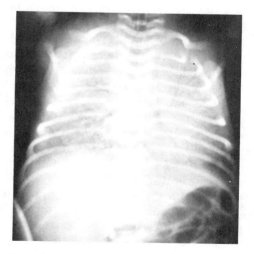

Figure 26–2. Radiograph of a newborn with severe acute respiratory distress syndrome. Note bilateral pulmonary consolidation with marked air bronchogram.

large diaphragmatic hernia, aspiration, heart failure, and pneumonia, should be properly ruled out. The prenatal diagnosis of lung immaturity and, therefore, prediction of which fetus is at risk of developing respiratory distress is by studying the amniotic fluid obtained by a special technique. Among several available methods, direct determination of surface-active material (especially the lecithin level and the **lecithin/sphingomyelin** ratio) and indirect estimation of its activity are most useful. The latter method, known as the shake test, depends on the ability of surfactant in the amniotic fluid to generate a stable foam in the presence of ethyl alcohol.

Management. With the understanding of the cause of neonatal respiratory distress syndrome, it is obvious that the prevention of premature births is the most important measure in reducing its incidence. In timing for Cesarean section or induction of labor, the determination of fetal age and the prediction of lung maturity are essential. The maternal administration of a synthetic corticosteroid for 2 to 3 days prior to delivery is known to increase fetal surfactant production.

The most important and critical problem in infants with RDS is hypoxemia, which necessitates immediate attention and correction by appropriate means. Close monitoring of the temperature, cardiorespiratory function, blood gases, and acid-base status is important to forestall clinical worsening and complications. It should be stressed that premature infants are prone to develop retinal lesion with high *arterial* oxygen tension, in addition to their susceptibility to pulmonary oxygen toxicity with high *inspired* oxygen tensions. An adequately staffed and equipped neonatal intensive care nursery is essential for the optimal treatment of these infants. Their thermal environment should be properly controlled to prevent increased oxygen consumption. Isolettes with heating systems controlled by the infant's skin temperature are commonly used.

In infants with mild to moderate hypoxemia, the administration of warm and humidified oxygen to bring the P_aO_2 to 60 to 80 torr is needed to improve oxygenation while minimizing the possibility of oxygen toxicity. In many cases, hypoxemia is more severe or progressive and measures to improve pulmonary oxygen transport are needed. The most effective measure in this regard is the application of *continuous distending airway pressure*. This is based on the knowledge of pathogenesis of the respiratory distress and hypoxemia. As discussed earlier, the lack of stability of the alveoli and their tendency to collapse and reduce the lung volume constitute the major problem. Maneuvers that result in increased resting lung volume would improve oxygenation. This is indeed the case in clinical trial of continuous distending airway pressure in this disease. This may be accomplished either by *continuous positive airway pressure* (CPAP) or by continuous negative pressure around the body.

CPAP may be applied through an endotracheal tube or, to avoid tracheal intubation, it may be used with a head hood, head chamber, tight-fitting mask, or special nasal prongs. *Constant negative* pressure also obviates the need for intubation. The baby's body is placed in a special chamber or box, sealed at two ends around the neck and pelvic area, and the desired negative pressure is applied by a vacuum pump. With either method of constant distending pressure, the baby is breathing spontaneously a proper mixture of oxygen. It is the combination of appropriate pressure and the administration of nontoxic oxygen mixture that provides the optimal oxygenation.

Very ill babies who show evidence of severe respiratory distress, intractable hypoxemia, hypercapnia, acidosis, or prolonged apneic episodes are candidates for mechanical ventilatory support. Either a positive pressure or a negative pressure respirator may be used. The superiority of high-frequency ventilation over the conventional method in management of RDS has not been proven.

Topical administration of surfactant is now possible with the availability of two preparations, namely a liquid formulation extracted from minced bovine lungs (Survanta) and a synthetic emulsified phospholipid compound (Exosurf). They have recently been approved for prevention and treatment of the neonatal RDS. These preparations are injected via an endotracheal tube into the neonate's airway. Prophylactic use immediately after intubation is intended to prevent atelectasis and edema in premature infants at a very high risk of developing RDS (those delivered before the 30th week of gestation). For treatment purpose, these preparations are administered promptly if the infant develops RDS. Surfactant therapy has been shown to be effective in reducing the risk of developing or worsening RDS and in decreasing its complications. Its long-term effects on morbidity and mortality are not entirely known.

Complications. Infants suffering from RDS are prone to develop a variety of pulmonary and extrapulmonary complications, which are in part due to therapeutic interventions. Severe hypoxemia, acidosis, and other factors increasing pulmonary artery resistance may prevent timely closure of **ductus arteriosus** through which significant shunting between pulmonary artery and aorta takes place. Although with the improvement of respiratory status, it may eventually close spontaneously, in some children it remains open (*patent ductus arteriosus*). The administration of high oxygen concentrations may result in *pulmonary oxygen toxicity*, which is enhanced by positive pressure ventilation. Infants requiring mechanical ventilation and high FIO_2s who survive the early acute stage of RDS may develop a chronic condition known as **bronchopulmonary dysplasia** (BPD). Instead of the usual improvement that most surviving infants show on the third or fourth day of their illness, these babies continue to have respiratory difficulty and require prolonged ventilatory support. The radiographic findings rapidly evolve from the consolidation of RDS to cystic changes, showing areas of atelectasis and hyperinflation with a sponge-like appearance. After a long hospitalization and intensive respiratory care, many infants with BPD will survive and may even recover completely; however, pulmonary fibrosis, chronic respiratory failure, and cor pulmonale may develop from this complication.

BIBLIOGRAPHY

Caminiti SP, Young SL. The pulmonary surfactant system. *Hosp Pract.* 1991; 26(1):94–117.

Dobbs LG. Pulmonary surfactant. *Annu Rev Med.* 1989; 40:431–446.

Golembeski D, Merritt TA. New strategies for prevention of neonatal respiratory distress syndrome: acceleration of fetal lung maturation and exogenous surfactant replacement. *Semin Respir Med*. 1990; 11:117–126.

Hallman M, Gluck L. Respiratory distress syndrome. *Prediatr Clin North Am*. 1982; 29(5):1057–1075.

Horbar JD, Soll RF, Sutherland JM, et al. A multicenter randomized, placebo-controlled trial of surfactant therapy for respiratory distress syndrome. *N Engl J Med*. 1989; 320:959–965.

Jefferies AL, Coates G, O'Brodovich H. Pulmonary epithelial permeability in hyaline-membrane disease. *N Engl J Med*. 1984; 311:1075–1080.

Kendig JW, Notter RH, Cox C. et al. A comparison of surfactant as immediate prophylaxix and as rescue therapy in newborns of less than 30 weeks' gestation. *N Engl J Med*. 1991; 324:788–794.

Merritt TA, Cochrane CG, Hallman M, et al. Reduction of lung injury by human surfactant treatment in respiratory distress syndrome. *Chest*. 1983; 83(suppl):27S–31S.

Moores RR, Abman SH. Bronchopulmonary dysplasia. *Semin Respir Med*. 1990; 11:140–151.

Phelps DL. Neonatal oxygen toxicity—is it preventable? *Pediatr Clin North Am*. 1982; 29(5):1233–1239.

Surfactant for premature infants with respiratory distress. *Med Lett Drugs Ther*. 1990; 32:2–3.

Wright JR, Clements JA. Metabolism and turnover of lung surfactant. *Am Rev Respir Dis*. 1987; 136:426–444.

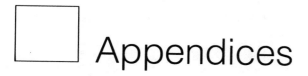

SECTION **XII**

Appendices

Certain Symbols and Abbreviations Used in Respiratory Physiology

A	alveolar gas	DCO	diffusing capacity for carbon monoxide
a	arterial blood		
$A\text{-}aDO_2$	alveolar-arterial oxygen gradient	D_LCO	diffusing capacity of lung for carbon monoxide
$ATPS$	ambient temperature and pressure saturated with water vapor	DO_2	diffusing capacity for oxygen
BSA	body surface area	E	expired gas
$BTPS$	body temperature and pressure saturated with water vapor	ERV	expiratory reserve volume
C	content; concentration; compliance	F	fractional concentration
		f	frequency of breathing
c	capillary blood	FEF	forced expiratory flow
$C(a\text{-}vDO_2)$	arteriovenous oxygen content difference	FEF_{25-75} or MMF	maximum mid-expiratory flow
C_aO_2	oxygen content in 100 mL of arterial blood	$FEF_{200-1200}$ or $MEFR$	maximum expiratory flow rate
C_cO_2	oxygen content in 100 mL of pulmonary capillary blood	FEV_T	forced expiratory volume over a given time
C_L	compliance of lungs (static)	FIO_2	fractional concentration of oxygen in inspired gas
$C(L + T)$	compliance of lungs and thorax	FRC	functional residual capacity
C_vO_2	oxygen content in 100 mL of mixed venous blood	FVC	forced vital capacity
		I	inspired gas
CVP	central venous pressure	IC	inspiratory capacity
D	diffusing capacity; dead-space gas	IRV	inspiratory reserve volume
		$MEFR$	maximum expiratory flow rate
		$MMEF$	maximum mid-expiratory flow rate

MPAP	mean pulmonary artery pressure	**R**	respiratory exchange ratio or respiratory quotient ($\dot{V}_{CO_2}/\dot{V}_{O_2}$)
MVV	maximum voluntary ventilation	**RA**	right atrium
P	gas pressure	**RAW**	airway resistance
P$_{50}$	blood oxygen tension at which 50% of the hemoglobin is saturated	**RV**	residual volume, right ventricle
		S	percent of saturation
PA	pulmonary artery	**STPD**	standard temperature (0°C), 760 mm Hg pressure, dry
P(A-aDO$_2$)	alveolar-arterial oxygen tension difference		
P$_a$CO$_2$	partial pressure of carbon dioxide in arterial blood	**T**	total; tidal; temperature
		TLC	total lung capacity
P$_A$CO$_2$	partial pressure of carbon dioxide in alveolar gas	**Torr**	Torricelli, mm Hg
		TV	tidal volume
P$_a$O$_2$	partial pressure of oxygen in arterial blood	**V**	gas volume
		$\dot{V}$	gas flow
P$_A$O$_2$	partial pressure of oxygen in alveolar gas	**v**	venous blood
		$\bar{v}$	mixed venous blood
PAP	pulmonary artery pressure	**V$_A$**	volume of alveolar gas
P$_E$CO$_2$	partial pressure of carbon dioxide in expiratory gas	**VC**	vital capacity
		$\dot{V}$CO$_2$	carbon dioxide elimination per minute
PE$_{max}$	maximum expiratory pressure (static)	**V$_D$**	volume of dead space
PFR	peak flow rate	**V$_D$/V$_T$**	ratio of dead space to tidal volume
PI$_{max}$	maximum inspiratory pressure (static)	**V$_E$**	volume of expired gas
P$_v$O$_2$	partial pressure of oxygen in venous blood	**$\dot{V}_{max\ 50}$**	maximum expiratory flow at 50% of expired vital capacity
P$_{\bar{v}}$O$_2$	partial pressure of oxygen in mixed venous blood	**$\dot{V}_{max\ 75}$**	maximum expiratory flow at 75% of expired vital capacity
PVR	pulmonary vascular resistance		
PWP	pulmonary artery wedge pressure	**$\dot{V}$O$_2$**	oxygen consumption or uptake per minute
Q	volume of blood	**$\dot{V}/\dot{Q}$**	ventilation-perfusion ratio
$\dot{Q}$	blood flow	**V$_T$**	tidal volume
$\dot{Q}_S$	blood flow through shunt	**$\dot{V}$O$_{2\ max}$**	maximum O$_2$ uptake
$\dot{Q}_T$	total blood flow (cardiac output)		

Predicted Normal Values for Pulmonary Function Tests

LUNG VOLUMES

There are significant variations in lung volumes in normal individuals. They vary not only with age, race, sex, height, body surface area, and position, but also among members of a homogeneous group under standard conditions. Age is particularly important in relation to residual volume and the ratio of residual volume to the total lung capacity. Body height influences the total lung capacity, vital capacity, and functional residual capacity.

The following is an example of typical values for a healthy young male; the figures are approximate and are shown for the purpose of comparison between various lung volumes and capacities.

Total lung capacity	6000 mL
Vital capacity	4800 mL
Inspiratory capacity	3600 mL
Functional residual capacity	2400 mL
Tidal volume	500 mL
Residual volume	1200 mL
Inspiratory reserve volume	3100 mL
Expiratory reserve volume	1200 mL

There are several equations and nomograms for calculation of *predicted* normal lung volumes from age, sex, height, weight, and body surface area. The following are some of the useful prediction formulas that are commonly used.

Vital Capacity

Predicted normal values for vital capacity (vc) may be calculated from the following formulas:

For adult males;

$$VC \text{ (liters)} = 0.052 \times \text{height (cm)} - 0.022 \times \text{age} - 3.6$$

For adult females;

$$VC \text{ (liters)} = 0.041 \times \text{height (cm)} - 0.018 \times \text{age} - 2.69$$

Total Lung Capacity

Total lung capacity is estimated by dividing the calculated predicted normal vital capacity by 0.8 for the age group 15–34, by 0.75 for 35–49 years, and by 0.65 for the group over 50. It may also be computed by one of the prediction equations, such as:

$$TLC \text{ (liters)} = 0.078 \times \text{height (cm)} - 7.30$$

for adult males.

$$TLC \text{ (liters)} = 0.0746 \times \text{height (cm)} - (0.013 \times \text{age}) - 6.2$$

for adult females.

Residual Volume

One of the prediction formulas for RV in adult males is:

$$RV \text{ (liters)} = 0.027 \times \text{height (cm)} + 0.017 \times \text{age} - 3.45$$

and for adult females:

$$RV \text{ (liters)} = 0.028 \times \text{height (cm)} + 0.016 \times \text{age} - 3.54$$

Dead-Space Volume

Average normal dead-space volume for a young adult male is about 150 mL and V_D/V_T ratio is 0.33. The regression of the dead-space—tidal volume ratio with age in seated normal subjects at rest is given by the following formula:

$$V_D/V_T = 24.6 + 0.17 \times \text{age}$$

FLOW RATES

From a simple forced expiratory spirogram, the most commonly used variables, including forced vital capacity (FVC), forced expiratory volumes (FEV_1, FEV_2, FEV_3), FEV_1/FVC, maximum mid-expiratory flow rate (FEF_{25-75}), and maximum expiratory flow rate ($FEV_{200-1200}$), are compared with predicted normal values for height, age, and sex, derived from available tables, formulas, or nomograms. Figures B–1 and B–2 are prediction nomograms and formulas for normal men and women. Normal predicted values are determined by laying a straight edge between the height and the age of the individual and reading the values from the corresponding scales. It should be emphasized that there are significant variations among normal individuals with the same sex, height, and age, depending on other factors such as race and body build. Normal individuals can expire 83% of their vital capacity in 1 s, 94 percent in 2 s, and 97 percent in 3 s.

DIFFUSING CAPACITY

The average normal diffusing capacity is about 25 mLCO/min/mm Hg. There are numerous prediction equations for carbon monoxide diffusing capacity (D_LCO). The following prediction formulas are more commonly used:

Adult males:

$$D_LCO \text{ (mL/min/mm Hg)} = 0.416 \times \text{height (cm)} - 0.219 \times \text{age} - 26.34$$

Adult females:

$$D_LCO \text{ (mL/min/mm Hg)} = 0.256 \times \text{height (cm)} - 0.144 \times \text{age} - 8.36$$

Multiplying D_LCO by a factor of 1.23 will give diffusing capacity for oxygen (D_LO_2).

ARTERIAL BLOOD GASES

Normal arterial blood gases and pH at sea level are

PaO_2	95 ± 5 mm Hg
$PaCO_2$	40 ± 5 mm Hg
SaO_2	$97 \pm 2\%$
pH	7.40 ± 0.02
HCO_3^-	24 ± 2 mEq

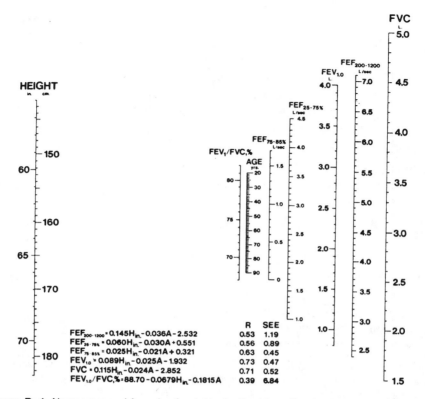

Figure B–1. Nomogram and formulas for determination of predicted values of expiratory flow rates for normal males. Reprinted by permission of the *Western Journal of Medicine*. (Morris JF. Spirometry in the evaluation of pulmonary function. *West J Med* 1976, August; 125: 110–118.)

In normal subjects the arterial blood PCO_2 does not change significantly with age. On the other hand, arterial blood PO_2 decreases with age according to the following regression formulas:

In supine position:
$$P_aO_2 = 103.5 - 0.42 \times \text{age}.$$
In seated position:
$$P_aO_2 = 104.2 - 0.27 \times \text{age}.$$

In young healthy adults the alveolar-arterial PO_2 difference is about 9 mm Hg. This increases with age according to the following formula:

$$P(A\text{-}aDO_2) = 2.5 + 0.21 \times \text{age}$$

COMPLIANCE

The normal values for static compliance are as follows:

Pulmonary compliance: 0.166–0.246 liters per cm of H_2O.

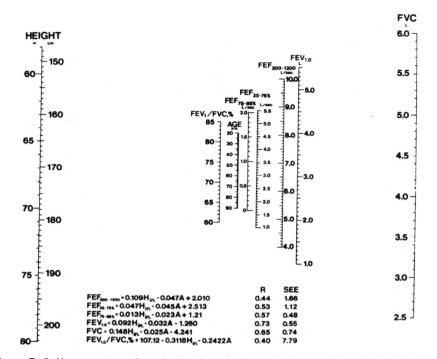

Figure B–2. Nomogram and formulas for determination of predicted values of expiratory flow rates for normal females. Reprinted by permission of the *Western Journal of Medicine*. (Morris JF. Spirometry in the evaluation of pulmonary function. *West J Med* 1976, August; 125: 110–118.)

Chest-wall compliance: 0.125–0.209 liters per cm of H_2O.
Total compliance: 0.072–0.110 liters per cm of H_2O.

MAXIMUM RESPIRATORY PRESSURES

The following are predicted normal values for maximum inspiratory and expiratory pressures in adults (between the ages of 19 and 49).

Adult males:

PI_{max}	−127 ± 28 (cmH_2O)
PE_{max}	216 ± 45 (cmH_2O)

Adult females:

PI_{max}	−91 ± 25 (cmH_2O)
PE_{max}	138 ± 39 (cmH_2O)

Normal Compensatory Responses to Simple Acid-Base Disturbances

The following are relationships between changes resulting from primary acid-base disorders and corresponding secondary or compensatory changes (simple acid-base disorders). It should be noted that these relationships are not applicable when the acid-base abnormalities are extreme.

Primary disorders	*Corresponding secondary changes*
Metabolic acidosis	$\Delta PCO_2(mm\ HG) = 1.1-1.3 \times \Delta HCO_3^-(mEq/L)$
Metabolic alkalosis	$\Delta PCO_2(mm\ Hg) = 0.6-0.8 \times \Delta HCO_3^-(mEq/L)$
Respiratory acidosis (acute)	$\Delta HCO_3^-(mEq/L) = 0.1 \times \Delta PCO_2(mm\ Hg)$
Respiratory acidosis (chronic)	$\Delta HCO_3^-(mEq/L) = 0.3-0.4 \times \Delta PCO_2(mm\ Hg)$
Respiratory alkalosis (acute)	$\Delta HCO_3^-(mEq/L) = 0.2 \times \Delta PCO_2(mm\ Hg)$
Respiratory alkalosis (chronic)	$\Delta HCO_3^-(mEq/L) = 0.5-0.6 \times \Delta PCO_2(mm\ Hg)$

The acid-base map in Figure C–1 shows, in different band forms, relationships between pH, PCO_2 and HCO_3^- in simple acid-base disturbances. Each band represents the 95% confidence limits with the particular acid-base disturbance as indicated. Mixed acid-base disorders are usually, but not always, located outside these bands.

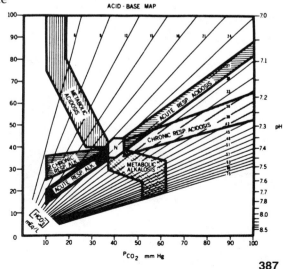

Figure C–1. Acid-base map. The bands show the six simple acid-base disorders. The numbered lines represent isopleths for bicarbonate levels. Mixed disorders are usually located outside the bands. Reproduced by permission from M. Goldberg et al. Computer-based instruction and diagnosis of acid-base disorders. (*JAMA* 1973, 223:269–275. Copyright 1973, American Medical Association.)

Alveolar Air Equation

When the inspired air enters the alveoli, it is warmed to the body temperature (37°C) and saturated with water vapor. At this temperature the water vapor pressure is 47 mm Hg. Therefore, at sea level, the total pressure of the alveolar O_2, N_2, and CO_2 is 760 minus 47, or 713 mm Hg.

If the number of molecules of O_2 absorbed were equal to that of CO_2 entering the alveoli, the $P_AO_2 = FIO_2$ (713) $- P_ACO_2$. However, because the respiratory exchange ratio (R, which is the ratio of the amount of CO_2 eliminated to the amount of O_2 consumed) is usually less than 1, a correcting factor of $[FIO_2 + (1 - FIO_2)/R]$ should be included in the above equation for accurate calculation of alveolar oxygen tension:

$$P_AO_2 = FIO_2 (713) - P_ACO_2 \times$$

$$\left(FIO_2 + \frac{1 - FIO_2}{R} \right)$$

A simplified form of the equation, which is commonly used for determining the alveolar oxygen tension, with an assumed R value of 0.8 is:

$$P_AO_2 = FIO_2 (713) - \frac{P_aCO_2}{0.8}$$

Calculation of Alveolar Ventilation

As all the CO_2 in the expired gas comes from alveolar gas, the volume of CO_2 will be equal to the alveolar ventilation multiplied by its fractional concentration (F_ACO_2):

$$\dot{V}CO_2 = \dot{V}_A \times F_ACO_2 \qquad (1)$$

$$\dot{V}_A = \frac{\dot{V}CO_2}{F_ACO_2} \qquad (2)$$

or

F_ACO_2 at atmospheric pressure of 760 torr will be equal to $P_ACO_2/760$. Substituting F_ACO_2 by P_ACO_2, equation (2) becomes

$$\dot{V}_A = \frac{\dot{V}CO_2 \times 760}{P_ACO_2} \qquad (3)$$

However, this equation, which is based on STPD (standard temperature of 0° C, 760 torr pressure, dry), should be corrected to BTPS (body temperature of 37° C and pressure saturated with water vapor). According to Charles's law, the volume of a gas increases proportionally to the absolute temperature. Therefore, equation (3) should be multiplied by a factor of $(273 + 37)/273$ or $310/273$. Thus

$$\dot{V}_A = \frac{\dot{V}CO_2 \times 863}{P_ACO_2} \qquad (4)$$

As P_ACO_2 is practically the same as P_aCO_2, the final equation will be

$$\dot{V}_A \ (mL/min) = \frac{\dot{V}CO_2 \times 863}{P_aCO_2} \qquad (5)$$

Calculation of Physiologic Dead Space: Bohr's Equation

Tidal volume (V_T) is composed of two portions:

1. The portion made up of physiologic dead space (V_D), which has the same concentration of carbon dioxide as inspired air, that is negligible and
2. the portion that participates in gas exchange and, therefore, is the source of carbon dioxide content of the expired tidal volume. The latter portion is equal to the difference between the tidal volume and the physiologic dead space ($V_T - V_D$).

Thus:

$$V_T \times F_E CO_2 = (V_T - V_D)F_A CO_2$$

in which $F_E CO_2$ and $F_A CO_2$ represent the concentration of carbon dioxide in expired air and alveolar air, respectively. The equation can be changed to:

$$V_D = V_T \frac{F_A CO_2 - F_E CO_2}{F_A CO_2}$$

By changing the fractional concentration (F) to the partial pressure (P), the equation becomes:

$$V_D = V_T \frac{P_A CO_2 - P_E CO_2}{P_A CO_2}$$

As the arterial PCO_2 is essentially the same as alveolar PCO_2, arterial PCO_2 ($P_a CO_2$) can be used to replace $P_A CO_2$. The final equation will be:

$$V_D = V_T \frac{P_a CO_2 - P_E CO_2}{P_a CO_2}$$

which is known as *Bohr's equation*.

Normal Hemodynamic Values in Recumbent Adults

Pressures (mm Hg)
  Systemic artery
    Systolic   90–140
    Diastolic   60–90
    Mean   70–105
  Pulmonary artery
    Systolic   15–28
    Diastolic   5–16
    Mean   10–22
  Pulmonary artery wedge
    Mean   6–15
  Right ventricle
    Systolic   15–28
    End-diastolic   0–8
  Right atrium   0–8
  CVP   0–8
Resistance (dyne. sec. cm^{-5})
  Total systemic   900–1400
  Total pulmonary   150–250
Flow
  Cardiac index (L/min/m²)
                         2.8–4.2

Venous-to-Arterial Shunt Equation

Arterial blood in a patient with venous-to-arterial shunt contains some mixed venous blood ($\bar{v}$) that bypasses the lungs and some well-oxygenated blood that passes through the pulmonary capillaries (c). The amount of O_2 in the arterial blood, therefore, equals the amount of oxygen in the pulmonary capillary blood plus the amount of this gas in the shunted venous blood:

$$\dot{Q}_T \times C_aO_2 = \dot{Q}_S \times C_{\bar{v}}O_2 + (\dot{Q}_T - \dot{Q}_S) \times C_cO_2 \quad (1)$$

$\dot{Q}_T$ = amount of total blood flow; $\dot{Q}_S$ = blood flow through shunt; $\dot{Q}_T - \dot{Q}_S$ = blood flow through pulmonary capillary; C_aO_2 = amount of O_2 in arterial blood; $C_{\bar{v}}O_2$ = amount of O_2 in mixed venous blood; C_cO_2 = amount of O_2 in pulmonary capillary blood.

Equation (1) can be rearranged to become:

$$\frac{\dot{Q}_S}{\dot{Q}_T} = \frac{C_cO_2 - C_aO_2}{C_cO_2 - C_{\bar{v}}O_2} \quad (2)$$

In situations in which P_aO_2 is high enough to ensure full saturation of hemoglobin (ie, P_aO_2 is 150 torr or higher), the equation can be written as:

$$\frac{\dot{Q}_S}{\dot{Q}_T} = \frac{P(A\text{-}aDO_2) \times 0.0031}{P(A\text{-}aDO_2) \times 0.0031 + C(a - \bar{v}DO_2)} \quad (3)$$

$P(A\text{-}aDO_2)$ is the alveolar-arterial oxygen tension difference, and $C(a\text{-}\bar{v}DO_2)$ is the arteriovenous oxygen content difference. The shunt is usually calculated while the patient is breathing 100% oxygen.

REFERENCES FOR APPENDICES

Boren HG, Kory RC, Syner JC. The Veterans Administration–Army cooperative study of pulmonary function: II. The lung volume and its subdivisions in normal men. *Am J Med.* 1966; 41:96–114.

Crapo RO. Reference values for pulmonary function tests. *Respir Care.* 1989; 34:626–634.

Crapo RO, Morris AH. Standardized single breath normal values for carbon monoxide diffusing capacity. *Am Rev Respir Dis.* 1981; 123:185–189.

Forster RE II, Dubois AB, Briscoe WA, Fisher AB. *The Lung,* 3rd ed. Chicago: Year Book Medical Publishers, 1986.

Goldberg M, Green SB, Moss ML, et al. Computer-based instruction and diagnosis of acid-base disorders: A systematic approach. *JAMA.* 1973; 223:269–275.

Kory RC, Callahan R, Boren HG, Syner JC. The Veterans Administration–Army cooperative study of pulmonary function: I. Clinical spirometry in normal men. *Am J Med.* 1961; 30:243–258.

Morris JF. Spirometry in the evaluation of pulmonary function. *West J Med.* 1976; 125:110–118.

West JB. *Pulmonary Pathophysiology,* 2nd ed. Baltimore: Williams & Wilkins, 1982.

Accessory. supplementary, added to, or helping another with the same function.

Acetylcholine. a chemical neurotransmitter operating in many parts of the nervous system and neuromuscular junction.

Acetylcholinesterase. an enzyme, present at the sites of acetylcholine activity, that hydrolyzes acetylcholine and thus controls its effect.

Acidemia. a decrease in pH of the blood.

Acidosis. a disorder of normal acid-base balance resulting from accumulation of acid and/or reduction of bicarbonate in the blood or tissue.

Acinus. the portion of the lung distal to terminal bronchiole comprising respiratory bronchioles, alveolar ducts, alveolar sacs, and alveoli.

Acrolein. an aldehyde (acrylic aldehide) generated by decomposition of glycerin.

Adrenergic. related to epinephrine (adrenaline) or substances with similar activity; pertaining to or affecting the sympathetic nervous system.

Adventitious. associated with or added to something in a nonessential and extrinsic fashion.

Aerobic. occurring in the presence of molecular oxygen.

Agammaglobulinemia. absence of gamma globulins in the blood.

Agglutination. the process of clumping together of antigen-bearing cells or substances in the presence of specific antibodies.

Air cyst or Bulla. a thin-walled radiolucent area surrounded by more or less normal lung.

Alkalemia. an increase in pH of the blood.

Alkalosis. a disorder of normal acid-base balance resulting from excessive accumulation of base or excessive loss of hydrogen ion (acid).

Allergen. a substance capable of causing allergy or hypersensitivity reaction.

Allergy. a hypersensitivity state developing as a result of exposure to a substance (allergen), reexposure causing an exaggerated reaction.

Alpha interferon. an interferon produced by leukocytes (see Interferon).

Alveolar (air space density). results from the presence of denser substances replacing the air in the alveoli. Alveolar edema gives rise to this type of radiographic change. Pulmonary consolidation is a confluent air-space density.

Alveolitis. inflammation at the alveolar sites.

Alveolus. a small saclike dilatation; the smallest gas exchanging unit of the lung outpouching from the respiratory bronchioles, alveolar ducts, or alveolar sacs.

Amyotrophic. pertaining to muscle atrophy.

Amyotrophic lateral sclerosis. a chronic neurologic condition resulting from degeneration of motor neurons in the spinal cord and brain stem causing progressive muscle weakness and atrophy.

Anaerobic. occurring in the absence of molecular oxygen.

Anaphylaxis. a severe, often life-threatening reaction resulting from an exaggerated allergic response to an antigen to which an individual is sensitized from previous exposure.

Angina pectoris. an acute, transient, and often recurring chest pain resulting from insufficient oxygen supply to the heart muscle to meet its metabolic demand.

Angiography. radiographic visualization of blood vessels following injection of contrast material.

Angiotensin. a polypeptide formed by the action of renin on its plasma precursor (angiotensinogen). Its activation by a converting enzyme results in formation of a potent substance known as angiotensin II.

Ankylosing spondylitis. inflammation of vertebrae that eventually results in their ankylosis.

Ankylosis. immobility of a joint resulting from fusion of component bones.

Anoxemia. lack of oxygen in the blood.

Anoxia. lack of oxygen in the tissue or cell.

Anthracite. hard coal.

Antibody. a specific protein molecule produced by special cells (plasma cells) as a result of their interaction with an antigen.

Anticholinergics. substances that block the passage of impulses through the parasympathetic nerves.

Antigen. any substance capable of inducing an immunologic response or production of an antibody.

Antiprotease. a substance that checks the effect of proteolytic enzymes.

Apnea. cessation of breathing.

Aromatic. characteristic of a chemical compound with a benzene ring.

Arthroconidia. spores formed asexually in close sequence in the hyphae of certain fungi.

Asbestosis. diffuse lung fibrosis resulting from exposure to asbestos fibers.

Atelectasis. incomplete or absence of expansion of a lung or part of it.

Atopy. a hereditary state of allergy predisposing to development of certain clinical conditions such as hay fever, asthma, and eczema.

Auscultation. the act of listening to the sounds produced within the body, usually with a stethoscope.

Autoantibody. an antibody against the body's own constituents.

Autoimmunity. a condition in which immunologic reaction occurs against the components of the body's own tissues or cells.

Bactericidal. capable of killing bacteria.

Bagassosis. lung disease due to exposure to moldy bagasse (the residue of sugar cane).

Barotrauma. injury resulting from changes in barometric pressure or high inflating pressure.

Bisulfite. an acid sulfite (salt of sulfurous acid).

Bituminous coal. soft coal.

Bleb. a blister; an air cyst in the lung adjacent to the pleura.

Blue bloater. a cyanotic patient with chronic respiratory failure, carbon dioxide retention, and right heart failure.

B lymphocytes. lymphocytes involved in humoral immunity (antibody production).

Bohr effect. facilitation of oxygen unloading at tissue sites by an increase in capillary blood PCO_2 (and decrease in pH).

Bradypnea. abnormally slow respiratory rate.

Bronchoconstriction. constriction or narrowing of the bronchi; bronchospasm.

Bronchogenic. originating in a bronchus.

Bronchogram. x-ray film demonstrating or outlining the bronchi, usually following instillation of a contrast material.

Bronchopulmonary dysplasia. a chronic lung disease of infants that usually develops following respiratory distress syndrome.

Bronchovesicular. pertaining to breath sounds with a quality between that of bronchial and vesicular sounds.

Buffer. a chemical system that prevents or attenuates changes in acid-base balance when an acid or base is added.

Bulla. an air cyst inside the lung.

Bullectomy. surgical excision of a bulla.

Calcification. hardening of tissues by deposition of calcium salts.

Carbamino compounds. chemical compounds resulting from combination of carbon dioxide with amino ($-NH_2$) groups of hemoglobin or plasma proteins.

Carbonic anhydrase. an enzyme that catalyzes the chemical reaction between carbon dioxide and water, thus facilitating the transfer of carbon dioxide from tissues to blood and to alveolar air.

Carboxyhemoglobin. chemical compound of hemoglobin with carbon monoxide.

Carcinogenic. producing cancer.

Carina. a ridge; a ridgelike structure at the end of the trachea between the openings of two main bronchi.

Caseous. cheeselike.

Catecholamine. group of compounds such as epinephrine and norepinephrine having a sympathomimetic action.

Cavity. a radiolucent lesion surrounded by denser tissue. It is due to a localized necrotic lung lesion that has sloughed off. It is the hallmark of the lung abscess. A fluid level may be seen inside a cavity.

Centrilobular. pertaining to the central portion of a pulmonary lobule or acinus; centriacinar

Chemoprophylaxis. use of chemotherapeutic agents to prevent development of a specific disease.

Chemoreceptor. a receptor that senses the presence of chemical substances.

Chemotherapy. treatment with chemical agents that have specific toxic effect on certain microorganisms (such as tubercle bacilli) or neoplastic cells.

Cheyne-Stokes respiration. a waxing and waning of breathing with changing in its depth and rate at regular intervals

Cholinergic. related to acetylcholine as applied to the nerve fibers with acetylcholine as their neurotransmitter, particularly the parasympathetic nerves; parasympathomimetic.

Cholinergic crisis. a critical worsening of muscular weakness in myasthenia gravis from excessive use of cholinergic drugs.

Chylothorax. presence of chyle (milky fluid of intestinal lymph) in the pleural cavity.

Cilia. hairlike, vibrating processes projecting from the free surface of cells lining the airways or other similar structures.

Circadian. pertaining to rhythmic biologic cycles repeated at 24-hour intervals.

Coalescence. growing or blending together into one body.

Compliance. a quality of yielding to pressure; increase in volume per unit of pressure change.

Congestion. excessive accumulation of blood in the vessels of an organ.

Consolidation. process of becoming solid, as the lung becoming airless with accumulation of exudative fluid and cells in pneumonia.

Consumption. a wasting away of the body as applied to advanced tuberculosis.

Contusion. a traumatic lesion of an organ or tissue without breaking the overlying skin; bruise.

Costal. pertaining to ribs.

Costophrenic. pertaining to ribs and diaphragm, as applied to the angle between the rib cage and diaphragm in the chest x-ray film.

Croup. a condition resulting from an acute inflammation of laryngeal structures causing characteristic barking cough.

Cyanosis. bluish or purplish discoloration of skin or mucous membrane usually from the presence of high concentration of reduced hemoglobin in the capillaries.

Cylindrical. shaped like a cylinder, describing a form of bronchiectasis.

Cyst. any saclike structure containing air or fluid.

Cytotoxic. having toxic effect against cells.

Decortication. removal of covering, usually applied to surgical excision of pleural peel from around the lung.

Deglutitory. pertaining to deglutition (swallowing).

Dermatomyositis. inflammation of skin and muscle.

Diffusion. random molecular movement by which a matter is transported from an area of higher to one of lower concentration until equilibrium is reached.

Ductus arteriosus. a fetal blood vessel that connects the pulmonary artery to the aorta (it normally closes shortly after birth).

Dyskinesia. difficult or abnormal movement.

Dysplasia. abnormality of growth or development of an organ, tissue or cell.

Dyspnea. difficulty in breathing.

Edema. accumulation of excessive amount of fluid in extracellular space resulting in swelling that usually pits upon pressure.

Effector. an organ, tissue, or cell that responds to a chemical mediator.

Effusion. escape of fluid from its natural vessels into a body cavity.

Egophony. a characteristic change in sound upon its transmission through the diseased lung and pleura; sound of a bleating goat.

Elastase. one of the proteases (enzymes that split the proteins) that preferentially attacks the elastic tissue.

Electrooculogram. a graphic tracing of the changes in electrical potentials resulting from eye movements.

Embolism. occlusion of a blood vessel by a matter (embolus) carried by the blood flow from another site.

Embolus. an undissolved matter carried in blood to be lodged in a vessel and to obstruct it.

Empyema. accumulation of pus in a body cavity, usually referring to pleural space.

Endemic. present among a particular people or in a specified locality.

Endogenous. originating or growing from within.

Endoscopy. visual inspection of a body cavity or hollow organ with the help of an appropriate instrument (endoscope).

Epiglottitis. inflammation of the epiglottis.

Epithelioid. resembling epithelium, applied to cells in granulomas (derived from monocytes or macrophages).

Ergometer. a device for measuring the amount of work performed.

Etiology. study of the causes of diseases.

Exacerbation. increase in severity of a disease, its symptoms, or signs.

Exocrine. secreting externally.

Exogenous. originating or growing from outside.

Expectoration. the act of coughing up and spitting out materials from within the thorax.

Expiratory reserve volume (ERV). the maximum volume of air that can be exhaled after expiration of tidal volume.

Extrinsic. originating or operating from without.

Exudate. a fluid with a high protein content, and often with a high cell count, that has exuded from blood capillaries, as a result of abnormal leakage, as with inflammation.

Fibroblast. a connective tissue cell that is involved in formation of fibrous tissue.

Fibroplasia. formation of fibrous tissue.

Fibrosis. development in an organ or tissue of excess fibrous and connective tissue.

Fibrothorax. a chronic pleural disease characterized by formation of thick fibrous tissue and adhesion of the two layers of pleura.

Fick method (principle). a method of measurement of cardiac output (L/min) by the oxygen consumption (mL/min) divided by the difference between the arterial and mixed-venous blood oxygen contents (mL/L).

Fremitus. a vibration felt by palpation.

Functional residual capacity (FRC). the volume of air remaining in the lungs at the end of expiration of tidal volume. *This is the resting end-expiratory position.*

Fusiform. shaped like a spindle.

Genioglossus. one of the muscles of the tongue originating from the inner surface of the mandible (mental spine) and attaching to the hyoid bone and the whole length of undersurface of the tongue.

Genomic. pertaining to a genome (the complete set of genetic factors).

Glossopharyngeal. pertaining to the tongue and pharynx, usually applied to the 9th cranial nerve.

Glottis. the opening between the vocal cords.

Glutathione. a reduced form of tripeptide that is an important antioxidant against harmful effects of many toxic substances.

Granulocytopenia. reduced numbers of granulocytes (mainly neutrophils) in blood.

Granuloma. a tumor-like pathologic structure composed of modified macrophages (epithelioid and giant cells) and usually surrounded by lymphocytes, resulting from chronic inflammation as in tuberculosis or sarcoidosis.

Haldane effect. facilitation of carbon dioxide loading at the tissue site by unloading of oxygen (changing from HbO_2 to Hb).

Heat exhaustion. extreme weakness or fatigue from water loss or salt depletion.

Hectic. related to having undulating fever with wasting away, as in advanced tuberculosis.

Hematoma. a localized swelling from accumulation of blood.

Hemithorax. one half (right or left) of the chest.

Hemodynamics. science or study of the movements of blood and related forces.

Hemopneumothorax. accumulation of blood and air in the pleural cavity.

Hemoptysis. expectoration of blood.

Hemothorax. accumulation of blood in the pleural cavity.

Heterozygous. having dissimilar pairs of genes for any hereditary characteristic; opposite of homozygous.

Homogenous density. characteristic of uniformly dense lesions, such as a solid tumor, fluid-containing cyst, or collection of fluid in the pleural space.

Honeycombing. coarse reticular density.

Hyaline. resembling glass; translucent or transparent.

Hydropneumothorax. collection of fluid and air in the pleural space.

Hydrothorax. collection of watery fluid in the pleural space; pleural effusion.

Hypercarbia. excess of carbon dioxide in blood; hypercapnia.

Hyperlucency. excessive radiolucency.

Hyperplasia. a nontumorous increase in the number of normal cells in normal tissue resulting in its enlargement.

Hyperreactivity. greater than normal responsiveness to stimuli.

Hypertrophy. a nontumorous increase in size of an organ or tissue as a result of the enlargement, but not increase in number, of its cells.

Hypocarbia. reduced carbon dioxide in blood; hypocapnia.

Hypopharynx. the lower part of the pharynx located between the upper edge of epiglottis and openings of larynx and esophagus.

Hypoxemia. low blood level of partial pressure of oxygen.

Hypoxia. reduced oxygen in the tissue or cell.

Iatrogenic. induced in a patient by a physician's action, usually of adverse effect.

Idiopathic. of unknown origin or cause.

Idiosyncrasy. a structural or functional characteristic peculiar to an individual; an abnormal susceptibility to the effect of a drug, not from allergy.

Immune complex. combination of an antigen with its specific antibody.

Immunocompetent. capable of developing an immune response to antigenic exposure.

Immunocompromised. having a diminished or absent immune response as a result of pathologic conditions or the effect of certain drugs.

Immunodeficiency. a state of defective immune response, either humoral or cell-mediated.

Immunosuppressive. an agent that prevents or reduces an immune response.

Immunotherapy. a treatment intended to alter the immune response by administration of a known antigen or allergen.

Indolent. causing little or no pain (or other symptoms or signs).

Induration. an abnormally hard lesion or reaction, as in positive tuberculin skin test.

Infarction. formation of an area of necrosis as a result of failure of local blood supply (infarct).

Infiltration. penetration and accumulation in a tissue of substances or cells; radiodensity in the lung fields as a result of such an accumulation in lung parenchyma.

Inspiratory capacity (IC). the maximum volume of air that can be inpired from the resting end-expiratory position.

Inspiratory reserve volume (IRV). the maximum volume of air that one can breathe in after inspiration of tidal volume.

Interferon. a substance produced and released by certain cells infected by viruses, viral replication in many cells throughout the body.

Interstitial. situated between essential parts or in the interspaces of a tissue.

Intractable. difficult to manage or alleviate.

Ischemia. local deficiency of blood supply due to vascular disorder.

Kussmaul breathing. deep regular respiration in metabolic acidosis (particularly diabetic ketoacidosis) in which the accessory muscles of respiration are often utilized.

Kyphosis. abnormal increase in curvature of the spine with backward convexity.

Kyphoscoliosis. combination of kyphosis with scoliosis; abnormal backward and lateral curvature of the spine.

Laryngopharynx. hypopharynx.

Lecithin. a phospholipid that is a major constituent of surfactant.

Leukocytosis. an increase above normal (greater than 11,000/mm³) in the number of white blood cells in the blood.

Leukotrienes. chemical mediators of immediate hypersensitivity that include the slow-reacting substance of anaphylaxis (SRS-A).

Lobectomy. surgical resection of a pulmonary lobe.

Lymphadenitis. inflammation of lymph nodes.

Lymphadenopathy. disease of lymph nodes, usually characterized by their enlargement.

Lymphokine. any of the chemical mediators released from the activated lymphocytes that affect other cells, especially during a cell-mediated immunologic reaction.

Lysis. disintegration of cells (red blood cells, bacteria, etc.) by dissolution.

Macrophage. any of the large mononuclear phagocytic cells that exist in many organs including the lungs (alveolar macrophages).

Macule. a small spot or blotch differing from its surroundings by virtue of its color.

Mediastinum. a partition containing intrathoracic structures between the lungs.

Melanoptysis. expectoration of black sputum, as in coal workers' pneumoconiosis.

Mesothelioma. a tumorous growth derived from the lining cells of serous cavities (pleura, pericardium, or peritoneum).

Miliary. characterized by lesions resembling millet seeds, as in miliary tuberculosis.

Mucosa. a mucous membrane.

Mucopurulent. containing mucus and pus, as applied to sputum.

Mucoviscidosis. an alternative name for cystic fibrosis, which characterizes the abnormally viscous mucus in this disease.

Myasthenia crisis. a critically severe worsening of muscular weakness in myasthenia gravis related to its exacerbation.

Mycelium. filamentous vegetative parts of a fungus; hyphae.

Mycosis. a disease caused by a fungus.

Myopathy. any disease of the muscle.

Nasopharynx. upper part of the pharynx located above the level of the soft palate.

Necrosis. death of a cell or tissue.

Necrotizing. causing necrosis, as in necrotizing pneumonia.

Neoplasm. a new growth of different or abnormal tissue, usually uncontrolled.

Nitrosamine. a compound formed by the combination of nitrates with amines with the type formula R2N-NO.

Nodule. a small node or round lesion that can be palpated or visualized in a radiographic film.

Nomogram. a graph containing a number of parallel scales showing variables so that when a straightline connects two known values, the other related values are directly read at the points of intersection with their corresponding scales.

Normobaric. pertaining to normal atmospheric pressure.

Nosocomial. pertaining to or originating from a hospital, as a nosocomial infection.

Obtundation. dullness or obtuseness of sensorium.

Opportunistic. characterizing a microorganism that ordinarily does not cause disease but, with weakened body defenses, results in disease; describing a disease or infection caused by such an organism.

Oropharynx. part of the pharynx located between the levels of the soft palate and epiglottis.

Orthopnea. difficulty breathing on lying down, being improved on sitting or standing.

Panlobular or panacinar. involving the entire lobule or acinus of the lung, as in panlobular emphysema.

Paradoxical. occuring contrary to normal rule, as paradoxical chest wall or abdominal movement with breathing.

Paraneoplastic. occurring with or beside a neoplasm but not due to its direct effect; applied to syndromes associated with cancer.

Parenchyma. essential functional elements of an organ.

Paroxysmal. occurring in sudden and usually violent attack, as in paroxysmal dyspnea.

Partial pressure. pressure exerted by each of the components of a gas mixture.

Pathogenesis. mechanism of development of a diseased condition.

Pathognomonic. diagnostic of a specific disease.

Pathophysiology. study or mechanism of disordered function in a disease.

Pectus. chest, thorax, or breast.

Pectus carinatum. excessive prominence of the sterum; pigeon breast.

Pectus excavatum. excessive depression of the sterum; funnel breast.

Perfusion. the act of pouring over or through, as perfusion of tissue with blood; local blood flow.

Pericarditis. inflammation of the serous membrane enclosing the heart (pericardium).

Pertussis. whooping cough.

Petechia. a pinpoint purplish discoloration of skin or mucous membrane caused by intradermal bleeding.

Phagocyte. a cell that ingests and destroys microorganisms, foreign particles, or other cells.

Phlebitis. inflammation of a vein.

Phrenic. pertaining to the diaphragm.

Pink puffer. a patient with COPD who maintains fairly normal blood gases despite significant dyspnea.

Plasmapheresis. removal of plasma from withdrawn blood and retransfusion of its cells with donor plasma or albumin; plasma exchange.

Platypnea. dyspnea occurring in upright position, but relieved by lying down.

Plethysmograph. an instrument for measuring and recording of changes in volume of an organ or limb with blood flow, or determining changes in body volume with ventilation (body plethysmograph).

Pleural density. a radiodensity due to pleural inflammation, fluid, tumor or scarring.

Pleuritis. inflammation of pleura; pleurisy.

Pleurodesis. creation of adhesion between the parietal and visceral pleurae by surgical or medical means.

Pneumoconiosis. pulmonary disease from exposure to aerosolized particulate matter (dust).

Pneumomediastinum. presence of air in the mediastinum; mediastinal emphysema.

Pneumonectomy. surgical resection of a lung.

Pneumonitis. inflammation of the lung; pneumonia.

Pneumotachograph. an instrument for recording the velocity of respired air.

Pneumotaxic. related to repiratory rate regulation.

Pneumothorax. accumulation of air in the pleural space.

Polyclonal. derived from different clones of cells.

Polycythemia. an abnormal increase in red cells in the blood.

Polymyositis. inflammation of many muscles at once.

Polynuclear. having several nuclei.

Polypnea. an increase in the respiratory rate; tachypnea.

Polysomnography. recording of several physiologic events during sleep.

Prodrome. forewarning symptom(s) indicating that a disease is imminent.

Prostaglandin. a group of naturally occurring chemicals that have multiple functions including contraction and relaxation of smooth muscles.

Prostration. extreme physical exhaustion; a state of total helplessness.

Protease. any enzyme that acts upon proteins; a proteolytic enzyme.

Proviral. related to provirus (the genome of a virus integrated into the chromosome of the host cell).

Psychogenic. originating from an emotional or psychologic process.

Pulmonary mass. a large, 6 cm or more in diameter, demarcated radiodensity. It often indicates a neoplastic lesion. Mediastinal mass is a similar shadow in the ediastinum.

Pulmonary nodule. a circumscribed density, which may be single and then is called a solitary pulmonary nodule or "coin" lesion.

Purulent. consisting of, containing, or discharging pus.

Pyogenic. producing or able to produce pus.

Pyopneumothorax. collection of pus and air in the pleural space.

Pyothorax. collection of pus in the pleural space; thoracic empyema.

Pyrolysis. decomposition of an organic substance upon exposure to very high heat in the absence of oxygen.

Radiodensity. state of being relatively resistant to the passage of x-radiation.

Radiolucency. property of permitting the passage of x-radiation.

Rale. an abnormal crackling respiratory sound; crackle.

Receptor. a specific chemical structure on the surface or within a cell that upon recognizing and binding with another chemical structure (such as a hormone) causes a set of reactions culminating in a specific cellular response; a sensory nerve terminal that is specialized to respond to stimulating agents.

Residual volume (RV). the volume of air that remains in the lungs after a maximum expiration.

Resonance. prolongation and echoing of sound resulting from percussion over a relatively hollow structure.

Retrolental. behind the crystalline lens of the eye.

Rhonchus. an abnormal respiratory sound resulting from bronchial narrowing; a wheeze.

Saccular. shaped like a sac, as saccular bronchiectasis.

Sclerosis. a hardening of a tissue or part.

Scoliosis. an abnormal lateral curvature of the spine.

Sigmoid. shaped like the letter S.

Sign. any objective evidence of a disease as detected by examination.

Situs inversus. transposition of the organs from right to left and vice versa.

Spectophotometry. measurement of the intensity of light of a definite wavelength transmitted by a substance in solution, by which the quantity of the substance in the solution is determined.

Spherule. a small sphere; a round structure of the parasitic stage of *Coccidioides immitis* containing multiple small endospores.

Spherulin. an antigenic substance extracted from spherules of *C immitis*, used for skin testing.

Sphingomyelin. a phospholipid present in alveolar surfactant.

Spondylitis. inflammation of vertebrae.

Squamous. scaly, as squamous epithelium.

Sternotomy. an incision through the sternum; sternal splitting.

Stridor. a harsh, grating sound heard during inspiration in association with upper airway obstruction.

Superoxide dismutase. an enzyme that catalyzes the conversion of the highly reactive oxygen radical (superoxide) to less toxic substances.

Suppurative. producing pus.

Supraglottitis. inflammation of structures above the glottis; epiglottitis.

Surfactant. a surface active agent; any substance that in solution lowers the surface tension between it and another liquid, usually referred to phospholipids in pulmonary alveoli.

Sympathomimetic. an agent producing effects similar to those produced by stimulation of sympathetic nerves.

Symptom. a subjective evidence of disease as perceived by the patient.

Syndrome. a set of symptoms and signs occurring together and characterizing a particular condition or disease.

Tachycardia. excessively rapid heart rate.

Tachypnea. excessively rapid respiratory rate.

Tactile. pertaining to touch.

Tamponade. pathologic compression of an organ resulting in its malfunction, as cardiac tamponade from pericardial effusion.

Taxonomy. classification of organisms.

Tension hydrothorax. large pleural effusion causing increased intrapleural pressure and affecting circulation and ventilation.

Tension pneumothorax. a large pneumothorax causing increased intrapleural pressure and affecting circulation and ventilation.

Tetraplegia. quadriplegia (paralysis of all four extremities).

Thermister. an electric thermometer able to measure extremely small changes in temperature.

Thoracentesis. puncture of chest wall and pleural space for removal of pleural fluid; pleural tap.

Thoracoplasty. collapsing of chest wall by surgical removal of ribs.

Thoracotomy. surgical opening of the thoracic cavity.

Thromboembolism. obstruction of a blood vessel with a clot carried by the blood flow from its site of origin.

Thrombophlebitis. inflammation of a vein associated with blood clot formation.

Thrombosis. formation of blood clot (**Thrombus**) inside a blood vessel.

Tidal volume (TV). the volume of air inspired and expired with each normal breath.

T lymphocyte. thymus-dependent lymphocyte, being the major effector cell in cell-mediated immunity.

Tomography. special radiographic study in which the x-ray picture of selected plane of the body is recorded.

Total lung capacity (TLC). the volume of air in the lungs at the end of a maximum inspiration.

Tracheomalacia. softening and dilatation of tracheal cartilages.

Transbronchial. through the bronchial wall, as transbronchial lung biopsy.

Transcriptase. an enzyme that helps the synthesis or polymerization of RNA (also known as RNA polymerase).

Transcutaneous. through the skin.

Transthoracic. through the chest wall.

Transtracheal. through the wall of the trachea, as transtracheal aspiration.

Transudate. a fluid with a low protein content that has passed from blood capillaries through a serous membrane as a result of alteration of hydrostatic and colloid osmotic pressure balance.

Trepopnea. more comfortable breathing upon lying on one side or the other.

Trigeminal. pertaining to the 5th cranial nerve.

Trophozoite. active, feeding, and motile stage of a protozoan.

Tubercle. a small granulomatous lesion resulting from infection with *M tuberculosis* (Tubercle bacillus).

Unremitting. not abating or diminishing, as an unremitting symptom.

Vagus nerve. the 10th cranial nerve, which supplies nerve fibers to the respiratory tract and other thoracic and abdominal viscera.

Varicose. related to a varix, usually of a vein; also describing a form of bronchiectasis.

Vesicular. related to vesicles or small sacs; quality of breath sounds considered to be originating from the alveoli.

Vital capacity (VC). the maximum volume of air that can be exhaled by forceful effort following a maximum inspiration.

Volume loss. reduction of volume of the whole lung or part of it as seen on a chest x-ray film.

Wheezing. whistling sound made while breathing, caused by airway narrowing.